Management of Cancer in Older People

Jean-Pierre Droz • Riccardo A. Audisio
Editors

Riccardo A. Audisio
Series Editor

Management of Urological Cancers in Older People

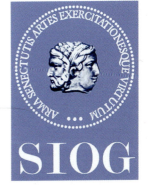

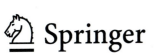

Editors
Jean-Pierre Droz, M.D., Ph.D.
Claude-Bernard-Lyon 1 University
Department of Medical Oncology
Centre Léon-Bérard
Lyon
France

Riccardo A. Audisio, M.D., FRCS
Department of Surgical Oncology
University of Liverpool
St Helens Teaching Hospital
St Helens
UK

Series Editor
Riccardo A. Audisio, M.D., FRCS
Department of Surgical Oncology
University of Liverpool
St Helens Teaching Hospital
St Helens
UK

ISBN 978-0-85729-986-4   ISBN 978-0-85729-999-4   (eBook)
DOI 10.1007/978-0-85729-999-4
Springer London Heidelberg New York Dordrecht

Library of Congress Control Number: 2012949473

Preface

As the population is aging to unprecedented levels, more and more older patients are referred to our clinics. It might be assumed that we do not need any specialized knowledge as we are all used to dealing with older patients in our daily practice. On the other hand, it has become very clear that older patients with cancer represent an entirely unique subset, presenting with special needs and requiring tailored care.

Genitourinary cancers represent a unique model in our practice, as the three major urological malignancies have different impacts on the risk of dying of cancer. Therefore, the conflict between the risk of dying of cancer and dying of other causes poses uncertainties in the design of a treatment plan. Conflicting risks of death are present in older patients, the most important being comorbidities, but dependence, malnutrition, fall, and even cognitive impairment may also play important roles. Tools are now available to assess the patients' health status, and they come under the name of Comprehensive Geriatric Assessment (CGA). These tools help to predict the individual likelihood of survival. This prediction is, however, only a probability and not a certainty.

Patients with low-risk prostate cancers are unlikely to die of their malignancy, while high-risk, life-threatening prostate cancers can develop. This is also the case with kidney cancer: small volume renal lesions and slow-growing masses are unlikely to be cancerous, and even when proved to be malignant, they generally do not develop into life-threatening conditions. Conversely, infiltrating bladder cancer presents with a completely different scenario, and this poor-risk condition requires surgical treatment.

The basic question is: what are the chances of living in relation to a health status evaluation? What is the chance of living with cancer rather than surviving the cancer treatment? This fine balance is more accurately estimated by weighing frailty (CGA) against cancer prognosis. Estimating these factors allows us to develop a patient-centered decision-making process for each individual patient.

It is important to appreciate how principles for the implementation of these decision-making processes are still needed. These aspects, cancer prognosis and the possibility to undergo treatment, as well as health status and need for a geriatric intervention, must be carefully considered.

No universal rule is available; hence our personal experience is essential in adapting the acquired knowledge into our clinical practice. The implementation of sophisticated geriatric tools into our oncology/urology practice is a big challenge. Different instruments have been developed to assist screening patients' health status and stratifying them into risk groups: i.e., fit, vulnerable, frail, and "too sick" patients. These tools have limited efficiency in decision making, but are extremely useful in clinical practice.

This book has been specifically designed and developed with the purpose to assist clinicians in optimizing their clinical proactivity when dealing with senior urological patients. Our aim was to review all different aspects of a geriatric oncology approach to urological cancers. Some sections might overlap, but they reflect the numerous and different schools of thought. It is indeed the reader's challenge to develop a critical interpretation of these different approaches. Eventually the reader will be inspired to build their own decision-making process on the basis of personal experience.

Genitourinary cancers are generally cancers of older patients, especially prostate and bladder cancers. The available literature is rich in experiences of treating older patients with prostate and bladder tumors as these cancers are highly prevalent among the elderly. Non-Hodgkin lymphomas are also relatively frequent in elderly patients, thus a chapter on this topic has been included.

Conversely, there are only minor differences evident in the prevalence of most other genitourinary cancers in older patients when compared with their prevalence in the general population. One exception is testicular cancer: germ cell tumors occur in patients younger than 50 years, and for this reason this tumor type is not included in this book. Other tumors show no age-related specificity, i.e., penile cancer, adrenal tumors, retroperitoneal sarcoma, or upper urinary cancers. It was nevertheless interesting to review the published data relevant to older patients, even though there was no specific decision-making processes to be developed.

We would like to congratulate all the authors and thank them for their enthusiasm in summarizing their experience. A special note of gratitude goes to Dr. Helen Boyle for her generous support on numerous areas across this editorial project.

It is our hope that this book might become a useful tool to assist the dissemination and implementation of geriatric oncology into urological practice.

Jean-Pierre Droz, M.D., Ph.D.
Riccardo A. Audisio, M.D., FRCS

Contents

Contributors

Hashim Uddin Ahmed, MRCS(Ed), BM, BCh (Oxon), B.A.(Hons) Department of Urology, University College Hospitals NHS Foundation Trust, London, UK

Gilles Albrand, M.D. Geriatric Evaluation Unit, Antoine-Charial Hospital— Lyon University Hospitals, Francheville, France

Riccardo A. Audisio, M.D., FRCS Department of Surgical Oncology, University of Liverpool, St Helens Teaching Hospital, St Helens, UK

Claire Benet, M.D. Department of Pathology, Hôpital Saint-Louis, Paris, France

Mohamed Omar Bishr, M.D., M.Sc. Division of Urology, Department of Surgery, Centre de Recherche du Centre Hospitalier de l'Université de Montréal (CRCHUM) and Institut du Cancer de Montréal, Montreal, Canada

Olivier Bouchot, M.D. Department of Urology, Nantes University Hospital, Nantes, France

Helen Boyle, M.D. Department of Medicine, Center Léon-Bérard, Lyon, France

Josette Briere, M.D., Ph.D. Department of Pathology, Hôpital Saint-Louis, Paris, France

Fabio Campodonico, M.D. Department of Urology, Galliera Hospital, Genova, Italy

Jan Willem Coebergh, M.D., Ph.D. Department of Research, Eindhoven Cancer Registry/Comprehensive Cancer Centre South, Eindhoven, The Netherlands

Department of Public Health, Erasmus MC, Rotterdam, The Netherlands

Stéphane Culine, M.D., Ph.D. Department of Medical Oncology, Hôpital Saint-Louis, Paris, France

Johann S. De-Bono, MBChB, M.Sc., Ph.D., FRCP Drug Development Unit and Prostate Targeted Therapy Group, The Royal Marsden Foundation Trust, Sutton, Surrey, UK

Louise Dickinson, M.B.B.S., B.Sc. (Hons), MRCS Department of Urology, University College Hospitals NHS Foundation Trust, London, UK

Jean-Pierre Droz, M.D., Ph.D. Department of Medical Oncology, Lyon-RTH Laënnec School of Medicine, Centre Léon-Bérard, Lyon, France

Sophie Duc, M.D. Department of Geriatric Medicine, University Hospital Bordeaux, Pessac, France

Mark Emberton, M.D., FRCS (Urol) Department of Urology, University College Hospitals NHS Foundation Trust, London, UK

John M. Fitzpatrick, MCh, FRCSI, FC Urol (SA), FRCSGlas, FRCS Irish Cancer Society and Mater Misericordiae Hospital, University College, Dublin, Ireland

Aude Fléchon, M.D., Ph.D. Department of Medicine, Center Léon-Bérard, Lyon, France

Paolo Gontero, M.D. Department of Urology, A.O.U. San Giovanni Battista Molinette, University of Turin, Turin, Italy

Brandon K. Isariyawongse, M.D. Department of Urology, Glickman Urological and Kidney Institute, Cleveland Clinic Foundation, Cleveland, OH, USA

Steven Joniau, M.D. Department of Urology, University Hospital Leuven, Leuven, Belgium

Michael W. Kattan, Ph.D. Department of Quantitative Health Sciences, Glickman Urological and Kidney Institute, Cleveland Clinic Foundation, Cleveland, OH, USA

Jean-Christophe Lifante, M.D., Ph.D. Department of General and Endocrine Surgery, Centre Hospitalier Lyon Sud, Pierre Bénite, France

Massimo Maffezzini, M.D. Department of Specialized Surgery, Galliera Hospital, Genova, Italy

Barry B. McGuire, M.D., IMRCS Department of Urology, The Mater Misericordiae University Hospital, Dublin, Ireland

Pierre Meeus, M.D. Department of Surgery, Center Léon-Bérard, Lyon, France

Cecile Mertens, M.D. Department of Geriatric Medicine, University Hospital Bordeaux, Pessac, France

Nicolas Mottet, M.D., Ph.D. Department of Urology, University Hospital of St. Etienne, St. Etienne, France

Deborah Mukherji, B.Sc., M.B.B.S., Ph.D., MRCP Drug Development Unit and Prostate Targeted Therapy Group, The Royal Marsden Foundation Trust, Sutton, Surrey, UK

Sylvie Négrier, M.D., Ph.D. Department of Medical Oncology, Centre Léon-Bérard, Lyon, France

Marco Oderda, M.D. Department of Urology, A.O.U. San Giovanni Battista Molinette, University of Turin, Turin, Italy

Jean-Louis Peix, M.D. Department of General and Endocrine Surgery, Centre Hospitalier Lyon Sud, Pierre Bénite, France

Carmel J. Pezaro, BHB, MBChB, FRACP, DMedSc Drug Development Unit and Prostate Targeted Therapy Group, The Royal Marsden Foundation Trust, Sutton, Surrey, UK

Pascal Pommier, M.D., Ph.D. Department of Radiation Oncology, Centre Léon Bérard, Lyon, France

Damien Pouessel, M.D. Department of Medical Oncology, Hôpital Saint-Louis, Paris, France

Muriel Rainfray, M.D., Ph.D. Department of Geriatric Medicine, University Hospital Bordeaux, Pessac, France

Jérôme Rigaud, M.D. Department of Urology, Nantes University Hospital, Nantes, France

Fred Saad, M.D., FRCS Division of Urology, Department of Surgery, Centre Hospitalier de l'Université de Montréal (CHUM), Montreal, Canada

Guru Sonpavde, M.D. Section of Medical Oncology, Department of Medicine, Genitourinary medical oncology, UAB Comprehensive Cancer Center, Birmingham, Alabama, USA

Cora N. Sternberg, M.D., FACP Department of Medical Oncology, San Camillo and Forlanini Hospitals, Rome, Italy

Catherine Terret, M.D., Ph.D. Geriatric Oncology Program, Department of Medical Oncology, University of Claude Bernard - Lyon 1, Center Léon-Bérard, Lyon, France

Jean Etienne Terrier, M.D. Department of Urology, University Hospital of St. Etienne, St. Etienne, France

Catherine Thieblemont, M.D., Ph.D. Department of Hemato-Oncology, Hôpital Saint-Louis, Paris, France

Hein Van Poppel, M.D., Ph.D. Department of Urology, University Hospitals Leuven, Leuven, Belgium

Rob H.A. Verhoeven, Ph.D. Department of Research, Eindhoven Cancer Registry/Comprehensive Cancer Centre South, Eindhoven, The Netherlands

Part I
Background and Epidemiology

Chapter 1
Background and Epidemiology

Jan Willem Coebergh and Rob H.A. Verhoeven

Abstract Epidemiological trends for urological malignancies are presented, as reported by population-based cancer registries from Europe and the United States.

Keywords Epidemiology • Prevalence • Comorbidity • Survival • Urological cancers

Introduction

Malignancies of the bladder, kidney, and prostate affect up to 10 % of older men in industrialized countries and a much lower proportion of older women. The major determinant is the degree of prostate cancer awareness, e.g., the tendency to be offered PSA testing, which is quite common in the USA, northern European countries, and France, despite a very limited effectiveness of mass screening as a recent update demonstrates [1]. However, bladder and, to a lesser extent, kidney cancer incidence is strongly related to the high level of smoking some decades ago and, to a lesser extent, due to occupational and chemical exposures, affecting less and less working class men in industrialized countries; this may be different across the industrializing phase. The current obesity endemic is likely to result in increases of

J.W. Coebergh, M.D., Ph.D. (✉)
Department of Research, Eindhoven Cancer Registry/Comprehensive Cancer Centre South, Eindhoven, The Netherlands

Department of Public Health, Erasmus MC,
Rotterdam, The Netherlands
e-mail: jw.coebergh@ikz.nl

R.H.A. Verhoeven, Ph.D.
Department of Research, Eindhoven Cancer Registry/Comprehensive Cancer Centre South, Eindhoven, The Netherlands
e-mail: r.verhoeven@ikz.nl

J.-P. Droz, R.A. Audisio (eds.), *Management of Urological Cancers in Older People*,
Management of Cancer in Older People,
DOI 10.1007/978-0-85729-999-4_1, © Springer-Verlag London 2013

kidney carcinoma in the near future. The increasing prevalence which can be estimated around 3–5 % annually will result in an increased workload for GPs, urologists, radiotherapists, and medical oncologists to monitor the condition as well as the treatment's side effects.

This chapter presents figures on trends in incidence, mortality, and survival in Europe and the United States, as derived from population-based cancer registries and population-based data on comorbidity at diagnosis of urological malignancies.

Data Sources
- Eindhoven Cancer Registry (ECR) collects data on incidence, mortality, and survival since 1955 and on comorbidity and quality of life since 1993 and 2005, respectively. (http://www.ikz.nl/page.php?id=97)
- GLOBOCAN provides incidence and mortality data from the major cancer types at national level for all countries in the world. Estimates for 2008 are available and used for this chapter. The most important source of information on cancer incidence are the successive volumes of Cancer Incidence in Five Continents CI5. Mortality statistics are made available by WHO. (http://globocan.iarc.fr)
- EUROCARE (European Cancer Registry-based study on survival and care of cancer patients): an epidemiological research project on survival of European cancer patients. The registry includes data of 12 countries since 1978 in four, soon five, projects up to 2007. (http://www.eurocare.it)
- NORDCAN collects cancer incidence, mortality, survival, and prevalence data from the Nordic countries: Denmark, Finland, Iceland, Norway, and Sweden. http://www-dep.iarc.fr/nordcan/English/frame.asp presents the incidence, mortality, prevalence, and survival statistics from 41 major cancers in the Nordic countries.
- SEER collects cancer incidence, mortality, and survival data from 18 geographic areas in the United States covering 26 % of the US population to date. (http://seer.cancer.gov)

Role of Comorbidity

Cancer treatment is often complicated by the presence of associated conditions (comorbidities or chronic disabilities), and the prognosis of cancer patients is obviously affected by the number, severity, and type of comorbidities, whether they are newly detected or long lasting [2]. The largest part of older cancer patients is affected by one or more comorbidities, cardiovascular disease being the most frequent one. In Table 1.1, the prevalence of the most important comorbidities are presented per tumor by age for the various comorbidities and for their combinations. A large proportion

Table 1.1 Percentage of patients with comorbidity by age category for tumors of prostate, kidney, and bladder between 2004 and 2009

	Prostate			Kidney			Bladder		
	55–69 years	70–79 years	80+ years	55–69 years	70–79 years	80+ years	55–69 years	70–79 years	80+ years
n	4,353	3,247	968	728	506	213	1,800	1,737	916
Number of comorbidities									
No comorbidity	39 %	24 %	16 %	24 %	18 %	10 %	30 %	16 %	10 %
One comorbidity	30 %	31 %	27 %	33 %	28 %	26 %	29 %	31 %	27 %
Two or more comorbidities	18 %	34 %	44 %	31 %	47 %	59 %	26 %	43 %	53 %
Comorbidity missing	13 %	11 %	13 %	11 %	8 %	5 %	15 %	11 %	10 %
Types of comorbidity									
Other malignancy	6 %	11 %	18 %	17 %	18 %	23 %	12 %	21 %	28 %
Hypertension	21 %	25 %	24 %	33 %	37 %	41 %	20 %	27 %	30 %
Cardiovascular disease	21 %	36 %	45 %	24 %	40 %	53 %	26 %	40 %	50 %
COPD	7 %	11 %	15 %	9 %	11 %	16 %	10 %	13 %	16 %
Diabetes mellitus	7 %	11 %	13 %	14 %	20 %	21 %	11 %	15 %	16 %
Most prevalent combinations of comorbidities									
Cardiovascular disease and hypertension	6 %	11 %	15 %	11 %	18 %	23 %	9 %	13 %	17 %
Cardiovascular disease and diabetes mellitus	2 %	5 %	8 %	5 %	11 %	12 %	5 %	8 %	10 %
Hypertension and diabetes mellitus	3 %	5 %	5 %	8 %	11 %	12 %	5 %	7 %	9 %
Other malignancy and cardiovascular disease	1 %	4 %	8 %	4 %	7 %	11 %	3 %	8 %	14 %
Cardiovascular disease and COPD	2 %	4 %	8 %	3 %	7 %	12 %	4 %	7 %	10 %

Source: Eindhoven Cancer Registry

of the 55–69-year-old patients present with known comorbidities: 48 % in prostate cancer patients, 64 and 55 % for kidney and bladder cancer, respectively. More on, this proportion raises to 73–80 % over the age of 80. It is well known that comorbidities further increase with age progression as chronic conditions are not likely to be resolved. Cardiovascular disease is present in about 50 % of the very old patients, and the prevalence of COPD and diabetes mellitus is remarkably similar to each other. The pattern of comorbidity is, to a certain extent, an indicator of the etiology of the tumor itself. Even more, comorbidity can be considered as an indicator of the complexity of care, whereas its precise prognostic value depends on the severity and related treatments and finally on the degree of synergetic collaboration between oncologists and other specialists. For this reason, dedicated cancer institutes may paradoxically be considered an inappropriate environment to treat older cancer patients, where there is no chest physician, cardiologist, or endocrinologist constantly present. It is becoming more obvious that bladder cancer patients tend to present higher rates of COPD and cardiovascular disease than prostate cancer patients; this obviously impacts on the rates of surgical management. A practical approach would suggest having specialized nurses available with a specific competence on other chronic conditions to offer the appropriate surveillance, beside the cancer itself. Diabetes in particular tends to be neglected in cancer patients, even by patients themselves. References [2–8] give more detailed interpretation and refer to other literature in this respect.

Trends in Incidence, Mortality, and Survival (Figs. 1.1, 1.2, 1.3, 1.4, and 1.5)

While the incidence of prostate cancer among the elderly seems to have stabilized in the USA since the mid-1990s, the incidence of prostate cancer among the Nordic European patients aged 65–74 kept rising until 2004. The mortality of prostate cancer decreased since the mid-1990s both in the USA and the Nordic countries. There is quite some variation among countries in 5-year relative survival of elderly prostate cancer patients; this is probably mainly due to differences in the use of methods for early detection of prostate tumors and therefore differences in the disease stage.

The incidence of bladder cancer was relatively stable during the last decade, and the mortality showed a slight decrease. The 5-year relative survival of bladder cancer generally varied between 60 and 80 %.

While, in the USA, the incidence of tumors of the kidney and the renal pelvis is clearly rising among the elderly, the incidence of kidney cancer in the Nordic European countries remains relatively stable. The trends of mortality are also conflicting, with a decreasing (65–74 years) and stable (75+ years) mortality rate in the Nordic countries and a stable (65–74 years) and increasing (75+ years) trend in the USA. Survival of kidney cancer patients among the different countries varied between 45 and 65 %.

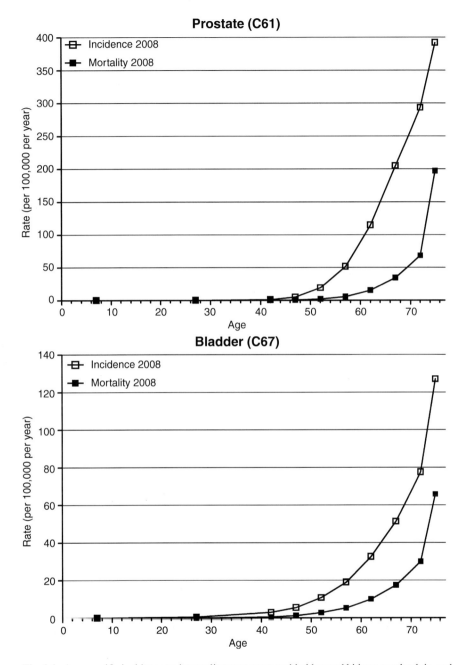

Fig. 1.1 Age-specific incidence and mortality rate: prostate; bladder; and kidney, renal pelvis, and ureter (*Source*: Globocan)

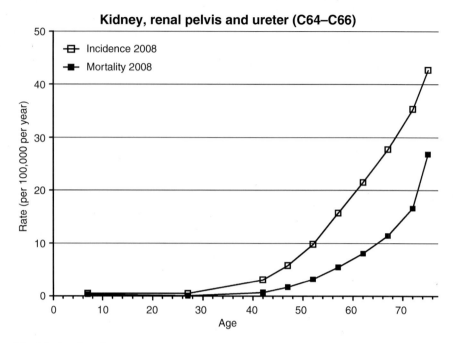

Fig. 1.1 (continued)

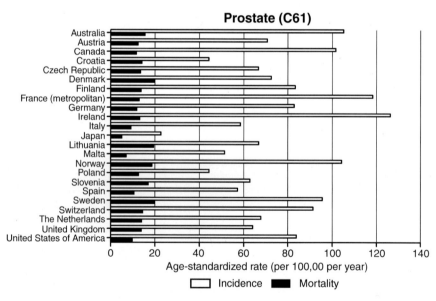

Fig. 1.2 Age-standardized incidence and mortality rate according to country: prostate; bladder; and kidney, renal pelvis, and ureter (*Source*: Globocan)

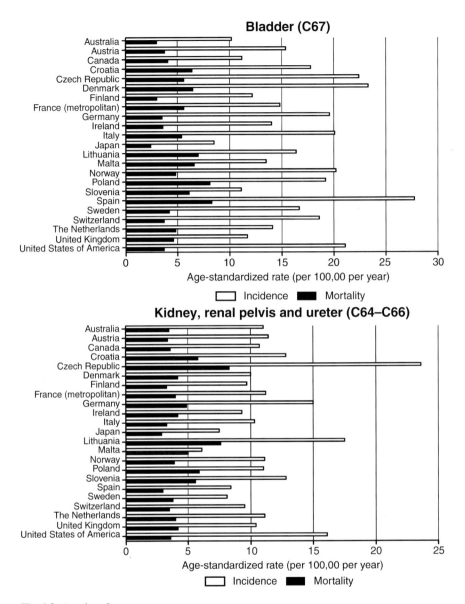

Fig. 1.2 (continued)

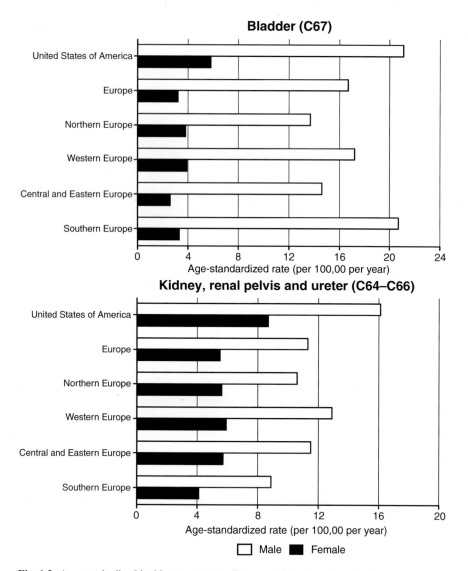

Fig. 1.3 Age-standardized incidence rate according to gender and region: bladder; kidney, renal pelvis, and ureter (*Source*: Globocan)

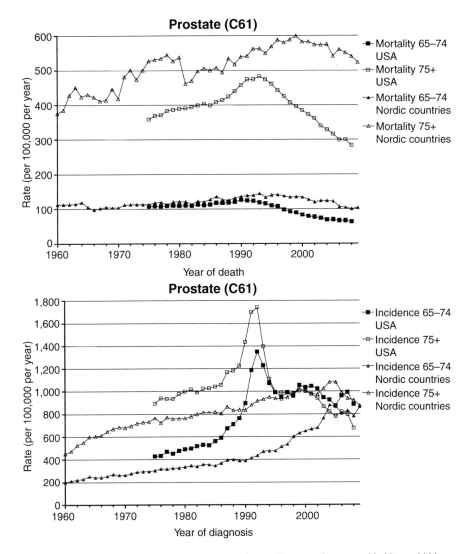

Fig. 1.4 Trends in age-standardized incidence and mortality rate of prostate, bladder and kidney cancer in the USA and the Nordic countries (*Source*: SEER and Nordcan)

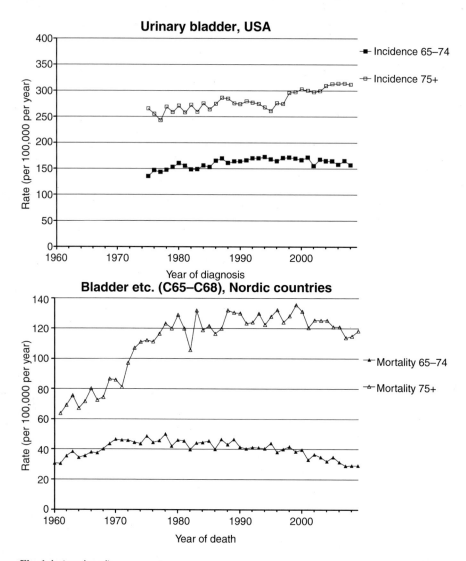

Fig. 1.4 (continued)

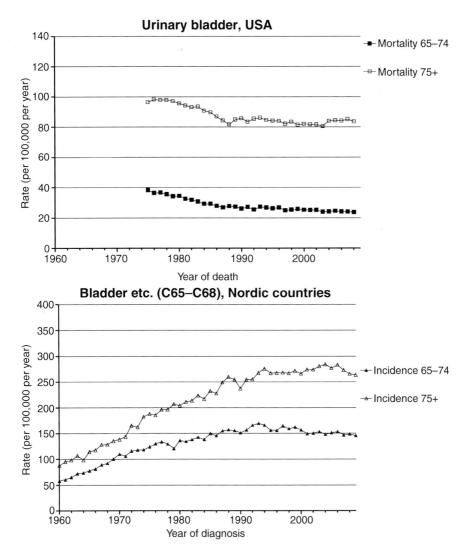

Fig. 1.4 (continued)

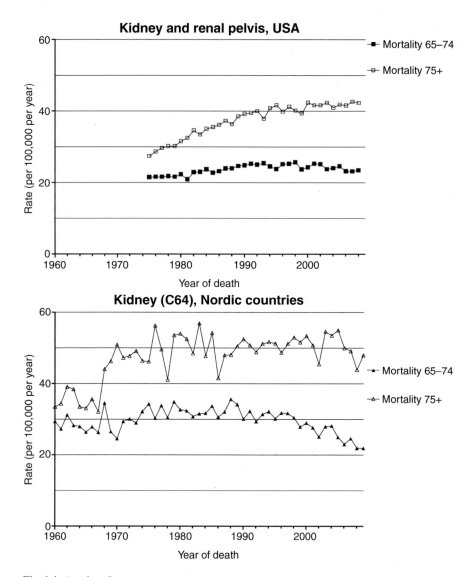

Fig. 1.4 (continued)

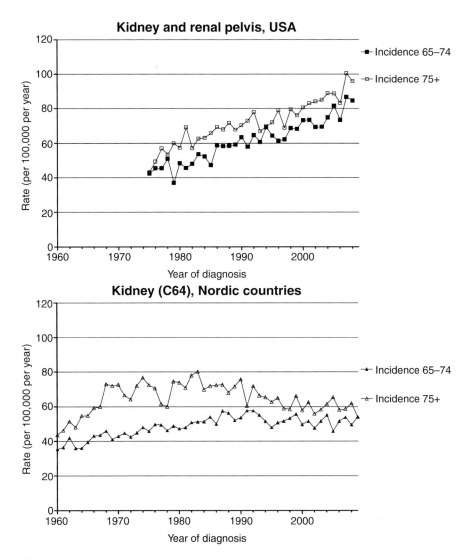

Fig. 1.4 (continued)

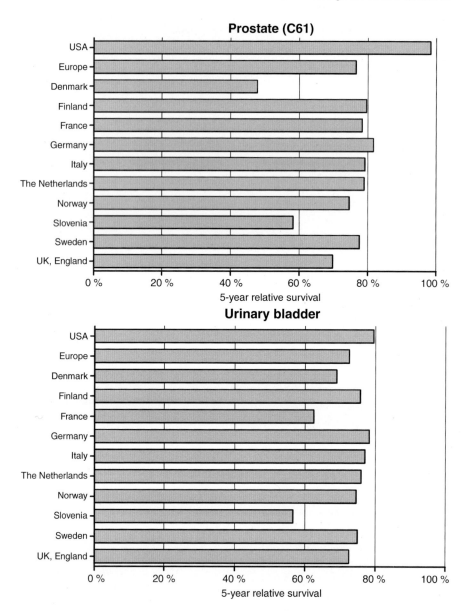

Fig. 1.5 Five-year relative survival of prostate, bladder and kidney, renal pelvis and ureter cancer according to country. For the European countries, the "other and unspecified urinary organs" (C68) are also included in the group of Kidney, renal pelvis and ureter cancers. *Source*: SEER and EUROCARE-4

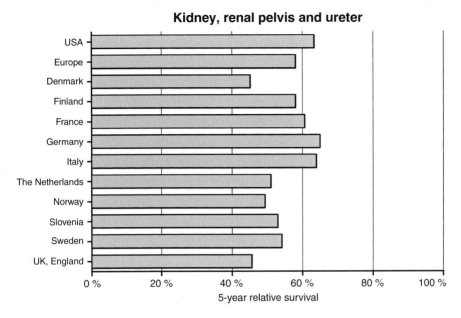

Fig. 1.5 (continued)

References

1. Miller AB. New data on prostate-cancer mortality after PSA screening. N Engl J Med. 2012;366(11):1047–8.
2. Janssen-Heijnen ML, Houterman S, Lemmens VE, et al. Prognostic impact of increasing age and co-morbidity in cancer patients: a population-based approach. Crit Rev Oncol Hematol. 2005;55:231–40.
3. Houterman S, Janssen-Heijnen ML, Hendrikx AJ, van den Berg HA, Coebergh JW. Impact of comorbidity on treatment and prognosis of prostate cancer patients: a population-based study. Crit Rev Oncol Hematol. 2006;58:60–7.
4. Houterman S, Janssen-Heijnen ML, Verheij CD, et al. Greater influence of age than co-morbidity on primary treatment and complications of prostate cancer patients: an in-depth population-based study. Prostate Cancer Prostatic Dis. 2006;9:179–84.
5. van de Schans SA, Janssen-Heijnen ML, Biesma B, et al. COPD in cancer patients: higher prevalence in the elderly, a different treatment strategy in case of primary tumours above the diaphragm, and a worse overall survival in the elderly patient. Eur J Cancer. 2007;43:2194–202.
6. Janssen-Heijnen ML, Szerencsi K, van de Schans SA, et al. Cancer patients with cardiovascular disease have survival rates comparable to cancer patients within the age-cohort of 10 years older without cardiovascular morbidity. Crit Rev Oncol Hematol. 2011;66:196–207.
7. Mols F, Aquarius AE, Essink-Bot ML, et al. Does diabetes mellitus as a co-morbid condition affect the health-related quality of life in prostate cancer survivors? Results of a population-based observational study. BJU Int. 2008;102:1594–600.
8. Louwman WJ, Aarts MJ, Houterman S, et al. A 50% higher prevalence of life-shortening chronic conditions among cancer patients with low socioeconomic status. Br J Cancer. 2010;103:1742–8.

Chapter 2
Health Status Evaluation of Elderly Patients with Genitourinary Tumors

Catherine Terret and Gilles Albrand

Abstract In addition to accurate cancer evaluation, aging people require geriatric assessment that explores non-cancer-related parameters with significant impact on the cancer treatment decision-making process and patient's outcomes. Emphasis should put specifically on the patient's performances in functional, cognitive, physical domains, as well as on his comorbidity and socio-environmental situation. To date, different kinds of geriatric assessment tools have been developed from the gold standard that is the comprehensive geriatric assessment approach to elementary screening tools. This chapter first reviews components, methods, and objectives of geriatric assessment in geriatric oncology. Then, we focus on areas that should be more specifically explored in older patients with genitourinary tumors according to the treatment option, surgery, radiation therapy, and/or medical therapy. This chapter provides additional tools, which could significantly improve the value of geriatric assessment in this setting.

Keywords Geriatric assessment • Screening tools • Cancer in the elderly Genitourinary cancer • Comorbidity • Functional status

C. Terret, M.D., Ph.D. (✉)
Geriatric Oncology Program, Department of Medical Oncology,
University of Claude Bernard - Lyon 1,
Center Léon-Bérard, Lyon, France
e-mail: catherine.terret@lyon.unicancer.fr

G. Albrand, M.D.
Geriatric Evaluation Unit, Antoine-Charial Hospital—Lyon University Hospitals,
Francheville, France
e-mail: gilles.albrand@chu-lyon.fr

J.-P. Droz, R.A. Audisio (eds.), *Management of Urological Cancers in Older People*,
Management of Cancer in Older People,
DOI 10.1007/978-0-85729-999-4_2, © Springer-Verlag London 2013

Introduction

Aging is a highly individual process which largely influences older people's health status. Age-linked physiological declines variably evolve among aging individuals. Furthermore, extrinsic factors, such as diet, exercise, personal habits, and psychosocial factors, heighten discrepancy between older persons [1]. Standard medical evaluations have failed to adequately approach the complexity of an aging individual's health status. Based on the work of Marjory Warren, geriatricians have progressively built appropriate evaluation and management of the elderly population [2].

Bladder tumors, prostate, and renal cancers mainly affect aging people. Incidence peaks around 75–80 years of age, except for bladder cancers which incidence increases continuously as a function of age. Active cancer treatments, particularly in early disease stages, involve various procedures with potential risks of adverse events. Consequently, cancer treatment decision making in such tumor types requires accurate assessment of individual's health status and survival likelihood.

Geriatric assessment in older patients with genitourinary tumors comprises core components corresponding to the main geriatric domains usually explored in every instrument. Additional investigations may be added depending on tumor types and projected cancer management plan

Common Geriatric Assessment Components

Comorbidity and Polypharmacy

Comorbidity has been defined as the coexistence or occurrence of any health-related condition or disease in reference to an index disease [3, 4]. Aging people are at risk of developing concomitant chronic conditions. Diabetes, respiratory diseases, cancer, cardiovascular problems, arthritis, hypertension are frequently encountered in older persons. Different measurement tools have been proposed depending on the population and research issues. Comorbidity instruments integrate data on different origins, medical record, and patient self-report, administrative database. Data collection represents a crucial step, in which errors can occur, especially in cognitively impaired patients who can underreport conditions [5]. The Charlson index weighs 19 conditions that significantly affect survival [6]. However, many diseases like hypertension are not rated although they may interfere with treatment regimen including targeted therapies. The Cumulative Illness Rating Scale for Geriatrics (CIRS-G) lists nonlethal diseases by organ system affected and rates them according to their severity and level of control by treatment [7]. The two indices have already been validated in older cancer patients with comparable prognostic performances [8].

Comorbidity impact has been largely studied in patients with localized bladder cancer [9–13] and prostate cancer [14, 15]. This index is also an appropriate prognostic tool for predicting postoperative complications [16].

Sensory impairments frequently lead to functional decline, increase risk for falls, and they worsen quality of life in older persons. As they may also interfere with patients' decisional capacity, they should be systematically screened in older cancer patients. Hearing loss may be easily detected with simple tests like the whispered-voice test [17]. Screening for vision disorders could lead to effective treatments that correct or prevent vision loss [18].

Older patients frequently receive medications prescribed by different physicians, leading to polypharmacy and increased risks of drug interactions. Therefore, patients' complete medication lists should be reviewed, as well as their observance. In case of potential severe drug adverse effect, treatment requires adaptation, including dosage changes and drug discontinuation.

Malnutrition

Malnutrition is a well-known indicator of poor health status and a strong prognostic factor for adverse outcomes [19, 20]. Older people with weight loss are twice likely to die than well-nourished people, regardless of their body mass index [21]. Nutritional disorders are frequently observed in elderly people, and up to 40 % of hospitalized cancer patients are at risk of malnutrition, if not already malnourished [22]. They originate from the combination of aging changes including reduced appetite, mouth dryness, tooth loss, dysgeusia, and cancer-related factors, like anorexia and treatment side effects. Cancer is probably the major cause of protein–calorie malnutrition in older patients

The Mini Nutritional Assessment developed in 1989 [23] is commonly used to evaluate older cancer patient's nutritional status. The test is composed of anthropometric parameters (weight, height, body mass index – BMI, and weight loss), brief questions related to lifestyle, medication, mobility, dietary questionnaire (number of meals, food, and fluid intake, and autonomy of feeding), and patient's self-perception of health and nutrition. It can be completed in less than 10 min. The MNA score distinguishes between elderly patients with adequate nutritional status, MNA $\geq$ 24; protein–calorie undernutrition, MNA < 17; and at risk for malnutrition, MNA between 17 and 23.5. MNA was found to be predictive of length of hospital stay and costs and of overall survival [24].

More generally, nutrition disorders, defined as weight loss, low body mass index, and low serum albumin level (<37 g/L), significantly predicted 90-day mortality and overall survival in bladder cancer patients undergoing radical cystectomy [25]. Similar results were shown in patients surgically treated for renal cell carcinoma [26].

Cognition

Cognitive impairment is increasingly encountered among aging patients. Since dementia causes disability and shortens patient's lifespan, the cancer treatment decision-making process must involve assessment of cognitive status. Cognitive decline actually interferes with the diagnosis step, reduces the spectrum of available treatment options, promotes treatment nonadherence, and increases the risks of severe adverse events. In geriatric oncology, assessment of decisional capacity defined as a person's abilities to understand, appreciate reason, and make a choice appears a mandatory step before cancer treatment decision making.

Detection of cognitive disorders frequently appeals to the Mini Mental State Examination. This 30-item interviewer-administered assessment explores several areas of cognitive functioning [27]. However, oncologists must keep in mind that MMSE is only a simple screening tool. Low scores do not always indicate a diagnosis of dementia, nor do normal results exclude the possibility of cognitive decline. Whenever a cognitive deterioration is suspected, patients may undergo further neuropsychological evaluation to confirm and precise the disorder.

A recent study showed that the diagnosis of prostate cancer was associated with a decreased survival of patients with preexisting dementia [28]. Demented patients were more likely to be diagnosed at an early or unknown stage of cancer. Approximately 28.5 % of patients with dementia and 4.3 % of nondemented patients died within 6 months of prostate cancer diagnosis. Dementia increased the risk of dying from all causes, predominantly from noncancer causes, whereas cancer stage did not substantially influence cancer-related or all-cause mortality, emphasizing the negative impact of dementia.

Affective Status

Mood disorders are commonly observed in the elderly population. The prevalence of depression in older patients ranges from around 40 % in hospitalized patients to 8–15 % in community settings [29, 30]. Chronic conditions like stroke, sensory impairment, cardiac disease, or chronic lung disease were risk factors for increased depression [31]. The occurrence of cancer psychologically affects elderly patients because it may cause disability and reduced lifespan. An appropriate assessment may reveal preexisting psychological and/or psychiatric disorders behind the additional distress brought about by the cancer itself. The 30-item Geriatric Depression Scale (GDS) was developed to facilitate the quick identification of depressive symptoms in older people without considering physical complaints [32]. A score between 0 and 10 indicates adequate emotional status, whereas a score higher than 10 suggests depression. This form has been validated in several settings worldwide. Among various shorter versions, the GDS-15 and GDS-4 forms are considered as adequate screening tools for depressive symptoms [33]. However, the reduction of items limits the clinical significance of the shortest version in terms of illness severity. Many other screening tools have been developed to detect depressive symptoms.

In patients with prostate cancer, studies showed that depressive symptoms significantly and consistently increase with age [34]. Similarly, patients with bladder cancer undergoing radical cystectomy frequently experience psychological distress during the perioperative period [35].

Psychological disorders in this population influence health-related quality of life.

Physical Capacities

Gait and balance disorders dramatically impact the general health of an individual since they are associated with a substantial increase in the risk of falls and of fall-related injuries (fractures, fear of falling, functional decline). Falls occur in 30–60 % of older adults each year, and 10–20 % of these result in injury, hospitalization, and/or death [36]. Various instruments are available that assess balance and gait. The Timed Up and Go test (TUG) is a timed measure of the patient's ability to rise from an arm chair, walk 3 m, turn, walk back, and sit down again; when time completion exceeds 20 s, patients deserve further evaluation [37]. The Performance-Oriented Assessment of Mobility instrument is a standardized instrument that measures gait and balance [38]. An aspect that is closely related to the emergence of balance and gait disorders is the safety of home environment. Hazard checklist may evaluate the risk of falls of older people [39].

Studies have shown a higher risk of falls and physical impairment in older prostate cancer patients treated with hormonal therapy [40].

Social Situation and Environment

The key component of social situation in geriatric oncology is the existence of effective support. It includes informal resources like family, friends, and neighborhood, as well as formal support like healthcare professionals. Social support may refer to reliance on relatives providing both emotional support and tangible aid in activities of daily living [41]. The availability of assistance from caregivers may influence cancer treatment decision making, cancer care strategy, and adverse events monitoring, especially in older people with cognitive impairment. It is worthy to identify the human resources available in case of sudden functional decline or difficulties to remain safely at home.

Two environment dimensions should also be assessed, the safety of home layout and the patient's accessibility to adequate personal and medical services, particularly for those with impaired physical capacities.

Functional Status

Functional status is a key indicator of health status. The patient's ability to perform routine tasks best describes the joint impact of individual's morbid conditions and age-related decline. In geriatric oncology, functional status provides useful prognostic information, but it is also increasingly considered as a major treatment outcome, even more relevant than survival in aging people whom lifespan might not be prolonged. Cancer care plan should integrate functional status assessment and targeted intervention to improve any impairment. Functional status can be evaluated in at least two areas. Basic activities of daily living (BADL) assess the patient's ability to perform basic self-care tasks (bathing, dressing, toileting, transferring, continence, and feeding) [42]. Instrumental activities of daily living (IADL) evaluate patient's competences to remain independently at home (i.e., meal preparation, groceries shopping, housework and/or handyman work, laundry, handling finances, taking medications, driving or using public transportation, and using the telephone) [43].

Geriatric Assessment Methodology

Comprehensive Geriatric Assessment (CGA)

The best biological and clinical markers for use in senior adult cancer patients are unknown. Geriatricians have developed a comprehensive geriatric assessment (CGA) tool to appraise the objective health status of elderly people.

Comprehensive geriatric assessment (CGA) is a multidisciplinary approach aiming at assessing and managing reserves and needs of aging people [44]. This instrument explores different key domains in geriatric medicine: cognition, comorbidity and pharmacy, mood, functional independence, nutrition, social and economic status, and environmental conditions. From this assessment, patient's resources and needs are carefully listed; recommendations and interventions are generated and integrated into an individualized care plan. It is noteworthy that the dynamic process of CGA involves also periodic reevaluation and adaptation of the care plan.

CGA has been performed in various settings from specific hospital wards called geriatric evaluation and management units (GEMU) to community-based locations like home assessment services (HAS). Randomized trials and meta-analysis demonstrated the positive effects of CGA on various outcomes, on mortality, living location, and on patients' physical and cognitive status [45–48]. A meta-analysis published in 1993 showed a 35 % decrease of 6-month mortality for GEMU and a 14 % decrease of 3-year mortality for HAS and an increased probability of living at home at 6 months [45]. This meta-analysis highlighted that CGA programs' effectiveness depended on the addition of proactive recommendations, implementation, and ambulatory follow-up. A second meta-analysis reported that older patients undergoing inpatient CGA were more likely to be alive at home after hospital admission as an emergency admission [46]. In a recent systematic review, CGA in GEMU provided lower rate of institutionalization and of functional decline than usual care [47], whereas effectiveness of preventive home visit programs appears dependent on the use of multidimensional geriatric assessment and follow-up [48].

The International Society of Geriatric Oncology (SIOG) published recommendations on the use of CGA-based instruments in geriatric oncology [49]. Experts advocate the integration of such instrument, with or without screening and with follow-up, in all cancer patients older than 70 years in order to detect unaddressed problems to improve their functional status and possibly also improve their survival. Recent studies showed that unsuspected conditions, mainly malnutrition, functional impairment, and depression, induced changes in cancer treatment decision making [50, 51]. Based on geriatric parameters, published indices may help estimate life expectancy or risk of morbidity and/or mortality related to cancer treatment [52–56].

Multidimensional Geriatric Assessment Instruments (MGA)

A geriatric assessment has been recommended as a basis for planning the treatment of older cancer patients [49]. The objectives of such an evaluation slightly differ in oncology in comparison with the general geriatric population. Geriatricians aim their process to determine comprehensive plans and long-term follow-up including interventions focused on the patient's problems, whereas oncologists have been looking for an instrument capable of discriminating older patients whose health problems may interfere with cancer treatment planning and monitoring.

Hence, multidimensional assessment tools (MGA) that exploit the CGA, first step of identification and description of patients' health problems, emerge as an appropriate approach in the geriatric oncology setting. However, most instruments consist of a set of different screening tools (i.e., MNA, MMSE, GDS,…). Though instruments generally cover similar domains, the screening tools they are composed of might differ from a study to another. Nevertheless, several studies showed that MGA instruments provide suitable data on older patients' noncancer health problems [50, 51, 57–62]. They may consequently constitute adequate tools in clinical research [62].

However, oncologists should keep in mind that those instruments do not provide accurate diagnosis and their results should be cautiously considered while they are not balanced by a geriatrician's judgment. Since MGA instruments were firstly developed in the geriatric setting, they optimally require specific resources such as a trained interdisciplinary team and geriatric skills that can hardly be available in conventional oncology units. Thus, the approach has been once again simplified with the implementation of a preliminary screening step before undertaking geriatric assessment.

Screening Tools

Screening instruments aim to help oncologists differentiate older cancer patients whose problems might interfere with cancer treatment and who require in-depth geriatric assessment. These tools share similar characteristics; they must be simply administered and quickly completed, without requiring geriatric resources or skills. Consequently, they provide basic information, and positive results indicate that patients need a geriatric evaluation. They should be considered as a preliminary step, and their results cannot be assimilated to those obtained with in-depth geriatric assessment.

Screening tools may be distributed in two groups. On the one hand, patients are asked to fill questionnaires up, sometimes with the assistance of a healthcare professional [63–66]. Items refer to common geriatric domains; they sometimes derive from longer validated screening tools. On the other hand, scoring systems have been evaluated in older cancer patients. For example, the Vulnerable Elderly Survey, the VES-13 tool was originally designed to identify vulnerable elderly people. Vulnerability is defined by the risk of functional decline or death over a 2-year period. A score greater than 3 corresponds to a high risk of vulnerability [67]. A pilot study has evaluated the performances of the VES-13 for identifying older prostate cancer patients at risk for impairment in the oncology clinic setting [68]. The investigators have found that the VES-13 tool is feasible in the oncology setting and predictive in identifying impairment when compared to a MGA procedure. Recently, a prospective trial, the ONCODAGE project, compared two screening tools (G8 and VES-13) to a standardized MGA instrument in France. The G8 scale incorporates seven items from the MNA test and age; it was initially aimed to identify older cancer patients with increased risks of death within a 6-month period after treatment initiation [69]. Preliminary data showed that G8 scores higher than 14 correctly distinguish patients with at least one impaired dimension in the MGA approach [70]. The ONCODAGE trial enrolled more than 1,500 cancer patients aged 70 years and older and confirmed these findings; G8 displayed sensitivity and specificity higher than 76 and 64 %, respectively [71].

Geriatric Evaluation Objectives

Treatment recommendations should balance, for each individual patient, the risk of cancer-related death against the risk of treatment adverse outcomes and the competing risks patients face from other causes.

Comprehensive geriatric assessment provides detailed evaluation of a given person's health status and an estimation of his/her expected lifespan. Such thorough procedure should be highly recommended in older patients with urological tumors when they are candidates to major surgery or complex combined treatment plan; i.e., when cancer treatment options impact on both patient's survival and quality of life and their balance between benefits and risks should be carefully determined.

On the other hand, simplified instruments, either MGA, or screening tools aimed to classify patients into health status groups in order to facilitate treatment decisions. Such instruments help developing clinical research dedicated to older cancer patients, allowing comparison between predefined age groups. SIOG guidelines for elderly prostate cancer patients provided an example of such classification effort (Table 2.1) [72]:

Table 2.1 SIOG classification for chemotherapy decision making in older prostate cancer patients [108]

Group	Characteristics	Treatment
Fit	Comorbidity (CIRS-G): grade 0, 1, or 2 IADL independency Adequate nutritional status (MNA > 23.5)	Standard regimen
Vulnerable (reversible problem)	Comorbidity (CIRS-G): at least one grade 3 Dependent in ≥ IADL At risk for malnutrition	Standard regimen after improvement of reversible conditions
Frail	Comorbidity (CIRS-G): several grade 3 or at least one grade 4 Dependent in ≥ IADL Severe malnutrition	Adapted regimen and targeted geriatric intervention plan
Too sick	Bedridden Life-threatening diseases Severe cognitive impairment	Palliative care

1. Patients considered fit, i.e., fully independent in IADL without any severe comorbidity or nutritional disorder. They should be offered cancer standard treatment.
2. Patients called "vulnerable," i.e., dependent in at least one IADL, or with at least one severe condition, or at risk for malnutrition. Appropriate geriatric interventions should improve reversible altered conditions, authorizing standard cancer treatment administration.
3. Patients called "frail," i.e., dependent in one or more IADL, or with two or more serious conditions, or one life-threatening comorbid condition, or severe malnutrition. Care plans should encompass targeted geriatric interventions and adapted cancer therapy options.
4. Patients called "too sick," i.e., impairments in several major health domains, without any possibility of long-lasting rehabilitation. Palliative and best supportive care is commonly offered to patients belonging to this group.

Screening tools may serve pedagogical purposes by alerting oncologists on possible health problems in their aging patients that they would not have suspected without screening tools.

Geriatric Evaluation in Older Patients with Urological Cancer

Core components of geriatric assessment remain relevant in urological cancers, regardless of the cancer type and treatment plan and intent. However, additional dimensions might be sometimes explored, using extra investigations or measurement tools, depending on the selected treatment plan.

Assessment Before Surgery

Surgery with curative intent in elderly people always raises the key issue of prognosis. Since aging people may die from various causes of death, accurate assessment of patient's potential lethal morbid conditions appears mandatory to establish a hierarchical listing and then to estimate the mortality risks of a given patient. Among mortality prediction indices developed in the geriatric setting, several tools exhibit potential advantage in geriatric oncology, exploring short- or longer-term outcome. Carey et al. developed a 2-year mortality index based on self-reported functional status, age, and gender [52]. The validation study determined six independent risk factors for 2-year mortality, male gender, age over 75 years, dependence in bathing and shopping, difficulty walking several blocks, and moving heavy objects. Points assigned to each item provide scores ranging from 0 to 10; patients were distributed to three risk groups according to their scores. Mortality rates varied between 5 % in the low-risk group (0–2 points), to 36 % in the high-risk group (7–10 points), and 12 % in the intermediate group (3–6 points). Another prognosis index including 12 variables, not only age, gender, and functional disability (bathing, managing money, walking several blocks, and moving heavy objects) but also morbid conditions (diabetes, cancer, lung disease, heart failure, current tobacco use, and body mass index less than 25), helps estimate 4-year mortality risk of older community-dwelling people [53]. Scores were associated with 4-year mortality that ranged from 4 % in older people with 0–5 points to 64 % in those with 14 or more points. Analogous 11-item index may predict 5-year mortality [54]. Because the benefits of treatment of early-stage bladder cancer or kidney tumor are not reached for 5 years, surgeons call for targeting surgical options to individuals with an expected lifespan of at least 5 years.

Conversely, guidelines recommend definitive therapy for localized prostate cancer in patient with survival likelihood of at least 10 years. Recent studies have shown that radical prostatectomy provides to older men gains in life expectancy comparable to those in younger men [73]. The ability of several instruments to predict 10-year mortality has been studied. The Charlson comorbidity index has been the most widely used, though this tool was developed in the 1980s and it does not involve recent progress in cardiovascular mortality control and updated disease definition. Because gait speed requests contribution from multiple organ systems, involving cardiovascular, respiratory and locomotor systems, as well as energy expenditures, it has been associated with older people survival and adverse outcomes in different studies [74–76]. Since cutoff turns around 0.8 m/s, older people with faster gait speeds may live longer than average life expectancy of their generation and gender. Conversely, persons with gait speeds lower than 0.6 m/s are more likely to develop functional decline and disability. Gait speed measure may be easily implemented in daily practice; it can be assessed by nonprofessional staff using a 4-m walkway and a stopwatch [76].

Besides survival probability, geriatric assessment helps determine risk factors for postoperative complications. The Physiological and Operative Severity Score for the Enumeration of Mortality and Morbidity (POSSUM) and the Portsmouth POSSUM were designed to evaluate risks for morbidity and mortality, respectively [77, 78]. These scores take into account 12 physiological variables, including white blood cell count and hemoglobin level, electrolytes, cardiovascular and respiratory signs, and 6 operative parameters (operation type, severity and presentation, number of procedures, blood loss). A new score was recently developed to specifically predict mortality and morbidity in elderly patients undergoing major colorectal surgery [79].

Delirium frequently occurs in older patients undergoing surgery with an incidence ranging widely from 8 to 70 %. Risk factors include low albumin level, anemia, functional decline cognitive impairment, and above all preexisting cognitive impairment [80]. A recent study showed that 3–4 ASA (American Society of Anesthesiologists) scores, impaired mobility (TUG > 20 s), and postoperative tramadol administration were independent risk factors for delirium after major abdominal surgery [81]. Postoperative delirium increases patient's risk of short- and long-term mortality. Adverse outcomes also include prolonged hospital stay, increased medical care costs, and early institutionalization. Previous history of delirium and hypotension episodes during surgery have been predictive variables for postoperative delirium in older patients undergoing urological surgery [82]. However, as surgery for urological tumor is generally an elective procedure, contributing factors like anemia, dehydration, hormonal disorders, psychoactive drugs, and opioids can be assessed and resolved before surgery.

Functional impairment increases the risk for postoperative complications [83]. Dependence in ADL was associated with postoperative complications in older patients undergoing thoracic surgery [84]. Impairment in IADL significantly increased postoperative complications in a sample of 460 older candidates to cancer surgery [85].

Cardiovascular complications are important causes of morbidity with major noncardiac procedures in aging patients [55]. A cohort study aimed to validate an index for risk of major cardiac complications after noncardiac elective surgery. Six factors with approximately equal prognostic importance were identified: high-risk surgery procedure, history of ischemic heart disease or of congestive heart failure, history of cerebrovascular disease, preoperative treatment with insulin, and preoperative serum creatinine >2.0 mg/dL. The presence of two or three and more of these factors identified patients with moderate (7 %) and high (11 %) complication rates, respectively.

Pulmonary complications represent a large part of postoperative morbidity, especially in older patients [86]. They include pneumonia, respiratory failure, and bronchospasm. Preoperative geriatric assessment may focus on patient-related factors include chronic obstructive pulmonary disease (COPD), recent cigarette use, high ASA scores, functional impairment. Clinical assessment may be completed with chest radiograph and laboratory tests investigating renal function and serum albumin level. Pulmonary function tests including spirometry might be recommended in patients with respiratory symptoms like cough or dyspnea or those who have COPD or asthma.

Specific attention should be paid to older patients undergoing surgery for bladder cancer as smoking is a well-known risk factor for this type of cancer [87] and for cardiovascular or pulmonary chronic conditions. Furthermore, studies have found that current smokers are two to six times more likely than noncurrent smokers to develop postoperative pulmonary complications as well as cardiovascular morbidity [88].

The burden of chronic kidney disease (CKD) increases with aging. Renal function should be then carefully assessed in older patients undergoing surgery for renal cancer [89]. A recent study determined that older age, tumor size, and baseline glomerular filtration rate (GFR) were significantly associated with postoperative onset of renal insufficiency. Another recent publication reported results of a comparative analysis of postoperative renal function after either radical nephrectomy (RN) or nephron-sparing surgery (NSS) in young and older patients with kidney cancer [90]. Around half of older patients, the older age group underwent decrease in GFR, regardless of the surgical procedure; 24 and 51 % of elderly patients developed new CKD after NSS and RN, respectively.

Hence, preoperative geriatric assessment should involve GFR estimation using adequate formula, like the Cockcroft–Gault (CG) and the Modification of Diet in Renal Disease (MDRD) formulas [91, 92]. It is noteworthy that these formulas may provide different GRF estimates depending on age, BMI, and serum creatinine level [93]. The measure of differential renal function by renal scintigraphy before nephrectomy may help treatment decision, especially in case of GFR <60 mL/min/1.73 m² [94].

Radiation Therapy

Radiation therapy (RT) is frequently administered to older patients with urological cancer. Definitive RT represents a relevant curative option for older patients with localized prostate cancer, with similar local control than for younger patients. RT also plays a crucial role in palliating symptoms in elderly patients due to progressive local and metastatic disease, especially painful bone metastasis.

Effectiveness of RT in older patients raises two key issues, technical feasibility and social resources [95].

Safe administration of RT implies repeated patient's immobilization in various positions, mainly in dorsal position, sometimes in ventral position, that may be totally unfeasible in some older patients. Chronic conditions like osteoarticular or neurological disorder and heart or lung disease may limit correct RT delivery. Immobilization devices may help patients to remain correctly positioned during sessions as far as they are able to endure them. Furthermore, RT requires adequate collaboration between patient and professionals who must be informed of existing cognitive decline or sensory impairment that may alter patient's ability to understand and respect instructions.

Social situation may also influence patient's availability to attend RT centers. Burden of travel, difficulties of living in accommodation, or financial concerns may negatively impact patient's willingness to undergo RT [96].

Concomitant comorbidity, nutritional disorders, physical and functional limitations might benefit from additional supportive care plan during RT, allowing its completion in adequate conditions.

Medical Treatment

Hormonal Therapy

Androgen deprivation therapy (ADT) remains the standard option of hormone-sensitive metastatic prostate cancer. However, adverse events should be carefully monitored in older patients [97]. Castration, regardless of its modality, induces several side effects. Baseline geriatric assessment aims to evaluate preexisting conditions that may promote or increase the prevalence of such side effects.

Surgical or chemical castration provokes weight gain and increased body fat mass, leading to increased risks of cardiovascular adverse events and diabetes [98]. Moreover, androgen suppression significantly increases the risk of loss of bone density and of fracture which have significant morbidity and mortality implications [99]. Dual-energy X-ray absorptiometry (DEXA) represents the most common way of evaluating born mineral density. In a cross-sectional study, 35.4 % men had osteoporosis before starting ADT [100]. Low BMI, alcohol or tobacco use, thyroid dysfunction, liver disease, and long-term corticosteroid therapy should be investigated before starting ADT. Effective preventive interventions include calcium and vitamin D supplementation and regular exercise program [101, 102]. Medical options include bisphosphonates and denosumab, a newly approved human recombinant monoclonal antibody that inhibits bone resorption by inhibiting osteoclast formation, function, and survival [103, 104].

Chemotherapy

Chemotherapy, regardless of the intent, exposes older patients to an increased risk of hematological and nonhematological side effects that may compromise their quality of life. Patients with urological tumors should undergo a geriatric assessment before starting treatment. Geriatricians should be informed of the selected regimen, its potential adverse events, and goals in order to adequately evaluate candidates to such therapy.

Geriatric assessment provides variables that have been recently correlated with the risk of severe toxicity [56, 57]. Two scoring models are now available: the Chemotherapy Risk Assessment Scale for High-age patients (CRASH) test and the

Cancer and Aging Research Group (CARG) model. Both of them integrate geriatric variables, MMS, MNA, and IADL scores on one hand [56], and hearing impairment, falls, difficulties in walking one block or taking medications, and decreased social activity on the other hand [57]. Furthermore, anemia (hemoglobin level <110 g/L for male; <100 g/L for female) and renal dysfunction (creatinine clearance <34 mL/min, according to Jelliffe formulae using ideal weight [105]) have also been integrated in the CARG model. Anemia has already been associated with increased risks for death in the elderly population [106]. Furthermore, anemia influences pharmacokinetics of drugs that are bound to red blood cells like epipodophyllotoxins, anthracyclines, and camptothecins with increased free plasma concentrations and enhanced drug effects, especially myelosuppression. Renal function alteration exposes older patients to increased toxicity linked to drugs that are renally excreted [107].

Variables from geriatric assessment have also shown their influence on the probability to complete chemotherapy in older patients [108]. Preexisting malnutrition (MNA score < 23.5) and cognitive decline (MMSE ≤ 24) were significantly associated with the risk of early chemotherapy discontinuation in a sample of 200 cancer patients aged 70 years and older.

In early-stage urological tumors, chemotherapy may be offered only in patients with bladder cancer in the neoadjuvant setting [109]. However, effectiveness of such treatment option has not been yet validated in people older than 75 years. Nevertheless, chemotherapy with curative intent only applies for those with a survival probability higher than risks of early recurrence [110]. Mortality indices, such as previously described, may help define candidates with expected lifespan long enough to observe benefits from chemotherapy. Neoadjuvant chemotherapy includes cisplatin-based regimen that requires adequate renal function (i.e., GFR higher than 60 mL/min) and cardiac function. Consequently, older bladder cancer patients should be carefully evaluated before receiving such regimen.

Moreover, in all patients with metastatic bladder cancer, renal function is the first factor limiting the administration of active chemotherapy regimens. Since chemotherapy generally has limited activity, the treatment of these patients should be at best palliative with specifically adapted chemotherapy and best supportive care. At present, the standard chemotherapy for patients with GFR > 60 mL/min and no frailty risk factors is the combination of gemcitabine and cisplatin; in patients with lower GFR and/or with geriatric disability, gemcitabine alone is considered to be the standard regimen. Prospective controlled trials should be conducted, based on accurate geriatric assessment, to define which regimen provides survival and quality of life outcomes with adequate toxicity profile. When palliative chemotherapy cannot be safely administered, patients should receive only symptom management and end-of-life care.

The International Society of Geriatric Oncology (SIOG) has already published guidelines on the use of chemotherapy in older patients with prostate cancer [72]. Experts recommended evaluation of three major geriatric domains, nutrition, functional status, and comorbidity. Based on a geriatric screening procedure, patients are distributed in four groups depending on their characteristics: fit, vulnerable, frail, and too sick patients (Table 2.1). Standard regimen of docetaxel given every 3 weeks may be offered to the two first groups. SIOG recommended proposing adapted regimen to frail patients i.e. suggesting weekly docetaxel, whereas palliative care will be considered in too sick patients.

Conclusions

Aging patients increasingly attend oncology clinics, jostling usual practice and conventional cancer treatment guidelines. Physicians face patients with multiple simultaneous health problems, and ordinary management shows limitations when applied to this heterogeneous population. Collaboration with professionals dealing daily with the geriatric population has been progressively developing worldwide. More and more oncologists acknowledge the need of accurate evaluation of older individual's resources and weaknesses and of comprehensive coordination of care enclosing cancer treatment plan. Interdisciplinary training will help both geriatric and oncology care providers to better collaborate, build up, and institute adequate standards of care in geriatric oncology.

References

1. Rowe JW, Kahn RL. Human aging: usual and successful. Science. 1987;237:143–9.
2. Warren MW. Care of chronic sick. Br Med J. 1943;2:822–3.
3. Feinstein AR. The pre-therapeutic classification of co-morbidity in chronic disease. J Chron Dis. 1970;23:455–69.
4. Yancik R, Erschler W, Satariano W, Hazzard W, Cohen HJ, Ferrucci L. Comorbidity: the ultimate geriatric syndrome: report of the national institute on aging task force on comorbidity. J Gerontol A Biol Sci Med Sci. 2007;62(3):275–80.
5. McCormick WC, Kukull WA, van Belle G, Bowen JD, Teri L, Larson EB. Symptom patterns and comorbidity in the early stages of Alzheimer's disease. J Am Geriatr Soc. 1994;42:517–21.
6. Charlson ME, Pompei P, Ales KL, MacKenzie CR. A new method of classifying prognostic comorbidity in longitudinal studies: development and validation. J Chronic Dis. 1987;40: 373–83.
7. Linn BS, Linn MW, Gurel L. Cumulative illness rating scale. J Am Geriatr Soc. 1968;16:622–6.
8. Extermann M, Overcash J, Lyman GH, Parr J, Balducci L. Comorbidity and functional status are independent in older cancer patients. J Clin Oncol. 1998;16:1582–7.
9. Prout Jr GR, Wesley MN, Yancik R, Ries LA, Havlik RJ, Edwards BK. Age and comorbidity impact surgical therapy in older bladder carcinoma patients: a population-based study. Cancer. 2005;104(8):1638–47.
10. Bostrom PJ, Kossi J, Laato M, Nurmi M. Risk factors for mortality and morbidity related to radical cystectomy. BJU Int. 2009;103(2):191–6.
11. Farnham SB, Cookson MS, Alberts G, Smith Jr JA, Chang SS. Benefit of radical cystectomy in the elderly patient with significant co-morbidities. Urol Oncol. 2004;22(3):178–81.
12. Bolenz C, Ho R, Nuss GR, Ortiz N, Raj GV, Sagalowsky AI, Lotan Y. Management of elderly patients with urothelial carcinoma of the bladder: guideline concordance and predictors of overall survival. BJU Int. 2010;106(9):1324–9.

13. Mendiola FP, Zorn KC, Gofrit ON, Mikhail AA, Orvieto MA, Msezane LP, et al. Cystectomy in the ninth decade: operative results and long-term survival outcomes. Can J Urol. 2007;14(4):3628–34.
14. Froehner M, Hentschel C, Koch R, Litz RJ, Hakenberg OW, Wirth MP. Which comorbidity classification best fits elderly candidates for radical prostatectomy? Urol Oncol. 2011 [Epub ahead of print].
15. Sanchez-Salas R, Prapotnich D, Rozet F, Mombet A, Cathala N, Barret E, et al. Laparoscopic radical prostatectomy is feasible and effective in 'fit' senior men with localized prostate cancer. BJU Int. 2010;106(10):1530–6.
16. Begg CB, Riedel ER, Bach PB, Kattan MW, Schrag D, Warren JL, et al. Variations in morbidity after radical prostatectomy. N Engl J Med. 2002;346(15):1138–44.
17. Bagai A, Thavendiranathan P, Detsky AS. Does this patient have hearing impairment? JAMA. 2006;295(4):416–28.
18. Chou R, Dana T, Bougatsos C. Screening older adults for impaired visual acuity: a review of the evidence for the U.S. Preventive Services Task Force. Ann Intern Med. 2009;151:44–58.
19. Sloane PD, Ivey J, Helton M, Barrick AL, Cerna A. Nutritional issues in long-term care. J Am Med Assoc. 2008;9:476–85.
20. Morley JE. Anorexia, sarcopenia, and aging. Nutrition. 2001;17:660–3.
21. Morley JE. Anorexia, weight loss, and frailty. J Am Med Dir Assoc. 2010;11:225–8.
22. Paillaud E, Caillet P, Campillo B, et al. Increased risk of alteration of nutritional status in hospitalized elderly patients with advanced cancer. J Nutr Health Aging. 2006;10:91–5.
23. Guigoz Y, Vellas B, Garry PJ. Mini nutritional assessment: a practical assessment tool for grading the nutritional state of elderly patients. Facts Res Gerontol. 1994;4 Suppl 2:15.
24. Guigoz Y. The mini nutritional assessment (MNA) review of the literature – what does it tell us? J Nutr Health Aging. 2006;10(6):466–85.
25. Morgan TM, Keegan KA, Barocas DA, Ruhotina N, Phillips SE, Chang SS, et al. Predicting the probability of 90-day survival of elderly patients with bladder cancer treated with radical cystectomy. J Urol. 2011;186(3):829–34.
26. Morgan TM, Tang D, Stratton KL, Barocas DA, Anderson CB, Gregg JR, et al. Preoperative nutritional status is an important predictor of survival in patients undergoing surgery for renal cell carcinoma. Eur Urol. 2011;59(6):923–8.
27. Folstein MF, Folstein SE, McHugh PR. Mini-mental state. A practical method for grading the cognitive state of patients for the clinician. J Psychiatr Res. 1975;12(3):189–98.
28. Raji Ma, Kuo Y-F, Freeman JL, Goodwin JS. Effect of a dementia diagnosis on survival of older patients after a diagnosis of breast, colon, or prostate cancer. Arch Intern Med. 2008;168(18):2033–40.
29. Leon FG, Ashton AK, D'Mello DA, Dantz B. Depression and comorbid medical illness: therapeutic and diagnostic challenges. J Fam Pract 2003; (Suppl.): S19–33.
30. Birrer RB, Vemuri SP. Depression in later life: a diagnostic and therapeutic challenge. Am Fam Physician. 2004;69(10):2375–82.
31. Chang-Quan H, Bi-Rong D, Zhen-Chan L, Ji-Rong Y, Qing-Xiu L. Chronic diseases and risk for depression in old age: a meta-analysis of published literature. Ageing Res Rev. 2010;9:131–41.
32. Yesavage JA, Brink TL, Rose TL, Lum O, Huang V, Adey M, Leirer VO. Development and validation of a geriatric depression scale: a preliminary report. J Psychiatr Res. 1983;17:37–49.
33. Almeida OP, Almeida SA. Short versions of the Geriatric Depression Scale: a study of their validity for the diagnosis of a major depressive episode according to ICD-10 and DSM-IV. Int J Geriatr Psychiatry. 1999;14:858–65.
34. Nelson CJ, Weinberger MI, Balk E, Holland J, Breitbart W, Roth AJ. The chronology of distress, anxiety, and depression in older prostate cancer patients. Oncologist. 2009;14(9):891–9.
35. Palapattu GS, Haisfield-Wolfe ME, Walker JM, BrintzenhofeSzoc K, Trock B, Zabora J, Schoenberg M. Assessment of perioperative psychological distress in patients undergoing radical cystectomy for bladder cancer. J Urol. 2004;172(5 Pt 1):1814–7.

36. Rubenstein LZ. Falls in older people: epidemiology, risk factors and strategies for prevention. Age Ageing. 2006;35 Suppl 2:ii37–41.
37. Podsiadlo D, Richardson S. The timed "Up & Go": a test of basic functional mobility for frail elderly persons. J Am Geriatr Soc. 1991;39:142–8.
38. Tinetti ME. Performance-oriented assessment of mobility problems in elderly patients. J Am Geriatr Soc. 1986;34:119–26.
39. Tideiksaar R. Preventing falls: home hazard checklists to help older patients protect themselves. Geriatrics. 1986;41:26–8.
40. Bylow K, Dale W, Mustian K, Stadler WM, Rodin M, Hall W, et al. Falls and physical performance deficits in older patients with prostate cancer undergoing androgen deprivation therapy. Urology. 2008;72(2):422–7.
41. Wortman CB. Social support and the cancer patient: conceptual and methodological issues. Cancer. 1984;63:2339–60.
42. Katz S, Ford AB, Moskowitz RW, Jackson BA, Jaffe MW. Studies of illness in the aged. The index of ADL: a standardized measure of biological and psychological function. J Am Med Assoc. 1963;185:914–9.
43. Lawton MP, Brody EM. Assessment of older people: self-maintaining and instrumental activities of daily living. Gerontologist. 1969;9:179–86.
44. Solomon D, Brown AS, Brummel-Smith K, Burgess L, D'Agostino RB, Goldschmidt JW, et al. National Institutes of Health Consensus Development Conference Statement: geriatric assessment methods for clinical decision-making. J Am Geriatr Soc. 1988;36(4):342–7.
45. Stuck AE, Siu AL, Wieland GD, Adams J, Rubenstein LZ. Comprehensive geriatric assessment: a meta-analysis of controlled trials. Lancet. 1993;342(8878):1032–6.
46. Ellis G, Whitehead MA, Robinson D, O'Neill D, Langhorne P. Comprehensive geriatric assessment for older adults admitted to hospital: meta-analysis of randomised controlled trials. BMJ. 2011;343:d6553.
47. Van Craen K, Braes T, Wellens N, Denhaerynck K, Flamaing J, Moons P, et al. The effectiveness of inpatient geriatric evaluation and management units: a systematic review and meta-analysis. J Am Geriatr Soc. 2010;58(1):83–92.
48. Stuck AE, Egger M, Hammer A, Minder CE, Beck JC. Home visits to prevent nursing home admission and functional decline in elderly people. JAMA. 2002;287:1022–8.
49. Extermann M, Aapro M, Bernabei R, Cohen HJ, Droz JP, Lichtman S, et al. Use of comprehensive geriatric assessment in older cancer patients: recommendations from the task force on CGA of the International Society of Geriatric Oncology (SIOG). Crit Rev Oncol Hematol. 2005;55(3):241–52.
50. Girre V, Falcou MC, Gisselbrecht M, Gridel G, Mosseri V, Bouleuc C, et al. Does a geriatric oncology consultation modify the cancer treatment plan for elderly patients? J Gerontol A Biol Sci Med Sci. 2008;63(7):724–30.
51. Caillet P, Canoui-Poitrine F, Vouriot J, Berle M, Reinald N, Krypciak S, et al. Comprehensive geriatric assessment in the decision-making process in elderly patients with cancer: ELCAPA study. J Clin Oncol. 2011;29(27):3636–42.
52. Carey EC, Walter LC, Lindquist K, Covinsky KE. Development and validation of a functional morbidity index to predict mortality in community-dwelling elders. J Gen Intern Med. 2004;19(10):1027–33.
53. Lee SJ, Lindquist K, Segal MR, Covinsky KE. Development and validation of a prognostic index for 4-year mortality in older adults. JAMA. 2006;295:801 8.
54. Schonberg MA, Davis RB, McCarthy EP, Marcantonio ER. Index to predict 5-year mortality of community-dwelling adults aged 65 and older using data from the National Health Interview Survey. J Gen Intern Med. 2009;24(10):1115–22.
55. Lee TH, Marcantonio ER, Mangione CM, Thomas EJ, Polanczyk CA, Cook EF. Derivation and prospective validation of a simple index for prediction of cardiac risk of major noncardiac surgery. Circulation. 1999;100(10):1043–9.
56. Extermann M, Boler I, Reich RR, Lyman GH, Brown RH, DeFelice J, et al. Predicting the risk of chemotherapy in older patients: the Chemotherapy Risk Assessment Scale for High-age patients (CRASH) score. Cancer. 2012:118(13):3377–86.

57. Hurria A, Togawa K, Mohile SG, Owusu C, Klepin HD, Gross CP. Predicting chemotherapy toxicity in older adults with cancer: a prospective multicenter study. J Clin Oncol. 2011;29(25):3457–65.
58. Kristjansson SR, Nesbakken A, Jordhøy MS, Skovlund E, Audisio RA, Johannessen HO, Bakka A, Wyller TB. Comprehensive geriatric assessment can predict complications in elderly patients after elective surgery for colorectal cancer: a prospective observational cohort study. Crit Rev Oncol Hematol. 2010;76(3):208–17.
59. Marenco D, Marinello R, Berruti A, Gaspari F, Stasi MF, Rosato R, et al. Multidimensional geriatric assessment in treatment decision in elderly cancer patients: 6-year experience in an outpatient geriatric oncology service. Crit Rev Oncol Hematol. 2008;68(2):157–64.
60. Terret C. Management and geriatric assessment of cancer in the elderly. Expert Rev Anticancer Ther. 2004;4(3):469–75.
61. Arnoldi E, Dieli M, Mangia M, Minetti B, Labianca R. Comprehensive geriatric assessment in elderly cancer patients: an experience in an outpatient population. Tumori. 2007;93(1): 23–5.
62. Kim YJ, Kim JH, Park MS, Lee KW, Kim KI, Bang SM, et al. Comprehensive geriatric assessment in Korean elderly cancer patients receiving chemotherapy. J Cancer Res Clin Oncol. 2011;137(5):839–47.
63. Brunello A, Sandri R, Extermann M. Multidimensional geriatric evaluation for older cancer patients as a clinical and research tool. Cancer Treat Rev. 2009;35(6):487–92.
64. Hurria A, Gupta S, Zauderer M, Zuckerman EL, Cohen HJ, Muss Hyman, et al. Developing a cancer-specific geriatric assessment. A feasibility study. Cancer. 2005;104:1998–2005.
65. Extermann M. Evaluation of the senior cancer patient: comprehensive geriatric assessment: screening tools for the elderly. In: Schrijvers D, Aapro M, Zakotnik B, Audisio R, van Halteren H, Hurria A, editors. Handbook of cancer in the senior patient. New York: Informa Healthcare; 2010. p. 13–21.
66. To THM, Okera M, Prouse J, Prowse RJ, Singhal N. Infancy of an Australian geriatric oncology program – characteristics of the first 200 patients. J Geriatr Oncol. 2010;1:81–6.
67. Saliba D, Elliott M, Rubenstein LZ, Solomon DH, Young RT, Kamberg CJ, et al. The vulnerable elders survey: a tool for identifying vulnerable older people in the community. J Am Geriatr Soc. 2001;49:1691–9.
68. Mohile S, Bilow K, Dale W, Dignam J, Martin K, Petrylak DP, et al. A pilot study of the vulnerable elders survey-13 compared with the comprehensive geriatric assessment for identifying disability in older patients with prostate cancer who receive androgen ablation. Cancer. 2007;109:802–10.
69. Soubeyran P, Rainfray M, Mathoulin-Pelissier S, Blanc-Bisson C, Mertens C, Blanc J, et al. Prediction of early death risk in the elderly with cancer: results of a prospective multicentric study of 364 patients under chemotherapy. J Clin Oncol. 2007;25(suppl):9040.
70. Bellera C, Rainfray M, Mathoulin-Pelissier S, Mertens C, Delva F, et al. Screening older cancer patients: first evaluation of the G-8 geriatric screening tool Ann Oncol 2012 [Epub ahead of print].
71. Soubeyran P, Bellera C, Goyard J, Heitz D, Cure H, Rousselot H, et al. Validation of the G8 screening tool in geriatric oncology: the ONCODAGE project. J Clin Oncol. 2011; 29(Suppl):9001.
72. Droz JP, Balducci L, Bolla M, Emberton M, Fitzpatrick JM, Joniau S, et al. Management of prostate cancer in senior adults: recommendations of a working group of the International Society of Geriatric Oncology (SIOG). BJU Int. 2010;106:462–9.
73. Richstone L, Bianco FJ, Shah HH, Kattan MW, Eastham JA, Scardino PT, Scherr DS. Radical prostatectomy in men aged ≥70 years: effect of age on upgrading, upstaging, and the accuracy of a preoperative nomogram. BJU Int. 2008;101:541–6.
74. Cesari M, Kritchevsky SB, Penninx BW, et al. Prognostic value of usual gait speed in well-functioning older people. J Am Geriatr Soc. 2005;53(10):1675–80.
75. Rolland Y, Lauwers-Cances V, Cesari M, Vellas B, Pahor M, Grandjean H. Physical performance measures as predictors of mortality in a cohort of community-dwelling older French women. Eur J Epidemiol. 2006;21(2):113–22.

76. Studenski S, Perera S, Patel K, Rosano C, Faulkner K, Inzitari M, et al. Gait speed and survival in older adults. JAMA. 2011;305(1):50–8.
77. Abellan van Kan G, Rolland Y, Andrieu S, Bauer J, Beauchet O, Bonnefoy M, et al. Gait speed at usual pace as a predictor of adverse outcomes in community-dwelling older people. J Nutr Health Aging. 2009;13(10):881–9.
78. Copeland GP, Jones D, Walters M. POSSUM: a scoring system for surgical audit. Br J Surg. 1991;78:355–60.
79. Prytherch DR, Whiteley MS, Higgins B, Weaver PC, Prout WG, Powell SJ. POSSUM and Portsmouth POSSUM for predicting mortality. Physiological and operative severity score for the enumeration of mortality and morbidity. Br J Surg. 1998;85:1217–20.
80. Tran Ba Loc T, Tezenas du Montcel S, Duron JJ, Levard H, Suc B, Descottes B, et al. Elderly POSSUM, a dedicated score for prediction of mortality and morbidity after major colorectal surgery in older patients. Br J Surg. 2010;97:396–403.
81. Robinson TN, Raeburn CD, Tran ZV, Angles EM, Brenner LA, Moss M. Postoperative delirium in the elderly: risk factors and outcomes. Ann Surg. 2009;249(1):173–8.
82. Brouquet A, Cudennec T, Benoist S, Moulias S, Beauchet A, Penna C, et al. Impaired mobility, ASA status and administration of tramadol are risk factors for postoperative delirium in patients aged 75 years or more after major abdominal surgery. Ann Surg. 2010;251(4):759–65.
83. Tognoni P, Simonato A, Robutti N, Pisani M, Cataldi A, Monacelli F, et al. Preoperative risk factors for postoperative delirium (POD) after urological surgery in the elderly. Arch Gerontol Geriatr. 2011;52(3):e166–9.
84. Fukuse T, Satoda N, Hijiya K, Fujinaga T. Importance of a comprehensive geriatric assessment in prediction of complications following thoracic surgery in elderly patients. Chest. 2005;127(3):886–91.
85. Audisio RA, Pope D, Ramesh HS, Gennari R, van Leeuwen BL, West C, et al. Shall we operate? Preoperative assessment in elderly cancer patients (PACE) can help. A SIOG surgical task force prospective study. Crit Rev Oncol Hematol. 2008;65(2):156–63.
86. Smetana GW. Preoperative pulmonary assessment of the older adult. Clin Geriatr Med. 2003;19(1):35–55.
87. Freedman ND, Silverman DT, Hollenbeck AR, Schatzkin A, Abnet CC. Association between smoking and risk of bladder cancer among men and women. JAMA. 2011;306(7):737–45.
88. Bluman LG, Mosca L, Newman N, Simon DG. Preoperative smoking habits and postoperative pulmonary complications. Chest. 1998;113(4):883–9.
89. Ohno Y, Nakashima J, Ohori M, Hashimoto T, Iseki R, Hatano T, Tachibana M. Impact of tumor size on renal function and prediction of renal insufficiency after radical nephrectomy in patients with renal cell carcinoma. J Urol. 2011;186:1242–6.
90. Roos FC, Brenner W, Jäger W, Albert C, Müller M, Thüroff JW, Hampel C. Perioperative morbidity and renal function in young and elderly patients undergoing elective nephron-sparing surgery or radical nephrectomy for tumours larger than 4 cm. BJU Int. 2010;107:554–61.
91. Cockcroft DW, Gault MH. Prediction of creatinine clearance from serum creatinine. Nephron. 1976;16:31–41.
92. Levey AS, Bosch JP, Lewis JB, Greene T, Rogers N, Roth D. A more accurate method to estimate glomerular filtration rate from serum creatinine: a new prediction equation. Modification of Diet in Renal Disease study group. Ann Intern Med. 1999;130:461–70.
93. Wieczorowska-Tobis K, Niemir ZI, Guzik P, Breborowicz A, Oreopoulos DG. Difference in estimated GFR with two different formulas in elderly individuals. Int Urol Nephrol. 2006;38(2):381–5.
94. Sanger JJ, Kramer EL. Radionuclide quantitation of renal function. Urol Radiol. 1992;14(2):69–78.
95. Durdux C, Boisserie T, Gisselbrecht M. Radiation therapy in elderly patients. Cancer Radiother. 2009;13:609–14.
96. Hegney D, Pearce S, Rogers-Clark C, Martin-McDonald K, Buikstra E. Close, but still too far. The experience of Australian people with cancer commuting from a regional to a capital city for radiotherapy treatment. Eur J Cancer Care. 2005;14(1):75–82.

97. Mohile SG, Mustian K, Bylow K, Hall W, Dale W. Management of complications of androgen deprivation therapy in the older man. Crit Rev Oncol Hematol. 2009;70(3):235–55.
98. Keating NL, O'Malley AJ, Smith MR. Diabetes and cardiovascular disease during androgen deprivation therapy for prostate cancer. J Clin Oncol. 2006;24(27):4448–56.
99. Shahinian VB, Kuo YF, Freeman JL, Goodwin JS. Risk of fracture after androgen deprivation for prostate cancer. N Engl J Med. 2005;352:154–64.
100. Morote J, Morin JP, Orsola A, Abascal JM, Salvador C, Trilla E, et al. Prevalence of osteoporosis during long-term androgen deprivation therapy in patients with prostate cancer. Urology. 2007;69(3):500–4.
101. Dawson-Hughes B, Harris SS, Krall EA, Dallal GE. Effect of calcium and vitamin D supplementation on bone density in men and women 65 years of age or older. N Engl J Med. 1997;337(10):670–6.
102. Pigozzi F, Rizzo M, Giombini A, Parisi A, Fagnani F, Borrione P. Bone mineral density and sport: effect of physical activity. J Sports Med Phys Fitness. 2009;49(2):177–83.
103. von Moos R. Bisphosphonate treatment recommendations for oncologists. Oncologist. 2005;10 Suppl 1:19–24.
104. Smith MR, Egerdie B, Hernández Toriz N, Feldman R, Tammela TL, Saad F, et al. Denosumab in men receiving androgen-deprivation therapy for prostate cancer. N Engl J Med. 2009;361(8):745–55.
105. Jelliffe RW. Estimation of creatinine clearance when urine cannot be collected. Lancet. 1971;1:975–6.
106. Culleton BJ, Manns BJ, Zhang J, Tonelli M, Klarenbach S, Hemmelgarn BR. Impact of anemia on hospitalization and mortality in older adults. Blood. 2006;107:3841–6.
107. Verbeeck RK, Musuamba FT. Pharmacokinetics and dosage adjustment in patients with renal dysfunction. Eur J Clin Pharmacol. 2009;65(8):757–73.
108. Aaldriks AA, Maartense E, le Cessie S, Giltay EJ, Verlaan HA, van der Geest LG, et al. Predictive value of geriatric assessment for patients older than 70 years, treated with chemotherapy. Crit Rev Oncol Hematol. 2011;79:205–12.
109. Advanced Bladder Cancer (ABC) Meta-analysis Collaboration. Neoadjuvant chemotherapy in invasive bladder cancer: update of a systematic review and meta-analysis of individual patient data advanced bladder cancer (ABC) meta-analysis collaboration. Eur Urol. 2005;48(2):202–6.
110. Extermann M, Balducci L, Lyman GH. What threshold for adjuvant therapy in older breast cancer patients? J Clin Oncol. 2000;18(8):1709–17.

Chapter 3
Nomograms and the Elderly: Applications in Genitourinary Oncology

Brandon K. Isariyawongse and Michael W. Kattan

Abstract Of all available clinical prediction tools, nomograms have been shown to provide the most accurate and practical individualized risk estimations, and for this reason, they have greatly grown in popularity in the modern era of medicine. These models function to replicate the clinical predictions of physicians in a reliable, unbiased, and evidence-based format that can provide patients with the necessary information to make a fully informed decision regarding treatment. The relevant clinical considerations – and, thus, the corresponding outcome predictions – may differ between populations of varying age, and nomograms predicting disease risk, quality of life, and mortality will likely be most relevant to an elderly population. The future of outcomes research should focus on the combination of multiple prediction models into comparative effectiveness tables which will serve as high-quality informed consent for the older patient contemplating therapy. While nomograms can help us to move beyond an era of age cutoff points, these and other prediction models will never be able to substitute for the clinical acumen and watchful eye of a thoughtful physician.

Keywords Elderly • Comparative effectiveness • Nomograms • Prediction tools

B.K. Isariyawongse, M.D.
Department of Urology, Glickman Urological and Kidney Institute, Cleveland Clinic Foundation,
Cleveland, OH, USA
e-mail: isariyb@ccf.org

M.W. Kattan, Ph.D. (✉)
Department of Quantitative Health Sciences, Glickman Urological and Kidney
Institute, Cleveland Clinic Foundation,
Cleveland, OH, USA
e-mail: kattanm@ccf.org

J.-P. Droz, R.A. Audisio (eds.), *Management of Urological Cancers in Older People*,
Management of Cancer in Older People,
DOI 10.1007/978-0-85729-999-4_3, © Springer-Verlag London 2013

Introduction

Prediction modeling has gained great popularity in medicine over the course of the past 15 years, and urologic oncology has identified itself as a field that has thrived on the development, validation, and implementation of models directly into clinical practice. The models that have been produced run the gamut of available prediction tools – from prediction tables to artificial neural networks to clinical nomograms – and we believe that the enthusiastic adoption of these models has resulted in great benefit to countless patients and providers alike. Given that the risk of many urologic malignancies increases proportionately with age, the application of such prediction tools in an elderly population is far from a stretch. However, recognizing that the relevant clinical considerations – and, thus, the appropriate outcome predictions – may differ between younger and older patients is essential when developing and applying nomograms in populations of varying age. Furthermore, the use of clinical prediction tools may obviate the need for age thresholds with regards to therapy by assessing the individual patient and his or her specific clinical parameters.

Why Nomograms?

Among all available clinical prediction tools, nomograms have been shown to provide highly accurate and individualized risk estimates for the purposes of clinical decision making and prognostic counseling [1]. Nomograms are, in essence, graphical representations of mathematical equations. Often based on multivariate models – including, but not limited to, Cox proportional hazards or competing risk analyses – nomograms can succinctly demonstrate the relationships between variables in a visual format. Each predictor is assigned a scale that is commensurate with its statistical impact, relative to other variables, on the specified outcome, and this scale is plotted such that the values (either continuous or categorical) correspond to numerical values. The tally of the values for all predictors will produce a risk estimate for the specified outcome.

There are many benefits to the use of nomograms in clinical practice. First and foremost, nomograms incorporate patient-specific variables into outcome predictions and, in so doing, offer patients individualized risk estimations based on their own clinicopathological data. Certainly, in this era of targeted therapies and individualized medicine, there is widespread recognition that a "one-size-fits-all" approach to medicine is not only archaic but also perhaps a bit unsophisticated, and patients crave information that is pertinent to them and only them. The overall simplicity of nomograms ensures relatively easy integration into modern clinical practice, and whether in electronic or hard copy format, they have become quite practical bedside counseling tools. Additionally, the nomogram itself can serve as a visual aid during patient counseling to identify which factors carry the most weight in terms of outcome prediction. Furthermore, the equations which are represented by the nomogram are founded on hard evidence, and so the use of nomograms can help to eliminate the inherent practitioner biases that result from the accumulation of anecdotal experiences. Provided that proper model validation has occurred, patients can be assured that the risk estimations provided via nomograms are based on the best information available at that time. And while the nomogram functions to replicate the clinical predictions of physicians in a reliable, unbiased, and evidence-based format, there is some evidence indicating that nomogram predictions may actually outperform the predictions of clinicians in certain circumstances [2, 3].

Utility of Nomograms in the Elderly

The purpose of prediction modeling is to improve upon the existing clinical decision making experience by providing patients with accurate risk estimations based on the most up-to-date knowledge. While some might argue that, as it stands right now, patients are already bombarded with an excess of information, there is evidence in the oncologic setting that has shown that these patients actually desire more information than has generally been provided to them [4, 5], and there is evidence in the breast cancer literature that further corroborates the fact that physicians often fail to meet the information needs and expectations of patients with cancer [6, 7]. Furthermore, it is well-recognized that patients who are better informed prior to therapy experience improved psychosocial outcomes following therapy [8, 9].

There should be little debate that the application of nomograms in an elderly population differs from their use in younger patients. Regardless of the topic of counseling, a provider must always take into account a patient's chronological and biological age, and with extended follow-up of several cohorts of patients, there is better understanding of the protracted natural history of genitourinary malignancies. A meta-analysis of ten reports of patients with small renal masses followed conservatively showed that these tumors have a low risk of clinical progression to metastatic disease [10]. Similarly, a large cohort of men with clinically localized prostate cancer managed in a conservative fashion demonstrated 10-year disease-specific mortality rates less than 10 % in patients diagnosed with well and moderately differentiated tumors [11]. Due in large part to our improved understanding of the natural history of these malignancies, in addition to the widespread recognition of the morbidity that is frequently associated with definitive therapies for genitourinary cancer, there has been a great deal of emphasis on the implementation of active surveillance protocols into clinical algorithms in urologic oncology. Given their risk of competing cause mortality, those with advanced age have understandably been targeted for these approaches. And while many elderly patients may still exhibit some aversion to the concept of cancer surveillance, outcome predictions for disease risk, quality of life, and mortality rates would likely be most relevant to this population during the treatment decision-making process.

Predicting Disease Risk

In order for patients to be considered appropriate candidates for surveillance, they in general must be felt to have low-risk disease and thus a presumed low likelihood of disease progression. However, not infrequently, disease risk cannot be accurately assessed until after surgery by means of the final surgical pathology. In the case of prostate cancer, disease risk is based on often unreliable measures such as serum prostate-specific antigen (PSA) and transrectal ultrasound-guided biopsy, which has inherent error of sampling, and rates of Gleason sum upgrading at radical prostate-ctomy pathology have been reported to be as high as 41 %, with advanced age serving as a significant risk factor [12]. Given the importance of the Gleason sum in characterizing the biologic potential of prostate cancer, the widely accepted initial step of an active surveillance protocol is a confirmatory biopsy to rule out higher risk disease.

As a result of this dilemma, several nomograms have been developed that predict the risk of Gleason sum upgrading from biopsy to radical prostatectomy pathology. Our group at the Cleveland Clinic generated a nomogram applicable to patients diagnosed by biopsy to have low- or intermediate-grade prostate cancer; the model incorporated a number of predictive variables including age, digital rectal examination, prostate volume, clinical stage, number of prior biopsies, serum PSA, number of positive cores, maximum percent cancer, and secondary Gleason score [13]. Significant predictors included age, PSA, perineural invasion, inflammation, secondary Gleason sum, clinical stage, and tumor volume, and the nomogram demonstrated reasonable accuracy with a concordance index 0.68 and graphically good calibration. The utility of this nomogram lies in the opportunity to counsel patients regarding the probability that their cancer may actually be a more biologically aggressive variant than was characterized by biopsy, and as surveillance becomes more and more widely utilized in the elderly population, it becomes essential to identify which patients may be at significant risk of pathologic upgrading at prostatectomy and potentially inappropriate candidates for active surveillance.

The prognosis of small renal masses is similarly difficult to predict as the criteria are almost exclusively gleaned from radiologic studies, most often without the benefit of any sort of tissue diagnosis. Even when a renal mass biopsy is employed, the results are frequently insufficient to produce a definitive diagnosis, and as a result, a large majority of enhancing renal masses had historically been excised surgically. Of these masses, approximately 20 % will exhibit benign pathology, and only about 25 % will show potentially aggressive kidney cancer [14, 15]. Furthermore, we know from a meta-analysis of several cohorts of patients that a small minority of small renal masses will progress clinically to overt metastasis [10]. Accordingly, many patients and urologists are now opting to follow these tumors radiographically over time rather than proceed directly to surgical extirpation. But because of the uncertainty regarding the risk of malignancy in these patients, several groups have undertaken the task of developing a nomogram predicting not only the overall risk of malignancy but also the probability of high-grade pathologic features. A group from Fox Chase Cancer Center produced just such a nomogram which incorporated RENAL nephrometry scores as a predictive variable [16]. The model showed good predictive accuracy, which was subsequently validated in an external cohort of patients. Because of the limitations of renal mass biopsy – and, often, the contraindications to it (e.g., anatomical factors, coagulopathy) – the use of such a nomogram which has shown reasonable predictive accuracy comprises the best counseling tool available to physicians when identifying those patients who may require definitive therapy.

Predicting Quality of Life

Quality of life outcomes are certainly not outcomes that are exclusively pertinent to an elderly population. However, given that the quantity of life is often limited in older patients, quality of life may comprise a disproportionate amount of consideration during the decision-making process. The morbidity associated with definitive therapies for prostate cancer has been well-reported; erectile function, urinary continence, and bowel function may all be affected as a result of radical prostatectomy, radiation, or interstitial brachytherapy. In the past, outcomes research has focused on oncologic results of therapy, but there is increasing focus on quality of life outcomes as patients have taken more ownership of their care and demonstrated the willingness to thoughtfully weigh the risks against the benefits of treatment. As a result, whereas nomograms were at one time predicting probabilities for cancer-specific mortality or extracapsular extension or nodal disease, we are now seeing an increased interest in nomograms that predict outcomes such as erectile dysfunction and rectal toxicity following definitive therapy for prostate cancer.

One such nomogram was produced by a group out of Italy which predicted late rectal toxicity following conformal therapy for prostate cancer [17]. The nomogram incorporates rectal radiation exposure as a prognostic variable and predicts the outcomes of fecal incontinence and grade 2–3 late rectal bleeding. This is one of the first nomograms designed to predict toxicity of therapy for prostate cancer, and we expect more groups to follow suit in the near future for other therapeutic modalities and their associated side effects. From a counseling standpoint, patients desire to know this information, but it is difficult to advise a man with low-volume Gleason 6 and a man with high-volume Gleason 8 prostate cancer regarding their chances of achieving a "trifecta" outcome of continence, potency, and cancer control following radical prostatectomy utilizing the exact same data. In reality, we accept the fact that the clinicopathological variables – including age – that are specific to each patient have a more than measurable effect on oncologic outcomes; quality of life outcomes are no different in this regard. Nomograms have the capacity to integrate these variables into a composite score and provide patients with the information that they need to make a fully informed treatment decision.

Predicting Mortality

The natural history of prostate cancer has been well-documented. The median time from biochemical recurrence to metastasis is 8 years; the median interval time between metastasis and death is 5 years [18]. In the past, this protracted course has limited outcomes research from predicting mortality due to an overall low event rate, and as a result, models have instead focused on more common outcomes such as biochemical recurrence and distant metastasis. However, the accumulation of patient data over the course of many years has now furnished the outcomes research community with the necessary information to analyze and accurately predict mortality outcomes.

A multi-institutional effort utilizing data from the Surveillance Epidemiology and End Results (SEER)-Medicare-linked database created nomograms predicting cancer-specific and other-cause mortality at 10 years following either radical prostatectomy or active surveillance [19]. The nomograms incorporate pretreatment information with oncologic predictive value, such as tumor stage and Gleason score; additionally, the models factor in overall health status by means of Charlson comorbidity index and patient age. Not surprisingly, the application of an active surveillance protocol has a negative impact on cancer-specific survival. More interestingly, however, surveillance also exhibits a negative impact on other-cause survival, with an overall effect comparable to having a Charlson comorbidity index of 1 or 2. The predictive accuracies of the models for 10-year cancer-specific and other-cause mortality were 73 and 69 %, respectively.

There is quite a bit of conflicting data regarding the benefit of local therapy for prostate cancer. Current evidence suggests that local therapy is associated with, at best, a 25 % reduction in prostate cancer-specific mortality, which adds a significant amount of complexity to the counseling discussion [20]. Nomograms that generate individualized mortality estimates for definitive therapy and active surveillance provide invaluable information that can aid patients in making the treatment decision that best suits their own risk profile. Elderly patients in particular may want to assess the risk of prostate cancer versus competing cause mortality, as increasing age and comorbidities may mitigate the benefits realized from local therapy. While keeping in mind that nomograms provide estimates of risk, the benefit of providing a prostate cancer patient with actual numbers specific to his clinical situation cannot be understated.

Nomograms predicting mortality risk estimates certainly embody a burgeoning area for outcomes research; there remains a void in this area for many urological cancers. Particularly in the area of prostate cancer, where there are a number of therapeutic options but no agreed-upon standard, the benefit realized by patients from more predictive models will be vast. But even in the cases of bladder and kidney cancers, where the population is typically older and oftentimes frail, an accurate assessment of mortality with and without therapies will allow patients to more readily make prompt and personalized decisions regarding treatment.

Table 3.1 Comparative effectiveness table

	Treatment X	Treatment Y
Benefits		
Benefit 1	B1 %	B1 %
Benefit 2	B2 %	B2 %
Harms		
Harm 1	H1 %	H1 %
Harm 2	H2 %	H2 %

Each cell is populated with individualized risk estimates produced via existing models based on either treatment choice X or treatment choice Y

Putting It All Together: Comparative Effectiveness

Comparative effectiveness is the side-by-side comparison of treatment options with respect to their expected benefits and harms. An example of a generic comparative effectiveness table is shown in Table 3.1. Ideally, the comparative effectiveness table would include not only oncologic outcomes but also quality of life outcomes such that the patient would have all predictions pertinent to his or her treatment decision in a single table. This can be accomplished by combining some of the aforementioned prediction tools into one table that incorporates all relevant patient data. Obviously, this is dependent on the availability of such prediction tools, which underscores the need for further development, validation, and implementation of mortality and quality of life models. Once all models are in place, they can be combined into a "mega-calculator" of sorts, which can often be formatted into an online tool available to providers and patients alike. Examples of individual nomograms that are available for public use are available at several websites, such as http://rcalc.ccf.org.

Ultimately, the combination of these nomograms into a comparative effectiveness tool would serve as high-quality informed consent for patients. Despite the fact that patients are bombarded with information following an oncologic diagnosis, we know that physicians are still falling short of appropriately meeting their information needs. Patients are sometimes so overwhelmed with their diagnosis that they cannot remember the options and the risk estimates cited by their doctors; a comparative effectiveness table is a counseling tool that patients can take home with them and refer back to whenever they are ready to fully digest the information.

The psychosocial benefits associated with this degree of counseling should not be underestimated. Particularly when dealing with an elderly population and cancers that may carry low malignant potential, the psychological outcomes may very well exceed in consequence the oncologic outcomes. There is certainly a subset of patients for whom the idea of therapy and its associated risk of morbidity is unacceptably high. At the same time, for others, the very thought of harboring active cancer within their bodies coupled with the risk of mortality is too much to bear. The point is that a comparative effectiveness table should provide each patient – regardless of his philosophic approach to malignancy, morbidity, and therapy – with the information that is most relevant to him. Furthermore, we believe that the presentation of this data will benefit patients from a psychosocial standpoint not only before therapy but also following therapy. Insofar as patients are able to make treatment choices based on the factors that they deem most important, they should theoretically feel more comfortable after the fact knowing that they had all the information required to make an informed treatment decision. Admittedly, this has not yet been studied prospectively to our knowledge.

Eliminating Age Cutoff Points

Not all elderly patients are created equally. The 70-year old (appearing much older than stated age) gentleman with a history of chronic obstructive pulmonary disease on 2 liters of oxygen at home and ischemic heart disease is not nearly the same candidate for therapy as the 70-year-old fit male with no associated comorbidities and parents who lived well into their tenth decade. Fortunately, when formulating the update of its clinical guidelines for the treatment of localized prostate cancer in 2007, the American Urological Association (AUA) guideline panel recognized this and specified that an assessment of the patient's life expectancy and overall health status should be undertaken prior to any treatment decisions [21]. Furthermore, the panel deemed life expectancy – as opposed to patient age – to be the critical factor when evaluating a patient for therapy, and as a result, they stated that a chronological age cutoff point was not specified.

However, there are certainly some factions who continue to adhere closely to age cutoff points. For example, many physicians believe that PSA screening should stop at age 75. While one can surely find merit on both sides of the argument, our objective is to demonstrate that we have tools at our disposal that may obviate the need for age cutoff points altogether. Rather than blanketing all men older than 75 as unfit for screening or for therapy, predictive models can incorporate comorbidities, disease risk factors, and other variables in addition to age to predict mortality. Taken one step further, models that feature quality-adjusted life years (QALY) as an outcome can quantify the capacity – in terms of both quality and longevity – to which patients may benefit from screening, therapy, surveillance, or whatever the clinical option may be. In this way, physicians would be able to advise all patients regarding potential advantages and disadvantages while taking life expectancy and quality of life into account, and patients would benefit from the opportunity to make a fully informed decision concerning screening or treatment regardless of their chronological age. While we do not doubt that most believe in utilizing an individualized patient approach to each encounter, we believe that presenting the patient with concrete data – as opposed to a more generalized and perhaps vague discussion – will optimize that individual's ability to more fully comprehend the factors that are implicit in the decision-making process. The approach of telling patients that they are simply too old to even enter into the decision-making process is exceedingly unsophisticated for the modern era of medicine and should be eliminated. Older patients have no desire to be treated differently than their younger counterparts. We have the capacity to construct and employ prediction tools that will allow us to counsel them in more concrete terms toward the decision that best suits them, and we believe that this should be a goal in evidence-based medicine moving forward.

Nomograms as a Counseling Tool

Although nomograms have greatly grown in popularity since their development, there has been some resistance to the widespread adoption of clinical algorithms and prediction models. Some clinicians might feel that increasing the number of evidence-based protocols may behave in a way that diminishes the significance of sound clinical judgment honed over years of practice. It is important to emphasize that nomograms act as a supplement to the clinical decision-making capacity of patients and providers. The practice of medicine is – and always will be – an art form. Whether an artist chooses to employ a brush, a pencil, or a piece of charcoal, the canvas remains blank until he or she interprets the subject matter, and this is very much how nomograms and other prediction models should be viewed. They serve primarily as tools that can help to characterize a disease state that requires interpretation and context that can only be offered by an experienced physician. Nomograms cannot replace clinical acumen when it comes to making clinical decisions; rather, they function primarily to mitigate the unintentional biases that are inherent in human estimations. They also incorporate an element of reproducibility among different patients that remains uninfluenced by anecdotal information. In this way, nomograms function to replicate the synthesization of clinical data carried out by physicians on a daily basis in an unbiased, reproducible, and evidence-based design, with an overarching goal of improving the patient decision-making process.

Conclusions

Of all available clinical prediction tools, nomograms likely provide the most accurate and practical risk estimations for the individual patient, and as a result, the popularity of nomograms has grown rapidly in the modern era of medicine. Nomograms mimic the synthesization of information performed by physicians on a daily basis, and they do so in a standardized, evidence-based format that mitigates the expected human error and biases. The development and application of nomograms predicting disease risk, quality of life, and mortality are most relevant to an elderly population and will provide the information necessary to make an informed medical decision. The next step in outcomes research should be to combine multiple prediction tools into comparative effectiveness tables in a way that will consistently offer older patients individualized high-quality informed consent. We should aim to move beyond an era of age cutoff points by employing nomograms predicting mortality outcomes, but there is no substitute for clinical expertise when it comes to the utilization and interpretation of prediction tools in the setting of the patient consultation.

References

1. Shariat SF, Capitanio U, Jeldres C, et al. Can nomograms be superior to other prediction tools? BJU Int. 2009;103(4):492–5.
2. Ross PL, Gerigk C, Gonen M, et al. Comparisons of nomograms and urologists' predictions in prostate cancer. Semin Urol Oncol. 2002;20(2):82–8.
3. Specht MC, Kattan MW, Gonen M, et al. Predicting nonsentinel node status after positive sentinel lymph biopsy for breast cancer: clinicians versus nomogram. Ann Surg Oncol. 2005;12(8):654–9.
4. Cassileth BR, Zupkis RV, Sutton-Smith K, et al. Information and participation preferences among cancer patients. Ann Intern Med. 1980;92(6):832–6.
5. Jenkins V, Fallowfield L, Saul J. Information needs of patients with cancer: results from a large study in UK cancer centres. Br J Cancer. 2001;84(1):48–51.
6. Rees CE, Bath PA. The information needs and source preferences of women with breast cancer and their family members: a review of the literature published between 1988 and 1998. J Adv Nurs. 2000;31(4):833–41.
7. Smyth MM, McCaughan E, Harrisson S. Women's perceptions of their experiences with breast cancer: are their needs being addressed? Eur J Cancer Care (Engl). 1995;4(2):86–92.
8. Butow PN, Dunn SM, Tattersall MH, et al. Computer-based interaction analysis of the cancer consultation. Br J Cancer. 1995;71(5):1115–21.
9. Rainey LC. Effects of preparatory patient education for radiation oncology patients. Cancer. 1985;56(5):1056–61.
10. Chawla SN, Crispen PL, Hanlon AL, et al. The natural history of observed enhancing renal masses: meta-analysis and review of the world literature. J Urol. 2006;175(2):425–31.
11. Lu-Yao GL, Albertsen PC, Moore DF, et al. Outcomes of localized prostate cancer following conservative management. JAMA. 2009;302(11):1202–9.
12. Isariyawongse BK, Sun L, Bañez LL, et al. Significant discrepancies between diagnostic and pathologic Gleason sums in prostate cancer: the predictive role of age and prostate-specific antigen. Urology. 2008;72(4):882–6.
13. Moussa AS, Kattan MW, Berglund R, et al. A nomogram for predicting upgrading in patients with low- and intermediate-grade prostate cancer in the era of extended prostate sampling. BJU Int. 2010;105(3):352–8.
14. Pahernik S, Ziegler S, Roos F, et al. Small renal tumors: correlation of clinical and pathological features with tumor size. J Urol. 2007;178(2):414–7.
15. Remzi M, Ozsoy M, Klingler HC, et al. Are small renal tumors harmless? Analysis of histopathological features according to tumors 4 cm or less in diameter. J Urol. 2006;176(3):896–9.
16. Kutikov A, Smaldone MC, Egleston BL, et al. Anatomic features of enhancing renal masses predict malignant and high-grade pathology: a preoperative nomogram using the RENAL Nephrometry score. Eur Urol. 2011;60(2):241–8.
17. Valdagni R, Kattan MW, Rancati T, et al. Is it time to tailor the prediction of radio-induced toxicity in prostate cancer patients? Building the first set of nomograms for late rectal syndrome. Int J Radiat Oncol Biol Phys. 2012;82:1957–66.
18. Pound CR, Partin AW, Eisenberger MA, et al. Natural history of progression after PSA elevation following radical prostatectomy. JAMA. 1999;281(17):1591–7.

19. Abdollah F, Sun M, Schmitges J, et al. Cancer-specific and other-cause mortality after radical prostatectomy versus observation in patients with prostate cancer: competing-risks analysis of a large North American population-based cohort. Eur Urol. 2011;60(5):920–30.
20. Bill-Axelson A, Holmberg L, Ruutu M, et al. Radical prostatectomy versus watchful waiting in early prostate cancer. N Engl J Med. 2011;364(18):1708–17.
21. Guideline for the management of clinically localized prostate cancer: 2007 update. 2007. http://www.auanet.org/content/clinical-practice-guidelines/clinical-guidelines/main-reports/proscan07/content.pdf. Accessed 20 Dec 2011.

Chapter 4
Renal Function in Elderly and in Relationship with Management of Genitourinary Tumors

Muriel Rainfray, Cecile Mertens, and Sophie Duc

Abstract Age-linked renal changes consist in a decrease in glomerular filtration rate (GFR) and limitations in sodium and water equilibrium. They predispose the old patients, over 75 years, to dehydration and acute renal failure. GFR estimation is always necessary and must be available before any drug prescription. Important variations are observed between the different methods of estimating GFR in elderly. Cockcroft and Gault and MDRD are the main formula used in bedside practice. The threshold of 60/ml/min/1.73 m^2 is relevant to define renal failure; this of 45 ml/min/1.73 m^2 is considered as a sign of frailty. Renal atherosclerosis is responsible of more than 50 % of chronic renal diseases in subjects over 65 years today, mostly in men. Considering the impact of genitourinary tumor treatment in elderly, radical nephrectomy remains an independent risk factor of chronic renal failure after surgery. Lower preoperative GFR, solitary kidney, older age, gender, tumor size, and longer ischemic interval predicted lower GFR after partial nephrectomy. Eligibility to cisplatin treatment depends on e-GFR, comorbidity, and oncological risk. As known and extensively studied for many years, the chief limit of cisplatin is nephrotoxicity which can be limited but not completely avoided by preventive procedures. Lastly, antiangiogenesis drugs need a broader evaluation of their effects on renal function in old people.

Keywords Elderly • Renal function • Genitourinary tumors • Chemotherapy Nephrectomy

M. Rainfray, M.D., Ph.D. (✉) • S. Duc, M.D.
Department of Geriatric Medicine, University Hospital Bordeaux,
Pessac, France
e-mail: muriel.rainfray@chu-bordeaux.fr; sophie.duc@chu-bordeaux.fr

C. Mertens, M.D.
Department of Geriatric Medicine, University Hospital Bordeaux,
Pessac, France
e-mail: cecile.mertens@chu-bordeaux.fr

J.-P. Droz, R.A. Audisio (eds.), *Management of Urological Cancers in Older People*,
Management of Cancer in Older People,
DOI 10.1007/978-0-85729-999-4_4, © Springer-Verlag London 2013

Anatomical and functional modifications of the kidney usually occur with aging in human as in animals. These age-linked changes are strongly correlated with vascular risk factors and chronic administration of cardiovascular drugs.

Anatomical changes consist in a reduction in size and weight of the kidneys to the detriment of the renal cortex. In subjects over 75 years, interstitial fibrosis, loss of 10–20 % of the glomeruli, and cystic transformation of the renal tubes are usual. The consequences of these changes on the renal functions concern the glomerular filtration rate (GFR) and the tubular abilities to maintain sodium, water, and acid–base equilibrium.

Functional Renal Changes with Aging

1. *Renal blood flow (RBF)* decreases about 10 % per decade, and glomerular vascular resistances progressively increase with aging.
2. *Functional renal reserve*, usually measured after a rich-protein diet, decreases but may remain normal in selected healthy old subjects [1]. The decline of functional renal reserve is the first step before those of GFR.
3. *Glomerular Filtration Rate (GFR)*

In transversal and longitudinal studies, GFR decreases with aging. However, this phenomenon is variable according to type of the studies, selection of the observed populations, and methods turned to account to measure or to estimate GFR.

Methods to Measure or to Estimate GFR

The physiological decline in lean muscle with aging, enhanced by malnutrition and poor physical activity, leads to a lower serum creatinine level. Therefore, a "normal" serum creatinine does not reflect renal function anymore and must not be utilized as the only way to adapt drug doses or to decide eligibility or not to a treatment. GFR estimation is always necessary and must be available before any drug prescription in the elderly. GFR can be measured by renal clearances of substances filtrated by the kidney (creatinine, inulin, cystatin C, DTPA, EDTA…) or estimated by creatinine-derived equations (e-GFR).

- The gold standard is the isotopic clearance of ^{51}Cr-EDTA or ^{99m}Tc-DTPA. This method gives an exact measurement of GFR and may be useful before radical nephrectomy to appreciate the remaining kidney function and predict the occurrence of acute renal failure in post-surgery. Nevertheless, it is a rather time-consuming and costly method which requires urine samples collection, which is not always easy and relevant in elderly because of frequent difficulties to completely void the bladder.
- Plasma cystatin C level, very utilized in children to estimate renal function, has not been validated in large samples of old subjects but is recognized to be a very good cardiovascular marker in this population [2].

Table 4.1 Chronic kidney disease definition and stages according to K/DOQI [7]

Stage	Description	GFR (ml/min/1.73 m^2)
1	Kidney damage with normal or increased GFR	≥90
2	Kidney damage with mild decreased GFR	60–89
3	Moderate decreased GFR	30–59
4	Severe decreased GFR	15–29
5	Kidney failure	<15 or dialysis

Kidney damage is defined by the existence of histological or biological or morphological defects for more than 3 months

- Estimation of GFR (e-GFR) by creatinine-derived equations has been proven to be a more sensitive method to estimate renal function than creatinine clearance measurement requiring timed urine samples [3]. However, important variations are observed between the different methods of estimating GFR in elderly. The older well-known Cockcroft and Gault formula integrating serum creatinine, age, sex, and weight is easy to calculate but has mostly been validated in selected populations of patients referred to nephrology clinics for symptoms related to renal diseases. Few old subjects have been tested. Modified Diet Renal Disease formula [4] does not integrate weight, which is an advantage in elderly, and has been validated in elderly subjects living in the community, not only in populations referred to nephrologists. A new close to MDRD formula is now available, recently proposed by the CKD-EPI group [5]. There is a debate about which formula is the better one in elderly. Nephrologists and biologists often recommend MDRD formula. A recent review of 12 studies comparing the Cockcroft and Gault and MDRD e-GFR to gold standards in subjects over 65 years [6] has shown that differences between e-GFR and gold standards vary with GFR level. For GFR > 60 ml/min/1.73 m^2, MDRD formula is closer to the gold standard than is Cockcroft and Gault formula, whereas for lower GFR < 60 or < 30 ml/min/1.73 m^2, Cockcroft and Gault formula is better to appreciate GFR. The threshold of 60/ml/min/1.73 m^2 is relevant to define renal failure according to CKD group guidelines [7]. Definition of chronic renal failure and different stages are given in Table 4.1. Concerning the necessary dose adaptation of the drugs having a renal metabolism, most of the studies have utilized Cockcroft and Gault formula to make recommendations. Therefore, it remains interesting to make use of this formula to prescribing.

Changes in Renal Function with Aging

In transversal studies including nonselected old subjects over 65 years, mean e-GFR, whatever the formula, decreases with age and is always lower in women than in men. In the French epidemiological survey "The Three-City" including nearly 10,000 subjects, mean age of 76.4 ± 18.2 years, living in the community, *e-MDRD* DFG is 78 (68–89) ml/min/1.73 m^2 in men and 74 (65–85) ml/min/1.73 m^2 in women. The prevalence of renal failure defined by DFG < 60 ml/min/1.73 m^2 is only 13 %. By contrast, in frail subjects living in nursing homes in Sweden, *e-MDRD* GFR is 67.2 ml/min/1.73 m² in men (82.8 years) and 64.9 ml/min/1.73 m² (85.7 years) in women [8].

DFG is related to vascular risk factors such as hypertension, diabetes, hypercholesterolemia, and ischemic cardiomyopathy; to cardiovascular treatments; and also to abilities in activities of daily living (ADL) or physical activity. An abundant literature concerns the role of environmental toxics, lead or cadmium, suspected of nephrotoxicity in community-living nonprofessional-exposed population, particularly in Asia. Longitudinal studies confirm the decrease of renal function with aging. In the above mentioned Three-City Study, 1,298 subjects are followed during 4 years. Mean GFR decline is 1.75 ml/min/1.73 m² in men and 1.41 ml/min/1.73 m² in women. Considering individual e-GRF evolution with time, Lindeman et al. [9] has individualized three different pathways: slight decrease in e-GFR representing usual renal aging, strong decline in e-GFR affecting subjects with authentic renal diseases, and stable e-GFR as a witness of successful renal aging.

Chronic Kidney Diseases in Aging

Vascular risk factors are the main determinants of decreased RBF and GFR in elderly. Even treated hypertension favors nephroangiosclerosis and renal atheromatosis. Type 2 diabetes leads, less often than type 1 diabetes, to glomerulosclerosis but favors also renal atherosclerosis. Thus, renal atherosclerosis is responsible of more than 50 % of chronic renal diseases in subjects over 65 years today, mostly in men. In various registers, renal atherosclerosis represents about 60 % of the diseases leading to end-stage renal failure and dialysis in western countries. Clinical manifestations of renal atheromatosis are hypertension and chronic renal failure related to bilateral renal stenosis or cholesterol emboli in renal parenchyma leading to partially reversible acute kidney injury (AKI).

Many drugs, usually prescribed in elderly patients, have a specific impact on renal vascularization (vasodilators, diuretics, angiotensin-converting enzyme (ACE) inhibitors), GFR autoregulation (ACE inhibitors, sartans) or direct toxicity on renal medullary [nonsteroidal anti-inflammatory (NSAID) drugs]. In very old patients, interstitial nephritis may be related to chronic nephrotoxic drug (phenacetin) self-administration in adult age. Chronic urological obstructions by voluminous prostatic adenomas get less frequent because of easier referral of old men with prostatism to urologists. However, bladder or ureteral obstructions by genitourinary or prostate cancers, lymph nodes, or specific retroperitoneal fibrosis still occur in advanced stages of cancers.

Sodium Metabolism

Final regulation of sodium resorption occurs in the distal collector under the influence of the renin–angiotensin–aldosterone system. Renin–aldosterone response to physiological stimuli (orthostatism, poor-salted diet) is blunted in the elderly due to vascular alterations of macula densa or decreased secretion of hormones interfering with renin secretion (angiotensinogen, progesterone, oestradiol, kallikrein). Basal plasma renin and aldosterone levels are normal which differs from hyporeninism to hypoaldosteronism occurring in diabetic patients. The main consequence is the inability of the aging kidney to maintain a perfect sodium regulation in all circumstances and to predispose old people to dehydration.

Water Metabolism

Renal water resorption occurs in the collecting duct under the influence of the antidiuretic hormone (ADH) along a cortico-medullary osmotic gradient created by sodium exchanges in the Henlé loop. During water restriction, maximal urinary osmolality (Uosmol) decreases with age. After 12 h of water restriction, Uosmol is 1,200 mosmol/l in young and 600–800 mosmol/l in older patients. Vascular alterations in the renal medullary or loop diuretics treatments disturb the osmolar gradient, and V2-ADH receptors changes deteriorate the process of water resorption. This phenomenon exposes the elderly to water losses and to hypernatremia especially if thirst sensation is blunted as it is observed in normal aging but often more in neurologic patients with strokes or dementia.

Acid–Base Equilibrium

Few changes in acid–base equilibrium occur with aging. A slower elimination of an acid load has been observed in many older patients without any remarkable consequence. However, in old diabetics, situations of hyporeninemic hypoaldosteronism may occur leading to type IV renal acidosis with decreasing titratable acidity.

Clinical Consequences of Usual Renal Aging

A Low e-GFR Is a Vascular Risk Factor

Many studies have shown that, as in younger adults, age-related decrease in e-GFR has a strong relationship with higher cardiovascular morbidity and mortality. However, the risk becomes significant for e-GFR < 45 ml/min/1.73 m^2 compared to 60 ml/min/1.73 m^2 in younger adults and increases with an even small albuminuria [10].

Age-Related Low e-GFR Is Not Often Associated to Renal Lesions and to Proteinuria, Hematuria, or Severe Hypertension as It Is in Younger Adults

In the Three-City Study, only 20 % of men and 10 % of women having an e-GFR between 45 and 60 ml/min/1.73 m² had symptoms of nephropathy – respectively 50 and 27 % for e-GFR lower than 45 ml/min/1.73 m² [11]. Moreover, competitive risk of death in subjects over 70 years having e-GFR between 30 and 60 ml/min/1.73 m² is very high: 49 % for the range 70–79 years and 84 % for the >79 years whereas the risk to reach end-stage renal failure is only 4 and 3 %, respectively [12].

Light consequences of age-related e-GFR decrease in elderly, and more precisely, very low risk of reaching end-stage renal failure by spontaneous evolution of the renal lesions explains that the usual guidelines of prevention strategy by ACE and low-protein diet do not concern patients over 75 years, in the absence of a broader validation of this preventive strategy. On the contrary, a low-protein diet is dangerous in the elderly leading to proteino-caloric malnutrition and its consequences: loss of muscle mass, falls, and fractures.

e-GFR < 45 ml/min/1.73 m² Is a Feature of Frailty

In several studies, e-GFR < 45 ml/min/1.73 m² is related to anemia, in men more than in women; disability; less physical activity; and depression in women [13]. Disability, fatigue, weakness, depression, and poor physical activity are criteria of frailty as defined by Linda Fried [14]. It is obvious that old patients with a low e-GFR must be considered as frail patients and treated with consideration to polypharmacy.

High Risk of Dehydration

Age-related changes in renal sodium and water balance predispose the elderly to global dehydration. Such circumstances as poor-salted diet, long period of anorexia, diuretics, diarrhea, and vomiting are dangerous for the elderly. Dehydration with hyponatremia occurs when sodium losses are predominant and when hyposmolar hydration is wrongly administered (water, glucose solute). Dehydration with hypernatremia occurs when water losses are predominant and associated with thirst defect. Thirst defect becomes frequent with aging especially in patients with neurological injuries (stroke, Parkinson disease, dementia)

High Risk of Acute Renal Failure or Acute Kidney Injury

Prerenal acute renal failure (ARF) is a frequent complication of acute states (dehydration, hypovolemia, sepsis, inflammation, cardiac failure) and polypharmacy in the elderly. If not diagnosed early, prerenal ARF leads to acute kidney injury (AKI). Early diagnosis of AKI is difficult because renal lesions may occur before serum creatinine increment and furthermore serum creatinine is not a good marker of renal function in acute catabolic states. Recently, novel biomarkers have been reported to detect early AKI [15]. These biomarkers reflect cellular injury, ischemia, or toxin-induced damage of tubular cells. The most promising one is NGAL which increases by 100-fold in the urine in the 2 h after acute renal cellular injury. It has been investigated in a variety of clinical contexts and is more sensitive than serum creatinine to detect AKI in postoperative states or kidney transplantation. It has not been investigated especially in elderly. Interleukin-18 (IL-18) is a pro-inflammatory cytokine activated in the proximal tubule cells and excreted in the urine after ischemic injury. Patients with acute tubular necrosis have increased IL-18 levels and urinary IL-18/ creatinine ratios. Further validation studies are necessary in old patients and in patients with preexisting chronic renal failure. Cystatin C and kidney injury molecule KIM-1 are also promising markers called to further development and validation in AKI. Detecting early AKI is challenging to test and validate ARF preventive strategies lying mainly on maintenance of an adequate circulating volume, an adequate perfusion pressure, and the avoidance of further insults to the kidney. In the context of AKI, nephrotoxic drugs such as aminoglycosides or amphotericin B must be avoided, or, if necessary, dose adjustments must be closely monitored by using plasma dosages. Radiocontrast-induced nephropathy must be prevented by using nonionic low and iso-osmolar contrast agents, by administering intravenous fluid prior to radiocontrast, and also by limiting as often as possible radiocontrast procedures.

ARF prevalence is underestimated because only the more severe forms with acute tubular necrosis are checked. AKI is estimated to occur in 5 % of hospitalized patients and in 25–30 % of critically ill patients. In urology, AKI is related to obstructive diseases, urosepsis, and nephrectomy. Tubular necrosis is the most severe complication of prerenal ARF. It occurs mainly in patients with preexisting chronic renal failure. The most frequent conditions of tubular necrosis in elderly are drug associations such as ACE inhibitors, NSAID, and diuretics or drugs with a renal elimination or direct nephrotoxicity (aminosides). Older age, sepsis, oliguria, respiratory failure, and needing dialysis are predictive factors of mortality in elderly patients in the acute care units.

Drug Prescriptions

Polypharmacy is usual in elderly and predisposes to many interactions and severe side effects. Guidelines for better prescribing in the elderly have been developed by geriatric societies, and several lists of inappropriate drugs in elderly are now available. Consequences of decreased GFR are mostly important concerning drugs with renal metabolism and narrow therapeutic index such as digitalis glycosides, valproate, gabapentin, aminosides, vancomycin, clavulanic acid and chemotherapy methotrexate, bleomycin, cisplatin, and melphalan. For every prescription of these drugs, a careful assessment of the renal function by e-GFR is necessary. Serum creatinine level is inadequate for estimating renal function for reasons mentioned above. In the Three-City Study, participants take an average of 4.4 drugs. Six-year mortality is increased by 40 % in subjects with e-GFR < 60 ml/min/1.73 m² exposed to drugs requiring dose adjustment and trends to increase in those with e-GFR < 60 ml/min/1.73 m² exposed to contraindicated drugs [16]. On another hand, in very old frail patients living in nursing homes, no link is really found between renal function, drug prescribing, and mortality emphasizing the utility of a geriatric formation for practitioners working in these institutions.

Relationship Between Renal Aging and GU Tumor Treatments

Nephrectomy

Nephrectomy is the recommended treatment of renal cell carcinoma. Partial nephrectomy is recommended for small tumors (≤4 cm) which represent 60–70 % of all diagnosed renal masses. Unfortunately, radical nephrectomy is still performed in more than 80 % cases of RCC all over the world.

Renal Function After Radical Nephrectomy

GFR usually decreases in adults after radical nephrectomy, and many patients, even those with normal e-GFR before surgery, experience chronic renal failure defined by e-GFR < 60 ml/min/1.73 m², as a consequence of radical nephrectomy. In Huang retrospective cohort study of 662 patients with renal tumors ≤4 cm, referred to a cancer center [17], 26 % had preexisting kidney disease before surgery though a "normal" serum creatinine and two functioning kidneys. This result has been already reported by other urologists and emphasizes the inadequacy of looking only on serum creatinine to assess renal function before surgery. After surgery, the 3-year probability of freedom from new onset of e-GFR < 60 ml/min/1.73 m² was 35 % [28–43, $p < 0.0001$] after radical nephrectomy versus 80 % [95 %CI 73–85] after partial nephrectomy. The 3-year probability of freedom from new onset of e-GFR < 45 ml/min/1.73 m² was 64 % [56–70, $p < 0.001$] after radical nephrectomy and 95 % [95 %CI 91–98] after partial nephrectomy. Thus, radical nephrectomy remains an independent risk factor of chronic renal failure after surgery.

Renal Function After Partial Nephrectomy

After partial nephrectomy, the risk of developing chronic renal failure is linked to the occurrence of AKI. In a prospective study of 1,169 patients undergoing partial nephrectomy for small RCC [18], the incidence of postoperative acute kidney injury was 3.6 % in the whole cohort, 0.8 % in patients with preoperative normal renal function, 6.2 % in those with stage 3 CKD, and 34 % in stage 4 CKD. Acute loss of renal function predicted lower ultimate GFR. Lower preoperative GFR, solitary kidney, older age, gender, tumor size, and longer ischemic interval predicted lower GFR after partial nephrectomy. As the duration of renal ischemia is the only modifiable surgical risk factor, efforts to limit ischemic time and injury should be pursued. In other studies, age > 60 years, basal GFR, hypertension, diabetes, and tumor >7 cm are independent risk factors of chronic renal failure after surgery.

Renal Function After Nephroureterectomy

Nephroureterectomy is indicated in upper-tract urothelial carcinoma. Because urothelial carcinomas are strongly related to tobacco, patients have more cardiovascular comorbidities and a higher risk of chronic kidney disease when facing the treatment. In a recent retrospective study of 470 patients with urothelial carcinomas [19], 336 patients underwent nephroureterectomy. Median age was 72 years (62–78), and 79 % had no or minimal comorbidity. Median presurgery MDRD e-GFR was 59 ml/min/1.73 m^2 (47–77), and 52 % of the patients were ineligible to adjuvant cisplatin-based combination chemotherapy (CBCC) on the basis of e-GFR < 60 ml/min/1.73 m^2. Median post-surgery MDRD e-GFR was 48 ml/min/1.73 m^2, and 78 % of the patients were ineligible for adjuvant CBCC. One hundred and forty-four high oncological risk patients might be considered for adjuvant CBCC. The proportion of ineligibility was 60 % before surgery and 76 % after surgery.

Cisplatin Therapy

Cancer patients appear to be particularly vulnerable to renal defects, and the older ones may be considered particularly at risk to develop renal failure. Eligibility to cisplatin treatment depends on e-GFR, comorbidity, and oncological risk. As known and extensively studied for many years, the chief limit of cisplatin is nephrotoxicity which can be limited but not completely avoided by preventive procedures. In the plasma, cisplatin is strongly bound to proteins, and the free portion of cisplatin is filtered in the glomeruli. A high renal uptake of the drug mediated by specific transport systems explains the particularly high kidney concentration of cisplatin. After oral administration, cisplatin is quickly excreted in the urine. Progressive renal function decline may appear with repeated cycles of cisplatin treatment in spite of initial dose reduction and other preventive measures, emphasizing the necessity of estimating GFR before each chemotherapy cycle. Tubular injury is often associated with the cisplatin-induced reduction in GFR, expressed by a minimal tubular proteinuria or rarely by a salt-wasting syndrome leading to orthostatic hypotension.

Tubular injuries are also expressed by defective transport of water, calcium, potassium, magnesium, and hydrogen ions leading to polyuria, hypocalcemia, hypokalemia, hypomagnesemia, and partial tubular acidosis. Recent works suggest that cisplatin may directly induce necrosis and apoptosis of renal tubular cells through toxic mechanisms implicating oxidative-stress processes for necrosis and p53 activation for apoptosis [20]. Renal function does not always recover to normal after withdrawal of the drug. Neither calcium channel blockers nor ACE inhibitors have demonstrated any reversal action in cisplatin-induced ARF which can be enhanced by gentamicin–cephalotin or other nephrotoxic coprescription.

European Society of Clinical Pharmacy Special Interest Group Recommendations for Prevention of Cisplatin Nephrotoxicity [20]

Before administration

- To estimate GFR by MDRD or Cockcroft and Gault formula
- To ensure that euvolemia is present
- To adjust cisplatin dosage according to the patient's renal function

Administration

- To administer the platinum slowly
- To use a saline solution infusion that produces a brisk dieresis
- To maintain a urine flow at 3–4 l/24 h the preceding day and for the next 2–3 days
- Not to use diuretics neither mannitol nor furosemide

After administration

- To determine, if feasible, serum creatinine 3–5 days after completion of the course
- To monitor magnesium levels routinely and supplement when necessary
- To avoid coadministration of nephrotoxic drugs such as aminoglycosides, NSAIDs, iodinated contrast media, and zoledronate
- To reevaluate renal function before the next course

Antiangiogenesis Therapy

Anti-vascular endothelial growth factor (VEGF) therapy has not been specially studied in elderly cancer patients with metastatic renal cell carcinoma. Elimination of anti-VEGF such as bevacizumab, sunitinib, temsirolimus, or everolimus is done by the liver. In patients with e-GFR equal or below 60 ml/min/1.73 m^2, reduction of doses is not recommended. However, those drugs induce an increment in vascular resistances, and hypertension occurs in 11 to 43 % of the treated patients. Mild to severe proteinuria and acute renal failure have also been reported independently of the pretreatment renal function or signs of renal injury [21]. In the absence of larger experience, these drugs need to be closely monitored in patients with mild renal impairment and in elderly patients.

References

1. Esposito C, Plati A, Mazzullo T, et al. Renal function and functional reserve in healthy elderly individuals. J Nephrol. 2007;20:617–25.
2. Shlipak MG, Sarnak MJ, Katz R, et al. Cystatin C and the risk of death and cardiovascular events among elderly persons. N Engl J Med. 2005;352:2049–60.
3. Stevens LA, Coresh J, Greene T, Levey AS. Assessing kidney function-measured and estimated glomerular filtration rate. N Engl J Med. 2006;354:2473–83.
4. Levey AS, Coresh J, Greene T, et al. Using standardized serum creatinine values in the Modification of Diet in Renal Disease study equation for estimating glomerular filtration rate. Ann Intern Med. 2006;145:247–54.
5. Levey AS, Stevens LA, Schmid CH, et al. A new equation to estimate glomerular filtration rate. Ann Intern Med. 2009;150:604–12.
6. Van Pottelbergh G, Van Heden L, Mathei C, Degryse J. Methods to evaluate renal function in elderly patients: a systematic literature review. Age Ageing. 2010;39:542–8. doi:10.1093/ageing/afq091.
7. National Kidney Foundation. K/DOQI clinical practice guidelines for chronic kidney disease. Evaluation, classification and stratification. Am J Kidney Dis. 2002;39(2 Suppl):S1–266.
8. Stengel B, Metzger M, Froissart M, Rainfray M, Berr C, Tzourio C, Helmer C. Clinical and prognostic significance of impaired kidney function in the elderly – the Three-City prospective cohort study. Nephrol Dial Transplant. 2011;26(10):3286–95.
9. Lindeman RD, Tobin J, Shock NW. Longitudinal studies on the rate of decline in renal function with age. J Am Geriatr Soc. 1985;33:278–85.
10. Chronic Kidney Disease Prognosis Consortium. Association of estimated glomerular filtration rate and albuminuria with all-cause and cardiovascular mortality in general population cohorts: a collaborative meta-analysis. Lancet. 2010;375:2073–81.
11. Eriksen BO, Ingebretsen OC. The progression of chronic kidney disease: a 10-years population-based study of the effect of gender and age. Kidney Int. 2006;69:375.
12. 3C Study Group. Vascular factors and risk of dementia: design of the Three-City study and baseline characteristics on the study population. Neuroepidemiology. 2003;22:316–25.
13. Roderick PJ, Atkins RJ, Smeeth L, Nitsch DM, Hubbard RB, Fletcher AE, Bulpitt CJ. Detecting chronic kidney disease in older people; what are the implications? Age Ageing. 2008;37:179–86.
14. Fried LP, Tangen CM, Walston J, et al. Frailty in older adults: evidence for a phenotype. J Gerontol A Biol Sci Med Sci. 2001;56:M146–56.
15. Thomas AA, Demirjian S, Lane BR, Simmons MN, Goldfarb DA, Subramanian VS, Campbell SC. Acute kidney injury: novel biomarkers and potential utility for patient care in urology. Urology. 2011;77:5–11.
16. Breton G, Froissart M, Janus N, Launay-Vacher V, Berr C, Tzourio C, Helmer C, Stengel B. Inappropriate drug use and mortality in community-dwelling elderly with impaired kidney function – the Three-City population-based study. Nephrol Dial Transplant. 2011;26:2852–9.

17. Huang WC, Levey AS, Serio AM, Snyder M, Vickers AJ, Raj GV, Scardino PT, Russo P. Chronic kidney disease after nephrectomy in patients with renal cortical tumours: a retrospective cohort study. Lancet Oncol. 2006;7:735–40.
18. Lane BR, Babineau DC, Poggio ED, Weight CJ, Larson BT, Gill IS, Novick AC. Factors predicting renal functional outcome after partial nephrectomy. J Urol. 2008;180:2363–9. doi:10.1016/j.juro.2008.08.036.
19. Lane BR, Smith AK, Larson BT, Gong MC, Campbell SC, Raghavan D, Dreicer R, Hansel DE, Stephenson AJ. Chronic kidney disease after nephroureterectomy for upper tract urothelial carcinoma and implications for the administration of perioperative chemotherapy. Cancer. 2010;116:2967–73. VC 2010 American Cancer Society.
20. Launay-Vacher V, Rey J-B, Isnard-Bagnis C, Deray G, Daouphars M. Prevention of cisplatin nephrotoxicity: state of the art and recommendations from the European Society of Clinical Pharmacy Special Interest Group on Cancer Care Cancer. Chemother Pharmacol. 2008;61:903–9.
21. Gupta S, Parsa V, Heilbrun LK, Smith DW, Dickow B, Heath E, Vaishampayan U. Safety and efficacy of molecularly targeted agents in patients with metastatic kidney cancer with renal dysfunction. Anticancer Drugs. 2011;22(8):794–800.

Part II
Prostate Cancer: General Considerations

Chapter 5
Prostate Cancer Screening or Early Diagnosis in Senior Adults?

Jean Etienne Terrier, Helen Boyle, and Nicolas Mottet

Abstract Prostate cancer is the most frequent cancer in older men. The benefit of mass screening is one of the hot topics in the urological community. The main question is related to the potential public health benefit of mass screening using PSA testing and digital rectal examination. The question is even more debatable in senior adults. Proponents of screening argue that mass screening leads to an early discovery of the tumor and more effective and less toxic curative treatment. Two large randomized studies have attempted to answer this question, which seems the only reasonable way to decide. But none have given a definitive answer.

At present, the interpretations of these two major studies diverge; early diagnosis remains the single most honest option to offer patients.

Keywords Prostate cancer • Screening • Early diagnosis • Senior adult • Lead time bias • Length time bias

Introduction

Prostate cancer (PCa) is the most frequent solid tumor (excluding skin cancer) [1] and the second cause of cancer death in men. Its incidence increases after the age of 60, reaching a maximum after 75 years. It is therefore logical to raise the question regarding a structured mass screening, especially in senior adults. This issue divides

J.E. Terrier, M.D. (✉) • N. Mottet, M.D., Ph.D.
Department of Urology, University Hospital of St. Etienne,
St. Etienne, France
e-mail: jetterrier@yahoo.fr; nicolas.mottet@chu-st-etienne.fr

H. Boyle, M.D.
Department of Medicine, Center Léon-Bérard,
Lyon, France
e-mail: helen.boyle@lyon.unicancer.fr

J.-P. Droz, R.A. Audisio (eds.), *Management of Urological Cancers in Older People*,
Management of Cancer in Older People,
DOI 10.1007/978-0-85729-999-4_5, © Springer-Verlag London 2013

since many years the urological community but also public health authorities all over the world. These divisions are explained by the high prevalence of PCa and its slow evolution that lead many patients to die with, not from their prostate cancer. In addition, the term "screening" is often used indiscriminately, most interlocutors mixing up "mass screening" with individual early diagnosis. These concepts are now well defined, and the requirements to determine whether they have an interest or not are pretty clear. In addition, recent trials from Europe (ERSPC) [2] and the USA (PLCO) [3] give some preliminary results that can push the discussion forward.

We will start by defining what are mass screening and early individual diagnosis. We will then consider which might be appropriate for the elderly, based on the available characteristics of both attitudes.

Definitions

The differences between both screening attitudes may be considered as purely academic. Mass screening (routine/general) offers all men in a predefined age group, regardless of symptoms, a screening test (such as PSA and digital rectal examination [DRE]). This was the policy used in the randomized trials we will discuss later. Early individual diagnosis (also called early detection) involves a voluntary patient who is asking his doctor for early diagnosis of prostate cancer using the same tests as above. The main difference between these two modes of testing is the patient's request.

At present, the practitioner is in the second situation. Choosing the appropriate attitude regarding screening requires being able to understand and master the paradoxes related to early diagnosis.

The Three Biases That Prevent Us from Understanding the Possible Paradox of Screening (Whether Mass or Individual)

The main argument of most proponents of mass screening for PCa seems: "The sooner the diagnosis, the better the cure." It is reinforced by the fact that we clinicians, unlike our fellow epidemiologists, are regularly confronted with patients with advanced diseases diagnosed late and sometimes leading to death. It should be borne in mind that this reasoning is simplistic and does not prove the benefit of early diagnosis. And three biases will compete to suggest an improved survival through an early detection, even if the proposed treatment was totally unnecessary, i.e., the volunteer effect, the lead time bias, and the length time bias:

- The volunteer effect: Patients who volunteer for screening are often in better shape than the ones who do not. Thus, in a study on breast cancer screening [4], it has been shown that among women who responded to screening (2/3 of the contacted population), deaths from any cause (including cardiovascular) were considerably lower than in the control population and even lower (half!) than in people contacted for screening and who refused it (1/3 of the contacted population).

- The lead time bias. Making the diagnosis a few months or years earlier will lead to artificially increase the "duration of diagnosis," regardless of the effect of treatment. PCa, due to the diagnostic power of PSA, is particularly likely to be affected by this type of bias.
- The length time bias relies on the fact that in general the less aggressive tumors have longer disease evolution. Thus, the "window of early diagnosis" will be likely to preferentially diagnose this type of tumor rather than more aggressive lesions. In this case, the analysis at the end of study will be biased by the fact that the tumor population will become heterogeneous between the early diagnosed arm and the other where there will be more aggressive lesions. Again, regardless of the effect of any treatment, a false impression of survival improvement in the early diagnosed arm will occur. As for the lead time bias, PCa is particularly likely to be affected by this type of bias based on its slow development. These methodological biases highlight the need for randomized trials to compare mass screening and early individual diagnosis.

Why Does the PCa's Natural History Lead to Considering Screening?

The theoretical interest of early diagnosis is to treat patients at an earlier stage, leading to a better disease control. This implies a known and regular disease growth. Even assuming this is not enough. It also requires that the "critical points" exist [5]. They represent points at which the treatments are easier or more efficient to implement than if they are used later in the course of the disease. This notion of "critical point" is particularly important in PCa based on its slow evolution. The PSA tests can effectively diagnose PCa before being clinically visible [6]. PCa is a very heterogeneous disease. Some indolent lesions do not require any form of treatment (or possibly a really delayed one) [7, 8], while others will lead to death 10 years after the diagnosis if no active treatment is considered. This might represent another important reason for screening.

PCa: Is It a Public Health Problem?

PCa is the most frequently diagnosed cancer in Western men: There were 71,577 new cases of prostate cancer and 8,791 deaths in France in 2010 and 218,890 new cases and 27,050 deaths in the United States in 2007 [1]. PCa is the second or third leading cause of cancer death, but these are usually late deaths occurring in about one third of men beyond 80 years. For men between 60 and 79 years of age, 54,959 deaths from lung cancer and 12,511 from PCa were observed in 2004, PCa being in third place behind colorectal cancer. Beyond the age of 80, 18,261 lung cancer compared to 15,341 PCa deaths were observed [1]. The number of lost years of life due to cancer is a more meaningful indicator, and PCa ranks only sixth behind lung, breast, colorectal, stomach, and pancreas. The SEER database indicates that the number of years of life lost per patient is 9.3 for PCa, compared to 15 for lung cancer [9].

The incidence of prostate cancer is increasing in all European countries, and France has the highest incidence with an estimated rate around 200/100,000 in 2010. In the USA, a doubling of the incidence from about 100 to more than 200/100,000 within 5 years was observed after 1991. However, in the United States, incidence has declined and tends to be stable now. This decline has so far not been observed in France. The effect of PSA testing and the enthusiasm for individual early diagnosis, however, gradually reach its maximum, and recent data suggest that incidence rates in different countries should stabilize or even decline outside USA.

What Performances Are Expected from Diagnostic Tools in Each of the Two Approaches (Individual Diagnosis or Early Mass Screening)?

To justify mass screening, a reduced mortality must be seen at a level that will offset the treatment-related morbidity.

For mass screening, tools should be simple and minimally invasive and be able to distinguish in large patient populations between men "not at risk" and men "at risk" for PCa. For men "at risk," prostate biopsies should be performed as they remain the reference diagnostic test. This explains why most studies were using biological tests only and increased their sensitivity at the highest possible value, with the associated risk of a poor specificity. On an individual basis, the negative predictive value must be as high as possible in order to rule out PCa. The combination of PSA testing and digital rectal examination (DRE) is the current available tool.

- Digital rectal examination (DRE) can detect cancers of the peripheral zone (the region where at least 60 % of lesions arise). It does not by itself detect all prostate cancers and must be associated with a measure of PSA. In the ERSPC trial based on 10,523 patients, the overall detection rate of cancers was 4.5 % when the DRE was associated with PSA and endorectal ultrasonography. The overall detection rate was 2.5 % when the DRE was used alone. The positive predictive value ranged between 4 and 11 % for a PSA below 2.9 ng/ml and 33 and 83 % when between 3 and 9.9 ng/ml or more. Out of the 473 PCa diagnosed, 82 (17.3 %) would have been missed by omitting the DRE [10]. Similar findings are observed in the PLCO study (16 %) [4] and in Friedman et al.'s study [11]. In summary, DRE is not a reliable tool for small lesions and is considered as invasive by many men. This is why it is less proposed for screening studies. However, it allows detecting 20 % of all PCa in patients with an otherwise normal PSA. Therefore, it must be systematically combined with PSA for an individual early diagnosis.

- The PSA blood test is currently widely used as a diagnostic test. Unfortunately, its specificity is very low. PSA is organ but not disease specific: PSA might be increased in benign situations such as benign prostatic hypertrophy, prostatitis, and other inflammatory conditions. Conversely, men with PCa may have a very low PSA. Its sensitivity varies with the threshold value. The most often used threshold is 4 ng/ml [12]. For a threshold of 4 ng/ml, a 93 % sensitivity and 24 % specificity are observed, leading to a positive predictive value of 25–35 % for a PSA between 4 and 10 ng/ml and 50–80 % for a PSA above 10 ng/ml. Recently, some authors suggest to lower this threshold [13]. This is mainly from the PCPT trial in which 18,882 patients were randomized to either placebo or finasteride for PCa prevention. An annual PSA and DRE were performed, and systematic prostate biopsies were done after 7 years on study. Out of the 9,459 patients receiving placebo, 2,950 had a PSA that remained below 4 ng/ml and a normal DRE. Among these 2,950 patients, 449 PCa were diagnosed (15.2 %), including 67 (14.9 %) with a Gleason score greater or equal to 7 [14]. In summary, PSA alone is sensitive but not specific. For individual early diagnosis, it must be associated with the DRE.

- Values of other diagnostic tools in the early individual diagnosis: The fraction of free PSA is lower in cancer than in benign disease. For PSA between 4 and 10 ng/ml, a free/total PSA less than 15 % is correlated with the presence of cancer, and its use leads to a sensitivity of 95 % and a specificity of 18 % [15]. However, its use is not recommended as first line, since a PSA above 4 ng/ml is considered high enough to justify a biopsy (at least 20 % probability to find a PCa). But it is interesting after a first set of negative biopsies. The use of PSA velocity (PSAV) or PSA density (PSAD) marginally improves the diagnostic probability [16]. Currently, research is turning to new tools such as urinary markers. PCA3 is the most studied. Its expression in prostate tumors is almost 66–144 times greater than in healthy tissue [17]. Several prospective studies have confirmed its superiority compared to PSA: slightly lower sensitivity (range 65–82 %), but a slightly better specificity (66–89 %), as well as better positive predictive value (48–75 %) and negative predictive value (80–90 %), the results being similar regardless of the PSA level [6, 18]. This marker may be of particular interest in patients with a first set of negative biopsies [19]. However, PCA3 is expensive and requires a prior prostatic massage. Therefore, even if promising, these data have to be confirmed on very large cohorts and at a cost-effectiveness level. Finally, no imaging techniques can be used as a mass screening tool.

If any of these tests are suspicious, prostate biopsies need to be performed. They are done transrectally under ultrasound guidance. But are they really harmless?

The real and detailed morbidity is poorly known except for prostatitis (around 2 %) [20]. Mortality primarily by septic shock is an issue, considered to be around 0.2 % [21]), even after correct prophylaxis.

Do We Have Curative Treatment for PCa in 2012?

As already explained in the preamble, the purpose of early diagnosis is to be more effective in curing patients or to lower morbidity. It is also a prerequisite in the context of the discussion on the possible interest of mass screening (WHO criteria).

There are three randomized trials comparing active treatment and observation in localized disease with a delayed palliative treatment for symptoms where overall survival was the main objective [22–24]. Only one has been published. In two trials, the active treatment was radical prostatectomy; in the other, it was old-fashioned radiotherapy. No randomized trial with brachytherapy or other modalities is available. Radical prostatectomy is associated with a mortality rate that can reach 5‰. The 30-day mortality rate increases with age (odds ratio = 2.04 per decade [25]). No specific mortality is associated with radiotherapy.

Six hundred and ninety-five patients with early prostate cancer were enrolled in a phase III clinical trial comparing radical prostatectomy to watchful waiting. Radical prostatectomy was associated with an increase in overall and specific survival by 15 and 38 %, respectively, compared to watchful waiting, the benefit being confirmed after a median 12.8 years of follow-up [22]. A clear benefit is seen in metastasis-free survival (41 % benefit), locoregional progression (64 % benefit), and hormonal treatment use (56 % benefit). However, this study has some limitations. The first is related to a subgroup analysis, where the survival benefit was observed only in patients younger than 65. The second refers to the population: Most patients had a palpable lesion and a mean PSA of 12.8 ng/ml. This does not represent the current screen-detected population. The second trial, not yet published, enrolled 731 screen-detected patients (50 % being T1c, 70 % with a Gleason below 7). At 10 years, no survival benefit, neither overall nor specific, was observed in the whole cohort. Considering subgroup analysis, the benefits were only seen for intermediate- or high-risk lesions. The full paper is awaited [23]. Regarding radiotherapy, the only available data from a randomized trial on 414 patients do not show any overall or specific survival at 15 years, but only a distant and recurrence-free survival benefit at 15 years; however, this was old-fashioned radiotherapy, using a low dose (64–68 Gy) [24].

Screening for Prostate Cancer and Randomized Trials

Recently, two randomized trials have attempted to answer the effect of PSA screening on mortality. A detailed review is far beyond the scope of this chapter. But some points have to be highlighted.

- The ERSPC trial (European Randomized Study of Screening for Prostate Cancer) [2] included seven European countries, initiated in the early 1990s, covering 182,000 patients aged 50–74. Eighty-two thousand eight hundred sixteen patients were in the screened group and 99,184 in the control group. Some differences exist between the different countries regarding PSA threshold leading to biopsies and screening intervals. After a median follow-up of nearly 9 years, 5,990 cancers were detected in the screened group and 4,307 in the control one, resulting in an increased incidence of 3.4 % compared with the control group. A prostate cancer death reduction by 20 % was observed, favoring screening. The absolute risk difference was 0.71 death per 1,000 men, meaning that 1,410 men would need to be screened to prevent one cancer death and that 48 additional patients would need to be treated to prevent one PCa death. The main drawback of this study was the huge overdiagnosis and overtreatment observed, acknowledged by the authors. Furthermore, when going into subgroup analysis, the overall survival benefit was only seen for those screened between 55 and 69 years old. It was never observed above 70, which represents the core of this chapter In the Swedish branch of the ERSPC representing 20,000 randomized patients with the same screening regimen [26] and 14 years of follow-up, the risk of PCa death was reduced by almost 50 %. It must be highlighted that this Swedish branch is driving the overall positive results of the entire ERSPC cohort. Finally, it must be acknowledged that even for the authors of the study, these results do not yet justify population screening [27].

- The other large randomized study is the American PLCO trial (Prostate, Lung, Colorectal, and Ovarian) [3]. Seventy-six thousand six hundred ninety-three men were randomized between 1993 and 2001, 38,343 in the screening group, and 38,350 in the control group. Patients were aged 55–74 years. After a median follow-up of 7 years, 2,820 PCa were diagnosed in the screened group compared to 2,322 in the control group, and 50 PCa deaths occurred in the screening group compared to 44 in the control group (RR: 1.11, 95 % CI, 0.83–1.50). The authors concluded that screening had no impact of survival. Compared to the ERSPC, the PLCO is homogeneous with a single PSA threshold. But again, no patient above 74 years was included.

- Recently a 20-year follow-up of a Sweden randomized trial was reported [28], again lacking to show any benefit of screening. However, it was only based on 9,026 men aged 50–69, and there was no PSA testing during the first two screening rounds. Therefore, no conclusion can be drawn from this negative study.

- Although these trials enrolled a very large number of patients, there are many limits. Besides considering only men below 70 year of age, one of the main limitations is represented by the contamination rate for noncompliance in the control group. Regarding screened patients, compliance is relatively easy to control, and a high rate (near 80 %) is observed. But in the control group, no PSA test or DRE would have been expected for 10 years in an ideal world. In the PLCO study, 40 % of patients had been screened prior to randomization, so it is unrealistic to imagine that they will refuse any form of screening for prostate cancer within 10 years. Zelen suggests a statistical correction to evaluate the effect of compliance on the effectiveness of a study [29] showing that compliance might be as important as having large number of patients. For the PLCO study, compliance was 85 and 50 % for the screened and control group, respectively, leading to an overall compliance of around 67.5 %. Applying the correction suggested by Zelen, the results are equivalent to a study with 9,300 men only. In the Swedish branch of the ERSPC, the proportion of patients who had already had a PSA measured at baseline was 3 % compared to 44 % in the PLCO. Furthermore, the lack of clear results from the PLCO trial might be related to a still short follow-up. In PCa, a potential curative treatment benefit is only seen beyond 10 years. With just a median time from randomization of 7 years, it is not a surprise that no benefit is seen, compared to a median 14 years in the ERSPC Swedish branch [26]. To conclude on available randomized trial results, convincing results are so weak that no country has accepted mass screening. On a population perspective, the risk-benefit balance appears to be too low for a usually slow-growing cancer. And overtreatment is a real issue, as highlighted at least by the ERSPC lead author [2]. A much longer follow-up is needed. But the contamination rate for noncompliance will remain a major limitation of both trials. Therefore, only individual early diagnosis is to be considered, with some precise age frame [13].

Individual Screening in Senior Adults: Any Special Points to Consider?

Individual screening is often considered only for men below 75. This limit is based on a misunderstanding of expected survival. A curative treatment is considered to be beneficial only beyond 10 years, especially for low- or intermediate-risk disease [24]. But the individual probability of survival is very heterogeneous, based mainly on comorbidity. This is known from the Walter and Covinsky study [30]. It is clearly shown that if 10 years survival is the considered threshold, then comorbidity must be considered first. Men at 75 with no or minimal comorbidities will have an individual life expectancy of nearly 15, 9 years for those with moderate, and 5 years for those with severe comorbidities (Fig. 5.1). Comorbidity is therefore the main point to consider, before chronological age (see chapter 2), to evaluate the overall individual life expectancy. It is also one of the main prognostic factors for survival in men with PCa, as recently shown in the SEER database [31]. Even for poorly differentiated disease, non-PCa-specific death remains the main cause of death in men with a Charlson score above 1.

Apart from comorbidity, senior adults have some differences regarding early diagnosis tools compared to younger men. For example, the biopsy-associated mortality is considered to increase with age, based on a Canadian study of mortality at 120 days after biopsy. It was found to be, respectively, 0.1, 0.3, 0.5, 0.7, and 1.7/1,000 for age categories ≤60, 65–70, 71–75, 76–80, and 81–85 years [21].

Finally, senior adults have an increased probability to have a high-risk lesion PCa. But controlling for treatment modality and risk category, age had no impact on specific survival as seen from the 11,790 men from the CaPSuRe database [32].

Regarding the benefit of treatment on survival, nothing has been shown in randomized trials, but no patient above 75 was included. In the SEER database

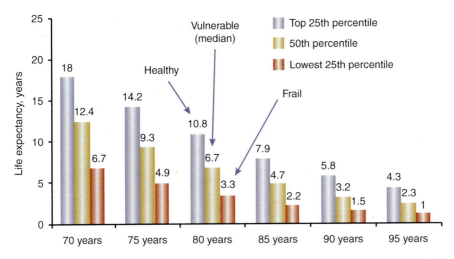

Fig. 5.1 Expected life survival for different "civil" age based on comorbidity (Adapted from Walter and Covinsky [30]). Vulnerable patients are defined as those with reversible impairment. Frail patients are defined as those with irreversible impairment

(retrospective comparison of treated vs. observed patients) reported by Wong et al. [33], a benefit of treatment was seen in a population of 44,630 patients aged 65–80 years with an organ-confined well- or moderately differentiated lesion, after a 12-year period. However, regarding the competitive mortality observed in other studies [7, 8], these results suggest that an individual early diagnosis leading to an early treatment will only be effective for the high-risk situations (30 % specific death rate at 10 years if untreated [8]) and for some intermediate-risk lesions with a long (>10 years) life expectancy, based on comorbidities (15–20 % specific death rate at 10 years for T2-untreated lesions [8]). Furthermore, the higher the risk (or the Gleason score) or the local lesion, the higher the risk of locoregional problems such as urethral obstruction, ureteral compression possibly leading to renal colic or renal insufficiency if bilateral, painful bone metastases, and so on.

Conclusions

It is clear that nowadays there is no place for mass screening in young or senior adults. An individual early diagnosis is a reasonable option for some senior adults with a significant individual life expectancy. This is the key point to evaluate before considering any form of screening. This evaluation must be based on comorbidity with the use of validated easy to use tools.

Early diagnosis is based on PSA testing and a DRE, both being mandatory to be effective. The aim of early diagnosis is to find an aggressive lesion (Gleason score above 7 or with a primary grade 4) and not any form of PCa. It must be repeatedly explained that finding a lesion does not systematically lead to an active treatment, especially for Gleason scores below 7. In case of a suspicious DRE, biopsies must be discussed whatever the PSA, considering the risk of local evolution especially with a high Gleason score. And this score is only available on histology. In symptomatic senior patients, a biopsy is required as long as a diagnosis of PCa will have an impact on the symptoms: an "early" diagnosis leading to an "early" treatment being of possible interest in aggressive lesions only.

References

1. Jemal A, Siegel R, Ward E, Murray T, Xu J, Thun MJ. Cancer statistics, 2007. CA Cancer J Clin. 2007;57(1):43–66.
2. Schröder FH, Hugosson J, Roobol MJ, Tammela TLJ, Ciatto S, Nelen V, et al. Screening and prostate-cancer mortality in a randomized European study. N Engl J Med. 2009;360(13):1320–8.
3. Andriole GL, Crawford ED, Grubb RL, Buys SS, Chia D, Church TR, et al. Mortality results from a randomized prostate-cancer screening trial. N Engl J Med. 2009;360(13):1310–9.
4. Shapiro S. Evidence on screening for breast cancer from a randomized trial. Cancer. 1977;39(6 Suppl):2772–82.
5. Hutchison GB. Evaluation of preventive services. J Chronic Dis. 1960;11:497–508.
6. Freedland SJ, Mangold LA, Walsh PC, Partin AW. The prostatic specific antigen era is alive and well: prostatic specific antigen and biochemical progression following radical prostatectomy. J Urol. 2005;174(4 Pt 1):1276–81; discussion 1281; author reply 1281.
7. Albersten PC, Hanley JA, Fine J. 20-year outcomes following conservative management of clinically localized prostate cancer. JAMA. 2005;293:2095–101.
8. Lu Yao GL, Albertsen PC, Moore DF, et al. Outcomes of localized prostate cancer following conservative management. JAMA. 2009;302(11):1202–9.
9. SEER cancer statistics review 1975–2006 – previous version – SEER cancer statistics [Internet]. [cité 2011 août 3]. Available at: http://seer.cancer.gov/csr/1975_2006/. Accessed on November 2011.
10. Schröder FH, van der Maas P, Beemsterboer P, Kruger AB, Hoedemaeker R, Rietbergen J, et al. Evaluation of the digital rectal examination as a screening test for prostate cancer. Rotterdam section of the European Randomized Study of Screening for Prostate Cancer. J Natl Cancer Inst. 1998;90(23):1817–23.
11. Friedman GD, Hiatt RA, Quesenberry CP, Selby JV. Case–control study of screening for prostatic cancer by digital rectal examinations. Lancet. 1991;337(8756):1526–9.
12. Catalona WJ, Smith DS, Ratliff TL, Dodds KM, Coplen DE, Yuan JJ, et al. Measurement of prostate-specific antigen in serum as a screening test for prostate cancer. N Engl J Med. 1991;324(17):1156–61.
13. NCCN guidelines: Available at: http://www.nccn.org/professionals/physician_gls/f_guidelines.asp.
14. Thompson IM, Pauler DK, Goodman PJ, Tangen CM, Lucia MS, Parnes HL, et al. Prevalence of prostate cancer among men with a prostate-specific antigen level < or =4.0 ng per milliliter. N Engl J Med. 2004;350(22):2239–46.
15. Roddam AW, Duffy MJ, Hamdy FC, Ward AM, Patnick J, Price CP, et al. Use of prostate-specific antigen (PSA) isoforms for the detection of prostate cancer in men with a PSA level of 2–10 ng/ml: systematic review and meta-analysis. Eur Urol. 2005;48(3):386–99; discussion 398–9.
16. Heidenreich A, Bellmunt J, Bolla M, PCa guidelines, et al. EAU guidelines on prostate cancer. Part 1: screening, diagnosis, and treatment of clinically localised disease. Eur Urol. 2011;59(1):61–71.

17. Vlaeminck-Guillem V, Ruffion A, André J, Devonec M, Paparel P. Urinary prostate cancer 3 test: toward the age of reason? Urology. 2010;75(2):447–53.
18. Deras IL, Aubin SMJ, Blase A, Day JR, Koo S, Partin AW, et al. PCA3: a molecular urine assay for predicting prostate biopsy outcome. J Urol. 2008;179(4):1587–92.
19. Haese A, de la Taille A, van Poppel H, Marberger M, Stenzl A, Mulders PFA, et al. Clinical utility of the PCA3 urine assay in European men scheduled for repeat biopsy. Eur Urol. 2008;54(5):1081–8.
20. Loeb S, Carter HB, Berndt SI, et al. Complications after prostate biopsy: data from SEER-Medicare. J Urol. 2011;186(5):1830–4.
21. Gallina A, Suardi N, Montorsi F, Capitanio U, Jeldres C, Saad F, et al. Mortality at 120 days after prostatic biopsy: a population-based study of 22,175 men. Int J Cancer. 2008;123(3):647–52.
22. Bill-Axelson A, Holmberg L, Ruutu M, Garmo H, Stark JR, Busch C, et al. Radical prostatectomy versus watchful waiting in early prostate cancer. N Engl J Med. 2011;364(18):1708–17.
23. Wilt TJ, Brawer MK, Jones KM et al. Radical prostactectomy for localized prostate cancer. N Engl J Med 2012;367:203–13.
24. Widmark A. ASTRO. 2011 (late breaking abstract).
25. Alibhai SMH, Leach M, Tomlinson G, Krahn MD, Fleshner N, Holowaty E, et al. 30-day mortality and major complications after radical prostatectomy: influence of age and comorbidity. J Natl Cancer Inst. 2005;97(20):1525–32.
26. Hugosson J, Carlsson S, Aus G, Bergdahl S, Khatami A, Lodding P, et al. Mortality results from the Göteborg randomised population-based prostate-cancer screening trial. Lancet Oncol. 2010;11(8):725–32.
27. Zhu X, Roobol MJ, Schröder FH. Screening for prostate cancer: have we resolved the controversy? Curr Opin Support Palliat Care. 2010;4(3):121–6.
28. Sandblom G, Varenhorst E, Rosell J, Löfman O, Carlsson P. Randomised prostate cancer screening trial: 20 year follow-up. BMJ. 2011;342:d1539.
29. Zelen M. Are primary cancer prevention trials feasible? J Natl Cancer Inst. 1988;80(18):1442–4.
30. Walter LC, Covinsky KE. Cancer screening in elderly patients: a framework for individualized decision making. JAMA. 2001;285(21):2750–6.
31. Albertsen PC, Moore DF, Shih W, et al. Impact of comorbidity on survival among men with localized prostate cancer. J Clin Oncol. 2011;29:1335–41.
32. Bechis SK, Caroll PR, Cooperberg MR. Impact of age at diagnosis on prostate cancer treatment and survival. J Clin Oncol. 2011;29:235–41.
33. Wong YN, Mitra N, Hudes G, et al. Survival associated with treatment vs observation of localized prostate cancer in elderly men. JAMA. 2006;296:2683–93.

Chapter 6
Androgen Deprivation in Elderly Prostate Cancer Patients: Side Effects and Their Prevention

Mohamed Omar Bishr and Fred Saad

Abstract Since the early 1940s, when Huggins and Hodges first demonstrated that prostate cancer was influenced by androgens, androgen deprivation therapy (ADT) became the standard therapy for metastatic prostate cancer. Later, ADT has been shown to improve survival times when given in combination with radiotherapy for locally advanced or high-risk disease and when given after radical prostatectomy for nodal metastasis. Recently, the use of ADT has expanded beyond these justified indications to include patients with biochemical relapse where ADT may be administered for years although there are no clear benefits in terms of survival. With this increasing trend of prescribing ADT in management of prostate cancer, early and long-term complications of ADT became more frequently confronted. In addition to the well-established side effects of ADT such as hot flashes, gynecomastia, decreased libido, and erectile dysfunction, a new continuum of adverse effects has emerged on the surface including decreased bone mass density with its consequences (osteoporosis and increased risk of bone fractures), neuropsychological adverse effects, sarcopenic obesity, and a host of metabolic changes including insulin resistance, hyperglycemia, hyperlipidemia, and metabolic syndrome which are thought to increase risk for diabetes and cardiovascular morbidity and mortality. In this chapter, we will try to provide an overview on common ADT adverse effects and highlight preventive and therapeutic choices for these adverse.

M.O. Bishr, M.D., M.Sc
Division of Urology, Department of Surgery, Centre de Recherche du Centre Hospitalier de l'Université de Montréal (CRCHUM) and Institut du Cancer de Montréal, Montreal, Canada
e-mail: drbishr76@yahoo.com

F. Saad, M.D., FRCS (✉)
Division of Urology, Department of Surgery, Centre Hospitalier de l'Université de Montréal (CHUM), Montreal, Canada
e-mail: fred.saad@umontreal.ca

J.-P. Droz, R.A. Audisio (eds.), *Management of Urological Cancers in Older People*,   77
Management of Cancer in Older People,
DOI 10.1007/978-0-85729-999-4_6, © Springer-Verlag London 2013

Keywords Prostate cancer • Androgen deprivation therapy • Osteoporosis • Hot flashes • Metabolic changes

Introduction

For over 70 years, androgen deprivation therapy (ADT) has been in continuous evolution. Since the early 1940s, when Huggins and Hodges first demonstrated that prostate cancer (PCa) was influenced by androgens [1], bilateral orchiectomy has been the most common and widely accepted modality to lower testosterone level in prostate cancer patients to castrate levels (<50 ng/ml) until the work of Schally and colleagues led to the development of synthetic luteinizing hormone–releasing hormone (LHRH) agonist which became more appealing to avoid the emotional trauma of surgical castration. A meta-analysis, involving more than 6,600 patients, found no significant difference in survival between LHRH agonist use and orchiectomy [2].

Enhancement in our understanding of tumor biology, the importance of androgen receptor signaling, and the mechanisms implicated in the development of androgen-independence after surgical or medical castration has revived the role of ADT in this subcategory of PCa patients and sparked the enthusiasm to search for more potent and well-tolerated modalities for ADT. Abiraterone acetate, a potent selective inhibitor of cytochrome P 17 (CYP17) enzyme which is a key pathway in the androgen biosynthesis, has shown in a recent phase III randomized controlled trial prolongation of the overall survival by 3.9 months (hazard ratio [HR]: 0.65; $P < 0.001$) among patients with metastatic CRPC who previously received chemotherapy [3].

In the setting of metastatic disease, ADT is the mainstay of management providing important quality-of-life benefits, including reductions of bone pain, pathological fracture, spinal cord compression, and ureteral obstruction and slight improvement of the overall survival [4]. Later, ADT has been shown to improve survival times when given in combination with radiotherapy for locally advanced or high-risk disease [5, 6] and when given after radical prostatectomy for nodal metastasis [7]. Although ADT is commonly used in patients with biochemical relapse, there is no clear evidence that ADT provides benefit in terms of survival [8]. With this expansion in the use of ADT, early and long-term treatment complications became more frequently confronted. In this chapter, we will try to provide an overview on common ADT adverse effects and highlight preventive and therapeutic choices for these adverse effects.

Musculoskeletal Complications

Bone Loss

A dynamic equilibrium between bone formation (mediated by osteoblasts) and bone resorption (mediated by osteoclasts) keeps the bone mass in a continuous turnover state. Testosterone stimulates bone formation directly by stimulating the osteoblasts proliferation, inhibiting the apoptosis of both osteoblasts and osteoclasts, and indirectly by being a precursor of estrogen which is also a powerful triggering factor for bone formation. These effects are abolished by the state of hypogonadism induced in patients with prostate cancer by orchiectomy or ADT [9].

Accumulating evidences from prospective trials have established the relation between ADT and low bone mass density (BMD) and osteoporosis. In one study including 390 patients with nonmetastatic prostate cancer followed for 10 years, none of the patients on ADT had normal BMD at the end of the study, and the prevalence of osteoporosis (diagnosed if T score < -2.5) was 35.4 % in hormone-naive patients and increased to approximately 50 % by 4 years and 80 % by 10 years in men on ADT [10]. Although the loss of BMD is more intense in the first year of ADT, the magnitude of BMD remains linked to the duration of therapy [11, 12].

Although fractures are an independent adverse predictor of survival in patients with PCa, no prospective data are yet available regarding the impact of ADT on fracture rates; nevertheless, several retrospective analyses provide significant evidence for increased fracture risk. Among 50,613 patients from the Surveillance Epidemiology and End Results (SEER) Medicare database, incidence of bone fractures, 5 years after the diagnosis of prostate cancer, was 19.4 % in patients receiving ADT compared to 12.6 % in hormone-naïve patients ($P < 0.001$). Another claims-based study also found a significant association between gonadotropin-releasing hormone (GnRH) agonist treatment and clinical fractures (relative risk [RR]: 1.21; $P < 0.001$) [13–15]. Decreased BMD and higher rates of bone fracture have been documented not only in patients receiving ADT but also in those undergoing surgical castration [14].

The use of intermittent ADT may be related to less significant bone loss compared with continuous ADT, but data are still limited, and prospective studies are presently ongoing [13].

Management Options

Lifestyle Changes

Smoking cessation and avoidance of excessive caffeine and alcohol intake should also be encouraged [16].

Regular exercise programs (20–45 min/session, 2–4 sessions/week) combining weight-bearing and muscle-strengthening exercises can increase BMD and muscle strength and thus improves stability and reduces fracture risk [17, 18]

In older patients, assessment of fall risk, home safety, and need for assistive devices is recommended [19].

Food Supplementation

It is generally recommended that patients receiving ADT be systematically started on oral vitamin D (800 IU daily) and calcium (500–1,500 mg daily). Yet the efficacy of this regimen alone in preventing ADT-related bone loss is not established [20].

Bisphosphonates

Bisphosphonates are potent inhibitors of osteoclast-mediated bone resorption, available in both oral and intravenous (IV) forms, and have been shown to significantly reduce the ADT-related bone loss in nonmetastatic prostate cancer patients in multiple randomized controlled studies [21–23]. Even a single dose of IV bisphosphonate (pamidronate or zoledronic acid) was sufficient to reduce BMD loss for at least 6 months [24, 25]. Among all bisphosphonates, zoledronic acid (4 mg IV every 3 months) is the only one that has shown significant increase in the BMD compared with baseline at all measured sites [22]. While up to date there are no studies that have demonstrated a role for bisphosphonates in prevention or reduction in risk of fractures in patients receiving ADT, zoledronic acid was the first bisphosphonate that has shown a protective effect against skeletal-related events (SRE) in patients with metastatic castration-resistant prostate cancer in terms of 48 % reduction in the mean annual incidence of SRE ($P=0.005$), 5 months prolongation of the median time to first SRE ($P=0.009$), and 36 % reduction in the ongoing risk of SRE in both the 15 and 24 months data sets [26, 27]. A large study is underway evaluating the effects of zoledronic acid on SRE incidence in patients with hormone-sensitive prostate cancer receiving ADT [28].

   Gastrointestinal toxicity is the most common adverse effect for oral bisphosphonate and not uncommonly affects patient compliance with therapy. Bisphosphonate-induced nephrotoxicity is a major concern especially with IV bisphosphonate; thus, slow IV administration over 15 min, renal function monitoring, and dose adjustment according to creatinine clearance are crucial to prevent significant deterioration in renal function. Other side effects can include self-limiting flu-like symptoms typically occurring with the first dose, hypocalcemia and osteonecrosis of the jaw (ONJ), which presents in the maxillofacial region as exposed bone that does not show signs of improvement after 8 weeks of therapy. ONJ is probably a very rare adverse event (<1/100,000–1/10,000 patient–treatment years) when bisphosphonates are used at therapeutic or prophylactic doses for osteoporosis, while in cancer patients the risk is much higher depending on the duration of therapy. Good oral hygiene, baseline dental evaluation for high-risk individuals, and avoidance of invasive dental surgery during therapy reduce risk of ONJ [29, 30].

Denosumab

Binding of the receptor activator of nuclear factor κ-B ligand (RANKL), secreted by the osteoblast, to its receptor (RANK) on the surface of osteoclast cells triggers maturation and activation of osteoclast and prolongs their survival resulting in bone resorption [31].

Denosumab is a fully human monoclonal antibody that specifically targets RANKL, thus preventing bone loss. In patients with nonmetastatic prostate cancer receiving ADT, denosumab (60 mg subcutaneously every 6 months) was associated with increased BMD at all sites (lumbar spines, the total hip, femoral neck, and distal third of the radius) at all time points and reduction in the incidence of new vertebral fractures (RR: 0.38; $P = 0.006$) [32]. In a randomized controlled trial comparing denosumab to zoledronic acid in metastatic castration-resistant prostate cancer, an improvement in the time to the first SRE was found with denosumab with a between-group difference of 3.6 months. Hypocalcemia was more common in the denosumab arm (13 %) than the zoledronic acid arm (6 %) ($P < 0.0001$) [33]. In a recent trial, denosumab significantly increased bone-metastasis-free survival by a median of 4·2 months compared with placebo (hazard ratio (HR):0·85, $P = 0.028$) [34].

Selective Estrogen-Receptor Modulators (SERMs)

Estrogen has functional receptors in both osteoblasts and osteoclasts, thus playing a pivotal role in bone homeostasis in men. SERMs, such as raloxifene and toremifene, selectively bind to estrogen receptors in bone and have been shown to increase BMD in patients on ADT [35, 36]. In a phase III trial, toremifene has also shown significant reduction in the incidence of vertebral fractures (HR: 0.50; $P < 0.05$) in patients on ADT. It is noteworthy that the venous thromboembolic events were more common in the toremifene arm (17 patients; 2.6 % incidence) than in the placebo arm (7 patients; 1.1 % incidence) [37].

Nonsteroidal Antiandrogen (NSAA)

Not all forms of hormone therapy are equivalent in terms of bone loss. NSAAs used as monotherapy, although nonstandard, do offer some bone protection due to the fact that androgen levels are not reduced. This may present an alternative option when bone loss is of particular concern [13].

Changes in Body Habitus

ADT causes changes in body habitus characterized by a very morbid combination of muscular atrophy (decreased lean body mass) and an increase in fatty deposits, a situation known as "sarcopenic obesity" [38]. In a review and meta-analysis of 16 studies (14 cohort and 2 randomized controlled trials), conducted to determine the effects of ADT on body composition in PCa patients, ADT was associated with increase in both body fat mass and weight by on average 7.7 and 2.2 %, respectively, and decrease in lean body mass by on average 2.8 % [39]. Fat deposition occurs mainly in the subcutaneous, while intra-abdominal fat generally does not change significantly. Changes in body habitus related to ADT are an early adverse effect for ADT which occur within the first 3 months of therapy. In the elderly, sarcopenia is a major contributing factor to falls, functional dependence, and frailty. Although resistance training programs had shown improvement in muscular fitness, fatigue, and quality of life in patients receiving ADT, however, no improvement in ADT-related changes in body habitus has been noted. Effective treatment strategies need to be defined for managing ADT-associated changes in body habitus [40, 41].

Hot Flashes

Hot flashes are a well-known adverse effect of ADT that had been reported by Huggins and Hodges during their pioneer work on the effect of castration on advanced PCa and were described as "profuse perspiration, often occurring at night, forcing the patient to throw off the bed covers" [1].

Fifty to eighty percent of patients receiving ADT experienced this side effect and up to 30 % consider it the most distressing adverse effect. Hot flashes are defined as sudden rush of warmth in the face, neck, upper chest, and back, followed by profuse sweating. The duration of these episodes could range from seconds to as long as an hour. They often occur spontaneously, but stress, poor sleep, hot weather, ingestion of hot liquid, and changes in body position could be triggering factors [42].

Although the exact etiology of hot flashes is not fully understood, a proposed hypothesis is alteration in the feedback mechanism of the hypothalamus due to decrease in the plasma sex hormones. This alteration results in an increase in hypo-thalamic catecholamine levels in response to a decrease in endorphins and catec-holestrogens and resets the nearby thermoregulatory center leading to the hot flashes [43].

Management Options

Pharmacologic Options

Hormonal Replacement Therapy

Since the ADT is contraindicated in PCa, estrogens and progesterone had been tested in treatment of ADT-related hot flashes. Estrogen compounds, such as diethylstilbestrol (DES) and transdermal estrogen, had shown dose-related effectiveness in controlling the symptoms of hot flashes [44, 45]; however, the enthusiasm for this therapy has been limited by its serious adverse effects which include cardiovascular complications (thromboembolic events, myocardial infarction, stroke), weight gain, edema, gynecomastia, and breast tenderness.

Similarly progesterone compounds, such as megestrol acetate and medroxyprogesterone acetate, had proved efficacy in reducing hot flashes in 80–90 % of patients on ADT but with a more favorable side effect profile [46, 47]. It should be mentioned that some trials had raised a concern about PCa progression on withdrawal of megestrol acetate; therefore, close monitoring is important [48]. Cyproterone acetate is a steroidal antiandrogen which has shown efficacy in management of ADT-related hot flashes due to its progestational effects. To avoid its hepatotoxicity, it should be started with low dose as 50–100 mg/day and titrated up to 300 mg/day if necessary [49].

Clonidine

It is a centrally acting α-receptor agonist that has shown effectiveness in treatment of postmenopausal hot flashes, but when evaluated in ADT-related hot flashes, no significant benefit has been reported [50].

Antidepressant Agents

Antidepressant agents such as sertraline and paroxetine (selective serotonin reuptake inhibitors) and venlafaxine (serotonin-norepinephrine reuptake inhibitor) had demonstrated efficacy in the treatment of hot flashes in patients on ADT. They are generally well tolerated and provide the additional benefit of correcting the psychological effects of ADT [43].

Other Agents

Toremifene, a selective estrogen-receptor modulator, seems to act as a partial agonist on the hypothalamic-pituitary axis and may decrease vasomotor flushing. The role of toremifene in treatment of ADT-related hot flashes is currently under evaluation in a phase III study [37].

Gabapentin, a structural analogue to the neurotransmitter γ- (gamma-) aminobutyric acid, has been shown to decrease hot flashes in women with breast cancer at high dose (300 mg three times daily). Yet there are no published randomized controlled studies evaluating its role in ADT-related hot flashes [51].

Non-pharmacological Options

In a prospective multicenter study, traditional acupuncture (TA) and electroacupuncture (EA) lowered the hot flashes score in approximately 70 % of patients on ADT, and this effect lasted up to 9 months after treatment ended [52]. TA and EA could be a therapeutic option in management of hot flashes, but further evaluation is needed.

Gynecomastia

Gynecomastia is a well-known adverse effect of ADT, and its incidence depends on the method used ranging from 10 to 15 % with GnRH analogue to 40–70 % with antiandrogen monotherapy. It is thought to be a consequence of the increased estrogen-to-androgen ratio often seen with ADT, which could explain the high incidence of gynecomastia with antiandrogen monotherapy which is associated with increased testosterone level and subsequent aromatization to estradiol, leading to high estrogen-to-testosterone ratio [43, 53]. Treatment options include prophylactic radiation therapy (RT), which has shown 70–90 % efficacy in prevention of gynecomastia. SERMs such as tamoxifen have been tested in patients receiving bicalutamide, a nonsteroidal antiandrogen, and the results suggest a beneficial effect in prevention of gynecomastia. In a randomized controlled trial, tamoxifen was more effective than prophylactic RT in prevention of bicalutamide-induced gynecomastia. Once gynecomastia is established, treatments include medical therapy or surgery, with a minor role for RT in reducing breast pain [43, 54, 55].

Sexual Dysfunction

Negative impacts of ADT on sexual function in terms of decreased libido and erectile dysfunction are directly related to the decline in testosterone levels. However, other confounding factors such as age, physical fitness, baseline testosterone levels, and previous exposure to radiation and/or surgery for localized disease could exacerbate the deterioration in sexual function [19].

In a study evaluating the quality-of-life outcomes after primary androgen deprivation, approximately 73 % of men ceased engaging in sexual activity after treatment, 69 % of men who were potent before treatment were impotent after treatment, and no significant differences were observed by type of AD therapy [56].

Medical management using oral phosphodiesterase type 5 inhibitors or intracavernosal injections of prostaglandin is considered the first choice therapy in well-selected patients. Other options include vacuum devices and penile prosthesis. Evaluation of the long-term efficiency of these agents in patient on ADT is still needed [57].

Neuropsychological Side Effects

Despite the small sample sizes and the variety of neuropsychological tests utilized in studies evaluating the impact of ADT on cognition in patients with PCa, most of these studies had reported a decline in at least one cognitive area. The most commonly affected areas are visuospatial abilities and executive functioning, while results regarding verbal memory are contradictory [58].

In a study including 45 men with prostate cancer receiving ADT, incidence of major depressive disorder was 13 % in men receiving ADT which is 8 times the national rate of depression in men, 32 times the rate in men over 65 years old [59].

In contrast to these results, one large population-based study evaluated the risks of depression and cognitive impairment and revealed no statistical difference between men on ADT and controls after adjustment for variables such as comorbidity, tumor characteristics, and age [60]. Further work is needed to clearly define the relation between ADT and neuropsychological problems and its clinical significance.

Metabolic Complications

Insulin Resistance and Hyperglycemia

A significant rise in fasting insulin levels has been noted with short-term ADT (3 months), indicating early development of insulin resistance. Although there was no significant change in fasting glucose levels, a statistically significant increase in glycosylated hemoglobin has been found which could be translated as a success of the compensatory hyperinsulinemia in preventing the development of diabetes [61]. In the same context, Basaria et al. reported that even after adjusting for age and body mass index (BMI), patients undergoing long-term ADT (≥ 12 months) had significantly higher fasting insulin levels than patients with prostatic cancer who did not receive ADT and healthy controls, suggesting that insulin resistance due to ADT occurs independently of BMI or age factors. The breakthrough in the study was the prevalence of fasting hyperglycemia in the ADT group. Moreover, 44 % of patients in the ADT group had a fasting glucose level of more than 126 mg/dl (a criterion defined by the American Diabetes Association for diagnosis of diabetes mellitus) compared with 12 and 11 % in the non-ADT and control groups, respectively [62]. In a recent population-based observational study, treatment with GnRH agonists was associated with statistically significantly increased risks of incident diabetes (adjusted hazard ratio [aHR] = 1.28) [63].

Based on recent data about the effect of ADT on insulin sensitivity and its association with diabetes, some authors recommend treating all men receiving ADT as high-risk individuals [40].

Dyslipidemia and Metabolic Syndrome

ADT significantly alters lipid profiles in men with PCa. Several studies had reported increase in serum total cholesterol, low-density lipoprotein (LDL) cholesterol, and triglycerides while on GnRH agonist. In one of these studies, 1 year of GnRH agonist therapy was associated with significant increase in total cholesterol (9.0 %, $P < 0.001$), triglycerides (26.5 %, $P = 0.01$), LDL (7.3 %, $P = 0.05$), and high-density lipoprotein (HDL) (11.3 %, $P < 0.001$). The clinical impact of these changes on cardiovascular risks is still not well defined [64].

The combination of sarcopenic obesity, increased triglycerides, and fasting blood glucose in patients on ADT fulfills the criteria for diagnosis of metabolic syndrome. In a cross-sectional study evaluating the prevalence of metabolic syndrome in men with PCa undergoing long-term ADT, 55 % of patients had metabolic syndrome. It is worth mentioning that ADT-related metabolic changes are different from the classically defined metabolic syndrome in the following: first, ADT increases subcutaneous rather than visceral fat and does not change waist-to-hip ratio. Additionally, ADT increases rather than decreases high-density lipoprotein cholesterol. Finally, ADT is associated with increased serum adiponectin levels and unchanged C-reactive protein levels, while the classic metabolic syndrome is characterized by low levels of adiponectin and increased C-reactive protein [65].

In addition to diet and lifestyle changes which are recommended as the first-line interventions to achieve target LDL level, statins are the mainstays of pharmacological management and have been shown to reduce all cause mortality. During testing toremifene for prevention of fractures in patients on ADT, an effect on serum lipid profile in the form of decreased LDL and triglycerides and increased HDL has been found.

Cardiovascular Morbidity and Mortality

ADT-related metabolic changes including obesity, insulin resistance, hyperglycemia, and dyslipidemia had raised concerns about the risk of cardiovascular morbidity and mortality in men with PCa undergoing ADT.

Higher risk of incident coronary artery disease in men undergoing ADT has been reported in several studies. In a recent retrospective population-based analysis including more than 37,000 men, Keating et al. noted that treatment with GnRH agonist was associated with significant increase in the risk of incident coronary heart disease (adjusted HR = 1.19), myocardial infarction (aHR = 1.28), sudden death (aHR = 1.35), and stroke (aHR = 1.22). Combined androgen blockade is significantly associated with an increased risk of incident coronary heart disease (aHR = 1.27), and orchiectomy is associated with coronary heart disease (aHR = 1.40) and myocardial infarction (aHR = 2.11). It is noteworthy that monotherapy with nonsteroidal antiandrogen was not associated with increased risk of incident coronary heart disease [63]. In contrast, a report of a Canadian database analysis of approximately 20,000 men 66 years old or older treated for prostate cancer showed no increase in the risk of acute myocardial infarction in men receiving ADT (HR: 0.91) [66].

Multiple studies had investigated the possible association between ADT and cardiovascular mortality, but results on ADT-attributable risk for cardiovascular mortality are contradictory. In a population-based observational study, Tsai et al. found that the incidence of cardiovascular death in the subset of men aged 65 years and older was 5.5 % with ADT and 2.0 % without ($P = 0.002$). Similar differences were observed in patients treated with radiation but were not statistically [67]. On the other side, the secondary analysis of 4 large randomized controlled trials of the Radiation Therapy Oncology Group (RTOG) and the European Organization for Research and Treatment of Cancer (EORTC) found no association between ADT and cardiovascular mortality [40].

Although the clinical impact of the ADT on cardiovascular morbidity and mortality is still not well defined, healthy lifestyle including balanced diet, smoking cessation, and regular physical activity should be encouraged. Control of cardiovascular risk factors such as obesity, hyperlipidemia, hyperglycemia, and hypertension and use of cardioprotective agents when indicated should be considered.

References

1. Huggins C, Hodges CV. Studies on prostatic cancer. I. The effect of castration, of estrogen and androgen injection on serum phosphatases in metastatic carcinoma of the prostate. CA Cancer J Clin. 1972;22(4):232–40.
2. Seidenfeld J, Samson DJ, Hasselblad V, et al. Single-therapy androgen suppression in men with advanced prostate cancer: a systematic review and meta-analysis. Ann Intern Med. 2000;132(7):566–77.
3. de Bono JS, Logothetis CJ, Molina A, et al. Abiraterone and increased survival in metastatic prostate cancer. N Engl J Med. 2011;364(21):1995–2005.
4. Walsh PC. Immediate versus deferred treatment for advanced prostatic cancer: initial results of the Medical Research Council trial. The Medical Research Council Prostate Cancer Working Party Investigators Group. J Urol. 1997;158(4):1623–4.
5. Bolla M, Collette L, Blank L, et al. Long-term results with immediate androgen suppression and external irradiation in patients with locally advanced prostate cancer (an EORTC study): a phase III randomised trial. Lancet. 2002;360(9327):103–6.
6. D'Amico AV, Manola J, Loffredo M, Renshaw AA, DellaCroce A, Kantoff PW. 6-month androgen suppression plus radiation therapy vs radiation therapy alone for patients with clinically localized prostate cancer: a randomized controlled trial. JAMA. 2004;292(7):821–7.
7. Messing EM, Manola J, Yao J, et al. Immediate versus deferred androgen deprivation treatment in patients with node-positive prostate cancer after radical prostatectomy and pelvic lymphadenectomy. Lancet Oncol. 2006;7(6):472–9.
8. Crawford ED. Early versus late hormonal therapy: debating the issues. Urology. 2003;61(2 Suppl 1):S8–13.
9. Riggs BL, Khosla S, Melton 3rd LJ. Sex steroids and the construction and conservation of the adult skeleton. Endocr Rev. 2002;23(3):279–302.
10. Morote J, Morin JP, Orsola A, et al. Prevalence of osteoporosis during long-term androgen deprivation therapy in patients with prostate cancer. Urology. 2007;69(3):500–4.
11. Greenspan SL, Coates P, Sereika SM, Nelson JB, Trump DL, Resnick NM. Bone loss after initiation of androgen deprivation therapy in patients with prostate cancer. J Clin Endocrinol Metab. 2005;90(12):6410–7.
12. Morote J, Orsola A, Abascal JM, et al. Bone mineral density changes in patients with prostate cancer during the first 2 years of androgen suppression. J Urol. 2006;175(5):1679–83; discussion 1683.
13. Saad F, Adachi JD, Brown JP, et al. Cancer treatment-induced bone loss in breast and prostate cancer. J Clin Oncol. 2008;26(33):5465–76.

14. Shahinian VB, Kuo YF, Freeman JL, Goodwin JS. Risk of fracture after androgen deprivation for prostate cancer. N Engl J Med. 2005;352(2):154–64.
15. Smith MR, Lee WC, Brandman J, Wang Q, Botteman M, Pashos CL. Gonadotropin-releasing hormone agonists and fracture risk: a claims-based cohort study of men with nonmetastatic prostate cancer. J Clin Oncol. 2005;23(31):7897–903.
16. Brown JP, Josse RG. Clinical practice guidelines for the diagnosis and management of osteoporosis in Canada. CMAJ. 2002;167(10 Suppl):S1–34.
17. Hertel KL, Trahiotis MG. Exercise in the prevention and treatment of osteoporosis: the role of physical therapy and nursing. Nurs Clin North Am. 2001;36(3):441–53.
18. Higano CS. Understanding treatments for bone loss and bone metastases in patients with prostate cancer: a practical review and guide for the clinician. Urol Clin North Am. 2004;31(2):331–52.
19. Mohile SG, Mustian K, Bylow K, Hall W, Dale W. Management of complications of androgen deprivation therapy in the older man. Crit Rev Oncol Hematol. 2009;70(3):235–55.
20. Lattouf JB, Saad F. Bone health in nonmetastatic prostate cancer: what's the big deal? Curr Oncol. 2010;17 Suppl 2:S49–54.
21. Smith MR, Eastham J, Gleason DM, Shasha D, Tchekmedyian S, Zinner N. Randomized controlled trial of zoledronic acid to prevent bone loss in men receiving androgen deprivation therapy for nonmetastatic prostate cancer. J Urol. 2003;169(6):2008–12.
22. Ryan CW, Huo D, Demers LM, Beer TM, Lacerna LV. Zoledronic acid initiated during the first year of androgen deprivation therapy increases bone mineral density in patients with prostate cancer. J Urol. 2006;176(3):972–8; discussion 978.
23. Greenspan SL, Nelson JB, Trump DL, Resnick NM. Effect of once-weekly oral alendronate on bone loss in men receiving androgen deprivation therapy for prostate cancer: a randomized trial. Ann Intern Med. 2007;146(6):416–24.
24. Diamond TH, Winters J, Smith A, et al. The antiosteoporotic efficacy of intravenous pamidronate in men with prostate carcinoma receiving combined androgen blockade: a double blind, randomized, placebo-controlled crossover study. Cancer. 2001;92(6):1444–50.
25. Michaelson MD, Kaufman DS, Lee H, et al. Randomized controlled trial of annual zoledronic acid to prevent gonadotropin-releasing hormone agonist-induced bone loss in men with prostate cancer. J Clin Oncol. 2007;25(9):1038–42.
26. Saad F, Gleason DM, Murray R, et al. A randomized, placebo-controlled trial of zoledronic acid in patients with hormone-refractory metastatic prostate carcinoma. J Natl Cancer Inst. 2002;94(19):1458–68.
27. Saad F, Gleason DM, Murray R, et al. Long-term efficacy of zoledronic acid for the prevention of skeletal complications in patients with metastatic hormone-refractory prostate cancer. J Natl Cancer Inst. 2004;96(11):879–82.
28. ClinicalTrials.gov. Available at: http://www.clinicaltrials.gov/ct/show/NCT00329797. Accessed 6 Feb 2012.
29. Conte P, Guarneri V. Safety of intravenous and oral bisphosphonates and compliance with dosing regimens. Oncologist. 2004;9 Suppl 4:S28–37.
30. Khosla S, Burr D, Cauley J, et al. Bisphosphonate-associated osteonecrosis of the jaw: report of a task force of the American Society for Bone and Mineral Research. J Bone Miner Res. 2007;22(10):1479–91.
31. Boyle WJ, Simonet WS, Lacey DL. Osteoclast differentiation and activation. Nature. 2003;423(6937):337–42.
32. Smith MR, Egerdie B, Hernandez Toriz N, et al. Denosumab in men receiving androgen-deprivation therapy for prostate cancer. N Engl J Med. 2009;361(8):745–55.
33. Fizazi K, Carducci M, Smith M, et al. Denosumab versus zoledronic acid for treatment of bone metastases in men with castration-resistant prostate cancer: a randomised, double-blind study. Lancet. 2011;377(9768):813–22.
34. Smith MR, Saad F, Coleman R, et al. Denosumab and bone-metastasis-free survival in men with castration-resistant prostate cancer: results of a phase 3, randomised, placebo-controlled trial. Lancet. 2012;379(9810):39–46.

35. Smith MR, Fallon MA, Lee H, Finkelstein JS. Raloxifene to prevent gonadotropin-releasing hormone agonist-induced bone loss in men with prostate cancer: a randomized controlled trial. J Clin Endocrinol Metab. 2004;89(8):3841–6.
36. Smith MR, Malkowicz SB, Chu F, et al. Toremifene increases bone mineral density in men receiving androgen deprivation therapy for prostate cancer: interim analysis of a multicenter phase 3 clinical study. J Urol. 2008;179(1):152–5.
37. Smith MR, Morton RA, Barnette KG, et al. Toremifene to reduce fracture risk in men receiving androgen deprivation therapy for prostate cancer. J Urol. 2010;184(4):1316–21.
38. Galvao DA, Spry NA, Taaffe DR, et al. Changes in muscle, fat and bone mass after 36 weeks of maximal androgen blockade for prostate cancer. BJU Int. 2008;102(1):44–7.
39. Haseen F, Murray LJ, Cardwell CR, O'Sullivan JM, Cantwell MM. The effect of androgen deprivation therapy on body composition in men with prostate cancer: systematic review and meta-analysis. J Cancer Surviv. 2010;4(2):128–39.
40. Saylor PJ, Smith MR. Adverse effects of androgen deprivation therapy: defining the problem and promoting health among men with prostate cancer. J Natl Compr Canc Netw. 2010;8(2):211–23.
41. Carmeli E, Coleman R, Reznick AZ. The biochemistry of aging muscle. Exp Gerontol. 2002;37(4):477–89.
42. Alekshun TJ, Patterson SG. Management of hot flashes in men with prostate cancer being treated with androgen deprivation therapy. Support Cancer Ther. 2006;4(1):30–7.
43. Guise TA, Oefelein MG, Eastham JA, Cookson MS, Higano CS, Smith MR. Estrogenic side effects of androgen deprivation therapy. Rev Urol. 2007;9(4):163–80.
44. Gerber GS, Zagaja GP, Ray PS, Rukstalis DB. Transdermal estrogen in the treatment of hot flushes in men with prostate cancer. Urology. 2000;55(1):97–101.
45. Miller JI, Ahmann FR. Treatment of castration-induced menopausal symptoms with low dose diethylstilbestrol in men with advanced prostate cancer. Urology. 1992;40(6):499–502.
46. Loprinzi CL, Michalak JC, Quella SK, et al. Megestrol acetate for the prevention of hot flashes. N Engl J Med. 1994;331(6):347–52.
47. Langenstroer P, Kramer B, Cutting B, et al. Parenteral medroxyprogesterone for the management of luteinizing hormone releasing hormone induced hot flashes in men with advanced prostate cancer. J Urol. 2005;174(2):642–5.
48. Sartor O, Eastham JA. Progressive prostate cancer associated with use of megestrol acetate administered for control of hot flashes. South Med J. 1999;92(4):415–6.
49. Kouriefs C, Georgiou M, Ravi R. Hot flushes and prostate cancer: pathogenesis and treatment. BJU Int. 2002;89(4):379–83.
50. Loprinzi CL, Goldberg RM, O'Fallon JR, et al. Transdermal clonidine for ameliorating post-orchiectomy hot flashes. J Urol. 1994;151(3):634–6.
51. Pandya KJ, Morrow GR, Roscoe JA, et al. Gabapentin for hot flashes in 420 women with breast cancer: a randomised double-blind placebo-controlled trial. Lancet. 2005;366(9488):818–24.
52. Frisk J, Spetz AC, Hjertberg H, Petersson B, Hammar M. Two modes of acupuncture as a treatment for hot flushes in men with prostate cancer – a prospective multicenter study with long-term follow-up. Eur Urol. 2009;55(1):156–63.
53. Thompson CA, Shanafelt TD, Loprinzi CL. Andropause: symptom management for prostate cancer patients treated with hormonal ablation. Oncologist. 2003;8(5):474–87.
54. Gagnon JD, Moss WT, Stevens KR. Pre-estrogen breast irradiation for patients with carcinoma of the prostate: a critical review. J Urol. 1979;121(2):182–4.
55. Di Lorenzo G, Perdona S, De Placido S, et al. Gynecomastia and breast pain induced by adjuvant therapy with bicalutamide after radical prostatectomy in patients with prostate cancer: the role of tamoxifen and radiotherapy. J Urol. 2005;174(6):2197–203.
56. Potosky AL, Knopf K, Clegg LX, et al. Quality-of-life outcomes after primary androgen deprivation therapy: results from the Prostate Cancer Outcomes Study. J Clin Oncol. 2001;19(17):3750–7.

57. Holzbeierlein JM. Managing complications of androgen deprivation therapy for prostate cancer. Urol Clin North Am. 2006;33(2):181–90.
58. Nelson CJ, Lee JS, Gamboa MC, Roth AJ. Cognitive effects of hormone therapy in men with prostate cancer: a review. Cancer. 2008;113(5):1097–106.
59. Pirl WF, Siegel GI, Goode MJ, Smith MR. Depression in men receiving androgen deprivation therapy for prostate cancer: a pilot study. Psychooncology. 2002;11(6):518–23.
60. Shahinian VB, Kuo YF, Freeman JL, Goodwin JS. Risk of the "androgen deprivation syndrome" in men receiving androgen deprivation for prostate cancer. Arch Intern Med. 2006; 166(4):465–71.
61. Shahani S, Braga-Basaria M, Basaria S. Androgen deprivation therapy in prostate cancer and metabolic risk for atherosclerosis. J Clin Endocrinol Metab. 2008;93(6):2042–9.
62. Basaria S, Muller DC, Carducci MA, Egan J, Dobs AS. Hyperglycemia and insulin resistance in men with prostate carcinoma who receive androgen-deprivation therapy. Cancer. 2006; 106(3):581–8.
63. Keating NL, O'Malley AJ, Freedland SJ, Smith MR. Diabetes and cardiovascular disease during androgen deprivation therapy: observational study of veterans with prostate cancer. J Natl Cancer Inst. 2010;102(1):39–46.
64. Saylor PJ, Smith MR. Metabolic complications of androgen deprivation therapy for prostate cancer. J Urol. 2009;181(5):1998–2006; discussion 2007–8.
65. Van Poppel H, Tombal B. Cardiovascular risk during hormonal treatment in patients with prostate cancer. Cancer Manag Res. 2011;3:49–55.
66. Alibhai SM, Duong-Hua M, Sutradhar R, et al. Impact of androgen deprivation therapy on cardiovascular disease and diabetes. J Clin Oncol. 2009;27(21):3452–8.
67. Tsai HK, D'Amico AV, Sadetsky N, Chen MH, Carroll PR. Androgen deprivation therapy for localized prostate cancer and the risk of cardiovascular mortality. J Natl Cancer Inst. 2007;99(20):1516–24.

Part III
Prostate Cancer: Localized Disease

Chapter 7
Prognostic Factors of Localized Prostate Cancer in Elderly Patients

Barry B. McGuire and John M. Fitzpatrick

Abstract Diagnosis of prostate cancer (PCa) in elderly men poses a serious challenge to most clinicians, with many of the opinion that radical treatment may result in complications affecting quality of life, and question whether if treated or untreated, the patient is likely to live long enough to die of the disease. However, there is good evidence that these cancers have worse tumor characteristics than those in younger men. In elderly patients, the number and severity of comorbid conditions and functional impairments are strong predictors of life expectancy. Recently, the International Society of Geriatric Oncology Prostate Cancer Working Group (SIOG) published guidelines on the management of PCa in men over the age of 70 and advises the approach should be the same as in younger men but tailored to their individual health status. To assist in decision-making, there are many tools available both in assessment of men in terms of comorbidity and eligibility for curative treatment, as well as nomograms to predict life expectancy in men with or without comorbidity following curative treatment. In this chapter, we describe the tumor and clinical characteristics of PCa's in this age group, the importance of comorbidity and not age in terms of assessment, and the tools available to the clinician; discuss life expectancy and predictors of survival; and report on the recent guidelines from SIOG.

Keywords Prostate cancer • Elderly • Nomogram • Guidelines • Comorbidity Charlson score • SIOG

B.B. McGuire, M.D., IMRCS
Department of Urology, The Mater Misericordiae University Hospital,
Dublin, Ireland
e-mail: barrymcguire@me.com

J.M. Fitzpatrick, MCh, FRCSI, FC Urol (SA), FRCSGlas, FRCS (✉)
Irish Cancer Society and Mater Misericordiae Hospital, University College,
Dublin, Ireland
e-mail: jfitzpatrick@irishcancer.ie

J.-P. Droz, R.A. Audisio (eds.), *Management of Urological Cancers in Older People*,
Management of Cancer in Older People,
DOI 10.1007/978-0-85729-999-4_7, © Springer-Verlag London 2013

Abbreviations

PCa   Prostate cancer
PCSM   Prostate cancer-specific mortality
RP   Radical prostatectomy
RT   Radiotherapy

Introduction

Prostate cancer (PCa) is a disease that encompasses a biological continuum ranging from a slow growing, indolent tumor to one that is highly aggressive and potentially fatal. Unfortunately, genetics and biomarker research have not yet discovered a marker which will define who will die from PCa and who will not. As there are competing causes of mortality in men over the age of 70, and because many PCa's in older men are indolent [1–4] (with the medium-term PCa-specific survival close to 100 % even in the absence of treatment [4]), PCa diagnosis in this age group poses a serious challenge to most clinicians. Many urologists are of the opinion that radical treatment in this age group may result in complications affecting quality of life and question whether if treated or untreated the patient is likely to live long enough to die of the disease [5].

The life expectancy of a contemporary US male is 75.4 years [6]. Worldwide, the median life expectancy is increasing due to factors such as increased fertility, increasing life span, and post-World War II "baby boom" [7]. It is estimated that the average life span is expected to extend another 10 years by 2050 [7]. As a result, the incidence of PCa is set to increase driven by cancer diagnosis in older people [8]. By 2020, it is anticipated that there will be a 30 % increase in PCa, of which 71 % of patients will be >65 years. In 2030, there will be a projected increase of 55 % in PCa diagnosis, of which 71 % will be greater than 65 years of age [8]. Increasingly, we will be witnessing many men over the age of 70 years with PCa and faced with the decision of whether to treat with curative intent or not.

The management of PCa in older men is controversial, deciphering who requires radical treatment or who should be managed conservatively. The mantra of "you will die with the disease, rather than from it" was often quoted to older patients but is now considered inaccurate, as men over the age of 70 can often have worse disease features and oncological outcomes compared to younger men [9–15]. In a series of 4,561 radical prostatectomies, it has been shown that men diagnosed with PCa over the age of 70 years have a higher risk of advanced pathological stage (pT3/pT4), more aggressive disease (Gleason sum greater than 7), and higher tumor volume compared to younger men (younger than 60, and 60–70 years old) [9] (Table 7.1). In a series of Asian men who underwent radical prostatectomy (RP), a large proportion of patients who were 70 years or older had a PSA < 4 ng/mL (10.4 %), which was comparable to younger men (10.6 %, $p=0.918$). However, the risk of locally advanced disease in patients whose PSA was < 4 ng/mL was nearly

Table 7.1 Men over the age of 70 years display worse disease-specific features compared to younger men [9]

Age	<60	60–70	>70	p value
pT3–4	33 %	44.3 %	52.1 %	<0.001
Pathological Gleason 7–10	9.5 %	13.4 %	17.2 %	<0.001
Tumor volume	3.7 cc	4.7 cc	5.2 cc	<0.001

Table 7.2 D'Amico risk groups: men aged 70+ with high-risk PCa have a significant risk of dying of it [5]

Prostate cancer risk group	Characteristics	10-year mortality in men 70+
Low	PSA < 10 and Gleason <7 and AJCC stage T1c, T2a	Overall ~20 % Due to prostate cancer ~0 %
Intermediate	PSA = 10–20 or Gleason 7 or AJCC stage T2b	Overall ~40 % Due to prostate cancer ~10 %
High	PSA > 20 or Gleason 8–10 or AJCC stage T2c, T3	Overall ~60 % Due to prostate cancer ~30 %

three times higher in older patients than in younger one [10]. Malaeb et al. examined a total of 689 patients who underwent RP and stratified patients into age groups: younger than 50, 50–70 years, and older than 70 years ($n = 39$) [11]. Although there was no difference among the three age strata in terms of clinical parameters (PSA, Gleason score, clinical stage, etc.), there was a higher rate of seminal vesicle invasion with the older age group (however, the number of men in the older cohort is quite small). Whitson et al. report that 71 % of Gleason 8–10 PCa tumors are diagnosed among men over the age of 65, and the proportion of tumors with low-risk features falls from 50 % among men diagnosed before the age 50 to just over 30 % among those in their 70s [15]. Furthermore, older men with D'Amico high-risk PCa (PSA > 20 ng/mL or Gleason 8–10 or AJCC stage T2c/T3) treated by radical radiotherapy (RT) or surgery still have a significantly high PCa-specific mortality (PCSM) of 30 % indicating the need for aggressive treatment in this age group, for this risk group [5] (Table 7.2).

However, many men aged >75 with low-risk disease are inappropriately receiving aggressive therapy [16, 17], and those with intermediate- to high-risk disease who undergo radical treatment nearly exclusively receive RT and not surgery [16]. A SEER-Medicare (Surveillance, Epidemiology and End Results Medicare Data) study reported that among older men (median age 77), 41 % of those not receiving local therapy were managed with primary androgen deprivation therapy as opposed to surveillance/watchful waiting [18]. Furthermore, men >75 years are 9 times as likely to choose watchful waiting and 34 times as likely to receive primary androgen deprivation therapy compared to those aged <60 years old [16]. The varied treatment modalities highlighted above likely reflects confusion due to absence of guidelines, entrenched opinion about PCa treatments for older men, lack of randomized controlled trials in this age group, heterogeneity within this age group in terms of comorbidities, and a relatively increasing phenomenon of "super healthy" elderly men.

Life Expectancy

The AUA, EAU, and NCCN guidelines advise that a patient would benefit from RP if the candidate has a life expectancy greater than 10 years and from RT with varied life expectancies depending on various clinical factors [19, 20]. Crucial decisions are made centered on the age of the patient, with most men over the age of 70 being managed by watchful waiting or primary androgen deprivation therapy [16]. However, a healthy 76-year-old man who exercises regularly and is independent in daily living may well be more suited to curative intervention than an unhealthy 60-year-old man. It is vitally important in this older age group that decisions are made on an individual basis, and this requires weighting quantitative information, such as risk of cancer death and likelihood of beneficial and adverse screening outcomes, as well as qualitative factors such as individual patient's values and preferences. Major clinical decisions often hinge on the median life expectancy for all men; however, median life expectancies have great variation within each age subgroup [21], and it is more beneficial to know life expectancies at various ages. For example, a healthy (i.e., in the top 25th percentile) 70-year-old man would be expected to live a further 18 years, a 75-year-old 14 years further, an 80-year-old 11 years further, and an 85-year-old 8 years further [22]. Bear in mind that even in seemingly low-risk localized disease, PCa-specific death dramatically increases after 15 years if left untreated [23]. Although it is impossible for physicians to predict the exact life expectancy of an individual patient, it is possible for physicians to make reasonably accurate estimates of whether a patient is likely to live substantially longer or shorter than an average person in his age group [24]. To formally assist in this estimation, there are many tools physicians can use to estimate whether older patients are typical of someone in the upper or lower quartiles of the age-specific median survival.

Comorbidity

Comorbidity is one of the major predictors of PCa survival [25–27], and there is a dose–response relationship between grades of comorbidity and death [28]. The number and severity of comorbid conditions and functional impairments are strong predictors of life expectancy in older people [29, 30]. Congestive heart failure, end-stage renal disease, oxygen-dependent chronic obstructive lung disease, or severe functional dependencies in activities of daily living are examples of risk factors that would cause an elderly person to have a life expectancy substantially below the average for his age [22]. Conversely, the absence of significant comorbid conditions or presence of functional status considerably better than age-group averages identifies older adults who are likely to live longer than average [22]. This argues in favor of considering life expectancy when making treatment decisions in older people.

However, an analysis from CAPSURE including over 2,000 men over the age of 75 found that whereas older men were less likely to receive treatment for PCa compared to younger men, there was little evidence that either tumor risk characteristics or patient comorbidities were adequately considered in decision-making for patients in this age group [31]. Similarly, in Canada, a population-based study reported inappropriate age bias, demonstrating that age was a strong inverse correlation with likelihood of local treatment; in particular, RP was less likely to be offered to older men compared to younger men with a similar relative life expectancy, accounting for comorbidity and tumor characteristics [32].

In men with clinically localized PCa treated by radiation or surgery, comorbidity measured by the Charlson comorbidity index (CCI) is a stronger predictor of non-PCSM, compared to biopsy grade, PSA, age, surgery, or radiation [26, 27] (Table 7.3). The CCI, however, only measures potentially lethal comorbid conditions. Recently, the International Society of Geriatric Oncology Prostate Cancer Working Group (SIOG) reviewed the recent literature and published their consensus opinion on PCa in the elderly [33, 34]. In the opinion of the SIOG, the best tool for predicting risk of death unrelated to PCa is the Cumulative Illness Score Rating-Geriatrics (CISR-G) [33, 35, 36] as in contrast to the CCI, this also rates nonlethal conditions.

Independence in daily living, or lack thereof, is an extremely important determinant of survival in older patients [28, 33]. Dependence can be easily assessed using the ADL [37] and IADL [38] scales. In brief, the ADL scale rates a patient's ability to accomplish basic activities of daily living, e.g., dressing, toileting, bathing, feeding, continence, and transferring. In older men with PCa, one ADL impairment is considered abnormal with the exception of incontinence. The IADL assesses activities that require a higher level of cognition and judgment. Four items apply to men with PCa: to manage medications, to use transportation, to use the telephone, and to manage money. Similarly, one IADL impairment is considered abnormal in older men with PCa.

Malnutrition is also an important determinant of survival with increased mortality in those displaying signs of malnutrition including weight loss, skinfold thickness, arm muscle circumference, serum albumin, and delayed cutaneous hypersensitivity reaction below the reference ranges, $p < 0.001$ [39]. Nutritional status can be estimated by calculating the variation of weight during the previous 3 months: (1) good nutritional status = <5 % weight loss, (2) risk of malnutrition = weight loss 5–10 %, and (3) severe malnutrition = weight loss >10 %.

Assessment of Older Patients with PCa

The SIOG working group recommends evaluating older patients with localized and advanced PCa using a mixture of the CISR-G scale, ADL and IADL, and nutritional status and has used this information to categorize men into one of four categories rather than using chronological age: (a) healthy, (b) vulnerable, (c) frail, and (d) too sick.

Table 7.3 Comorbidity is the strongest predictor of non-prostate-cancer mortality [27]

| | All-cause mortality | | PCSM | | Non-PCa mortality | |
	RR [95 % CI]	p value	RR [95 % CI]	p value	RR [95 % CI]	p value
RP	0.41 [0.31–0.54]	<0.001	0.35 [0.19–0.54]	0.001	0.44 [0.32–0.62]	<0.001
RT	0.90 [0.70–1.15]	NS	0.41 [0.22–0.74]	0.001	1.10 [0.84–1.45]	NS
Age at diagnosis	1.04 [1.02–1.06]	<0.001	1.04 [0.99–1.06]	0.14	1.05 [1.03–1.07]	<0.001
Charlson score 2+	2.63 [2.08–3.32]	<0.001	1.43 [0.79–2.56]	0.23	3.03 [2.35–3.92]	<0.001
Biopsy grade	1.28 [1.08–1.53]	0.005	2.08 [1.41–3.06]	<0.001	1.15 [0.94–1.41]	0.15
Log baseline PSA	1.55 [1.28–1.87]	<0.001	2.51 [1.85–3.41]	<0.001	1.22 [0.96–1.54]	0.10

Permission from Elsevier [27]

RP radical prostatectomy, *RT* radical radiotherapy, *RR* relative risk, *PCSM* prostate cancer-specific mortality

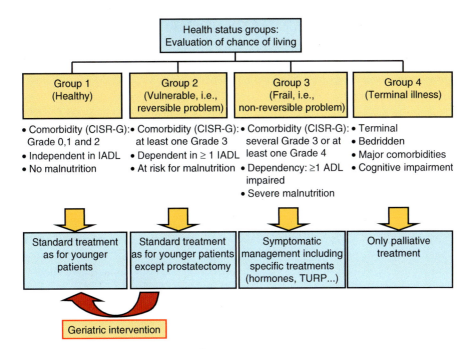

Fig. 7.1 The International Society of Geriatric Oncology algorithm for treating patients over the age of 70 years with localized disease (Ref. [33]. Used with permission from John Wiley & Sons Ltd.)

The SIOG PCa Working Group has developed evidence-based recommendations for the management of the older man with PCa which are summarized as follows:

- The approach to PCa in the older man should be the same as in the younger man.
- Older men diagnosed with PCa should be managed according to their individual health status, which is driven by the severity of associated comorbid conditions, dependence and nutritional status and not according to chronological age.
- Screening for health status should include evaluation of comorbid conditions (CISR-G scale), dependence status (IADL and ADL scales), and nutritional status (weight loss estimation). This allows the classification of men into one of four groups, and the SIOG has published a treatment algorithm (Fig. 7.1):

  1. "Fit" or "healthy": should receive the same standard treatment as younger patients. Specifically they should receive curative therapy in cases of high-risk localized PCa and standard chemotherapy in cases of CRPC.
  2. "Vulnerable" (i.e., reversible impairment): should receive standard treatment after resolution of any geriatric problems through geriatric interventions.
  3. "Frail" (i.e., irreversible impairment): should receive an adapted treatment.
  4. Patients who are "too sick" with "terminal illness" should receive only symptomatic palliative treatment.

Predictors of Prostate Cancer-Specific Mortality

The major predictors of death due to PCa are Gleason score, preoperative PSA, and tumor stage. Decisions for treatment in older men with localized PCa should take into consideration the risk of dying from PCa (which depends on the grade and stage of the tumor), the risk of dying from another cause (which depends more on the severity of the patient's comorbid illness than chronological age), and potential adverse effects of treatment and patient preferences [33].

In one of the largest series of watchful waiting, Albertsen et al. [1] performed a retrospective analysis in 767 men diagnosed with clinically localized PCa and treated with either observation or delayed androgen therapy, with a median follow-up of 24 years. In this study, there were 330 men diagnosed at age 70–74 years, and biopsy Gleason score and CCI were strongly related to mortality [1]. Of those with biopsy Gleason ≤ 6, 73 % had a CCI of 0–1 and 27 % ≥ 2 and 22 % died of PCa and 73 % of other causes (5 % unknown). Of those with biopsy Gleason 7, 75 % had a CCI of 0–1 and 25 % ≥ 2 and 41 % died of PCa and 56 % of other causes. In men with Gleason 8–10 disease, 82 % had a CCI of 0–1 and 18 % ≥ 2 and 64 % died of PCa. This data indicates that men of this age group with intermediate or high-grade PCa treated with watchful waiting have an extremely high likelihood of dying of PCa.

Johansson and colleagues report that older men with Gleason 8–10 disease who are managed conservatively (observation or androgen deprivation therapy) have a high PCSM [1, 23]. Considering that RP may reduce PCSM by up to half [40], then older patients should not be automatically excluded from this modality of treatment.

Using SEER data, Wong and colleagues examined overall survival in men aged 65–80 with organ-confined well- or moderately differentiated PCa who underwent treatment (RP or RT) versus observation [41]. They reported improved overall survival in the treatment group, including older men (75–80 years at diagnosis) [41].

In another retrospective study, Sweat et al. [25] examined survival outcomes in men between the ages of 55–74 following RP. The only significant predictor of PCa-specific death was biopsy Gleason score ($p < 0.001$), while only age and CCI were significant independent predictors of non-PCa death ($p < 0.001$). They also report that men with a score of 7–10 were at 29–42 % at risk of PCa-specific death even when PCa was diagnosed as late as age 74 and treated surgically [25].

Froehner et al. also observed a poor overall survival in men aged 70 years or older with Gleason 8–10 disease (33 % overall survival) or lymph node involvement (30 % overall survival) in men who underwent RP [26].

Nomograms and Risk-Stratification Tools

Risk-stratification tools are available for predicting pathological stage and outcomes after treatment [42–44] and provide accurate estimates of PSA failure on the basis of pretreatment parameters after RP or RT for patients with clinically localized disease. However, most pretreatment algorithms and prospective randomized controlled trials do not encompass comorbid illness limiting interpretation in the older age group [27].

Tewari and colleagues [27] have developed comprehensive lookup tables for estimating survival probability stratified by patient age, race, clinical variables, comorbidities, and treatment type in 1,611 men with clinically localized PCa. In these easy-to-use tables, 10-year overall survival is estimated according to preoperative PSA and Gleason grade and according to age and whether RP or RT is selected.

Cowen et al. developed a model that predicted life expectancy in men with clinically localized PCa [45] from a retrospective cohort of 506 men and report that overall life expectancy can be predicted with a moderate degree of accuracy.

Albertsen et al. measured the impact of comorbidity classifications on all-cause mortality and identified that comorbidity was a stronger predictor of survival than age, Gleason score, and stage [46].

However, the accuracy of the Tewari, Cowen, and Albertsen models was low, ranging from 69 to 73 %. Walz et al. developed a nomogram to predict 10-year life expectancy in men with PCa treated by RP or RT in a series of 9,131 men [47], which incorporated age and CCI as variables. This demonstrated much improved accuracy of 84.3 %, and when externally validated achieved 82 % accuracy [48]. Although the median age of the cohort was 68, advanced age and elevated CCI were independent predictors of poor 10-year life expectancy ($p < 0.001$). In a subsequent validation of this nomogram, Froehner et al. show an excellent performance of the nomogram in predicting life expectancy (in a very different cohort) [48].

In men with localized PCa not suitable for curative therapy, overall survival is slightly better with immediate androgen deprivation therapy, but there is no difference in PCSM or symptom-free survival between the two groups [49]. Androgen therapy in older men should be considered carefully, as there is increased risk of fracture [50] and diabetes [51]. There is an increased risk of all-cause mortality, including in patients with high-risk PCa in chronic heart failure, history of myocardial infarction, and history of stroke [52–54].

Summary

We are witnessing an increase in PCa diagnosis in men over the age of 70, and there is good evidence that the tumor characteristics can be worse than in younger men. The SIOG has published guidelines on the management of PCa in men over the age of 70, and the approach should be the same as in younger men but tailored to their individual health status. Finally, to assist in decision-making, there are many tools available both in assessment of men in terms of comorbidity and eligibility for curative treatment, as well as nomograms to predict life expectancy in men with or without comorbidity following curative treatment.

References

1. Albertsen PC, Hanley JA, Fine J. 20-year outcomes following conservative management of clinically localized prostate cancer. JAMA. 2005;293(17):2095–101.
2. Albertsen PC, Hanley JA, Gleason DF, Barry MJ. Competing risk analysis of men aged 55 to 74 years at diagnosis managed conservatively for clinically localized prostate cancer. JAMA. 1998;280(11):975–80.
3. Chodak GW, Thisted RA, Gerber GS, et al. Results of conservative management of clinically localized prostate cancer. N Engl J Med. 1994;330(4):242–8.
4. Bill-Axelson A, Holmberg L, Ruutu M, et al. Radical prostatectomy versus watchful waiting in early prostate cancer. N Engl J Med. 2005;352(19):1977–84.
5. D'Amico AV, Moul J, Carroll PR, Sun L, Lubeck D, Chen MH. Cancer-specific mortality after surgery or radiation for patients with clinically localized prostate cancer managed during the prostate-specific antigen era. J Clin Oncol. 2003;21(11):2163–72.
6. Arias E. United States life tables, 2007. Natl Vital Stat Rep. 2011;59(9):1–60.
7. Centers for Disease Control and Prevention (CDC). Trends in aging – United States and worldwide. MMWR Morb Mortal Wkly Rep. 2003;52(6):101–4, 106.
8. Smith BD, Smith GL, Hurria A, Hortobagyi GN, Buchholz TA. Future of cancer incidence in the United States: burdens upon an aging, changing nation. J Clin Oncol. 2009;27(17): 2758–65.
9. Sun L, Caire AA, Robertson CN, et al. Men older than 70 years have higher risk prostate cancer and poorer survival in the early and late prostate specific antigen eras. J Urol. 2009;182(5): 2242–8.
10. Kim JK, Cho SY, Jeong CW, et al. Patients aged more than 70 had higher risk of locally advanced prostate cancers and biochemical recurrence in Korea. BJU Int. 2012;110(4): 505–9. DOI:10.1111/j.1464-410X.2011.10927.x. Epub 2012 Feb 7.
11. Malaeb BS, Rashid HH, Lotan Y, et al. Prostate cancer disease-free survival after radical retropubic prostatectomy in patients older than 70 years compared to younger cohorts. Urol Oncol. 2007;25(4):291–7.
12. Obek C, Lai S, Sadek S, Civantos F, Soloway MS. Age as a prognostic factor for disease recurrence after radical prostatectomy. Urology. 1999;54(3):533–8.
13. Magheli A, Rais-Bahrami S, Trock BJ, et al. Prostate specific antigen versus prostate specific antigen density as a prognosticator of pathological characteristics and biochemical recurrence following radical prostatectomy. J Urol. 2008;179(5):1780–4; discussion 1784.
14. Bechis SK, Carroll PR, Cooperberg MR. Impact of age at diagnosis on prostate cancer treatment and survival. J Clin Oncol. 2011;29(2):235–41.
15. Whitson JM, Konety BR. Should men over the age of 65 years receive PSA screening? Argument in favor. Nat Clin Pract Urol. 2008;5(5):230–1.
16. Hamilton AS, Albertsen PC, Johnson TK, et al. Trends in the treatment of localized prostate cancer using supplemented cancer registry data. BJU Int. 2011;107(4):576–84.
17. Cooperberg MR, Lubeck DP, Meng MV, Mehta SS, Carroll PR. The changing face of low-risk prostate cancer: trends in clinical presentation and primary management. J Clin Oncol. 2004;22(11):2141–9.
18. Lu-Yao GL, Albertsen PC, Moore DF, et al. Survival following primary androgen deprivation therapy among men with localized prostate cancer. JAMA. 2008;300(2):173–81.
19. Thompson I, Thrasher JB, Aus G, et al. Guideline for the management of clinically localized prostate cancer: 2007 update. J Urol. 2007;177(6):2106–31.
20. Heidenreich A, Bellmunt J, Bolla M, et al. EAU guidelines on prostate cancer. Part 1: screening, diagnosis, and treatment of clinically localised disease. Eur Urol. 2011;59(1):61–71.
21. Welch HG, Albertsen PC, Nease RF, Bubolz TA, Wasson JH. Estimating treatment benefits for the elderly: the effect of competing risks. Ann Intern Med. 1996;124(6):577–84.
22. Walter LC, Covinsky KE. Cancer screening in elderly patients: a framework for individualized decision making. JAMA. 2001;285(21):2750–6.

23. Johansson JE, Andren O, Andersson SO, et al. Natural history of early, localized prostate cancer. JAMA. 2004;291(22):2713–9.
24. Froehner M, Koch R, Litz RJ, Hakenberg OW, Wirth MP. Which patients are at the highest risk of dying from competing causes ≤ 10 years after radical prostatectomy? BJU Int. 2012;110(2): 206–10. DOI:10.1111/j.1464-410X.2011.10693.x. Epub 2011 Nov 1.
25. Sweat SD, Bergstralh EJ, Slezak J, Blute ML, Zincke H. Competing risk analysis after radical prostatectomy for clinically nonmetastatic prostate adenocarcinoma according to clinical Gleason score and patient age. J Urol. 2002;168(2):525–9.
26. Froehner M, Koch R, Litz RJ, Hakenberg OW, Oehlschlaeger S, Wirth MP. Survival analysis in men undergoing radical prostatectomy at an age of 70 years or older. Urol Oncol. 2010;28(6):628–34.
27. Tewari A, Johnson CC, Divine G, et al. Long-term survival probability in men with clinically localized prostate cancer: a case–control, propensity modeling study stratified by race, age, treatment and comorbidities. J Urol. 2004;171(4):1513–9.
28. Rockwood K, Stadnyk K, MacKnight C, McDowell I, Hebert R, Hogan DB. A brief clinical instrument to classify frailty in elderly people. Lancet. 1999;353(9148):205–6.
29. Covinsky KE, Justice AC, Rosenthal GE, Palmer RM, Landefeld CS. Measuring prognosis and case mix in hospitalized elders. The importance of functional status. J Gen Intern Med. 1997;12(4):203–8.
30. Inouye SK, Peduzzi PN, Robison JT, Hughes JS, Horwitz RI, Concato J. Importance of functional measures in predicting mortality among older hospitalized patients. JAMA. 1998;279(15): 1187–93.
31. Konety BR, Cowan JE, Carroll PR. Patterns of primary and secondary therapy for prostate cancer in elderly men: analysis of data from CaPSURE. J Urol. 2008;179(5):1797–803; discussion 1803.
32. Alibhai SM, Krahn MD, Cohen MM, Fleshner NE, Tomlinson GA, Naglie G. Is there age bias in the treatment of localized prostate carcinoma? Cancer. 2004;100(1):72–81.
33. Droz JP, Balducci L, Bolla M, et al. Management of prostate cancer in older men: recommendations of a working group of the International Society of Geriatric Oncology. BJU Int. 2010;106(4):462–9.
34. Droz JP, Balducci L, Bolla M, et al. Background for the proposal of SIOG guidelines for the management of prostate cancer in senior adults. Crit Rev Oncol Hematol. 2010;73(1):68–91.
35. Extermann M. Measuring comorbidity in older cancer patients. Eur J Cancer. 2000;36(4): 453–71.
36. Linn BS, Linn MW, Gurel L. Cumulative illness rating scale. J Am Geriatr Soc. 1968;16(5):622–6.
37. Katz S, Ford AB, Moskowitz RW, Jackson BA, Jaffe MW. Studies of illness in the aged. The index of ADL: a standardized measure of biological and psychosocial function. JAMA. 1963;185:914–9.
38. Lawton MP, Brody EM. Assessment of older people: self-maintaining and instrumental activities of daily living. Gerontologist. 1969;9(3):179–86.
39. Cederholm T, Jagren C, Hellstrom K. Outcome of protein-energy malnutrition in elderly medical patients. Am J Med. 1995;98(1):67–74.
40. Holmberg L, Bill-Axelson A, Helgesen F, et al. A randomized trial comparing radical prostatectomy with watchful waiting in early prostate cancer. N Engl J Med. 2002;347(11):781–9.
41. Wong YN, Mitra N, Hudes G, et al. Survival associated with treatment vs observation of localized prostate cancer in elderly men. JAMA. 2006;296(22):2683–93.
42. D'Amico AV, Whittington R, Malkowicz SB, et al. Biochemical outcome after radical prostatectomy, external beam radiation therapy, or interstitial radiation therapy for clinically localized prostate cancer. JAMA. 1998;280(11):969–74.
43. Eggener SE, Scardino PT, Walsh PC, et al. Predicting 15-year prostate cancer specific mortality after radical prostatectomy. J Urol. 2011;185(3):869–75.
44. Freedland SJ, Humphreys EB, Mangold LA, et al. Risk of prostate cancer-specific mortality following biochemical recurrence after radical prostatectomy. JAMA. 2005;294(4):433–9.

45. Cowen ME, Halasyamani LK, Kattan MW. Predicting life expectancy in men with clinically localized prostate cancer. J Urol. 2006;175(1):99–103.
46. Albertsen PC, Fryback DG, Storer BE, Kolon TF, Fine J. The impact of co-morbidity on life expectancy among men with localized prostate cancer. J Urol. 1996;156(1):127–32.
47. Walz J, Gallina A, Saad F, et al. A nomogram predicting 10-year life expectancy in candidates for radical prostatectomy or radiotherapy for prostate cancer. J Clin Oncol. 2007;25(24):3576–81.
48. Froehner M, Koch R, Litz RJ, Wirth MP. Nomogram underestimates 10-year survival in healthy men selected for radical prostatectomy at age 70 years or older. Urology. 2009;73(3):610–3; discussion 613–14.
49. Studer UE, Whelan P, Albrecht W, et al. Immediate or deferred androgen deprivation for patients with prostate cancer not suitable for local treatment with curative intent: European Organisation for Research and Treatment of Cancer (EORTC) Trial 30891. J Clin Oncol. 2006;24(12):1868–76.
50. Shahinian VB, Kuo YF, Freeman JL, Goodwin JS. Risk of fracture after androgen deprivation for prostate cancer. N Engl J Med. 2005;352(2):154–64.
51. Keating NL, O'Malley AJ, Smith MR. Diabetes and cardiovascular disease during androgen deprivation therapy for prostate cancer. J Clin Oncol. 2006;24(27):4448–56.
52. D'Amico AV, Denham JW, Crook J, et al. Influence of androgen suppression therapy for prostate cancer on the frequency and timing of fatal myocardial infarctions. J Clin Oncol. 2007;25(17):2420–5.
53. Hayes JH, Chen MH, Moran BJ, et al. Androgen-suppression therapy for prostate cancer and the risk of death in men with a history of myocardial infarction or stroke. BJU Int. 2010;106(7):979–85.
54. Nguyen PL, Chen MH, Beckman JA, et al. Influence of androgen deprivation therapy on all-cause mortality in men with high-risk prostate cancer and a history of congestive heart failure or myocardial infarction. Int J Radiat Oncol Biol Phys. 2012;82:1411–6.

Chapter 8
Prostatectomy in Elderly Prostate Cancer Patients

Hein Van Poppel

Abstract As modern medicine will continue to prolong life expectancy, urologists can expect to encounter an increasing number of healthy septa- and octogenarians with newly diagnosed prostate cancer (PCa). Outcome data of radical prostatectomy (RP) in this population group is sparse, and controversy exists over the appropriate treatment of these patients with localized PCa. In this chapter, we review the survival rates for patients aged 70 years or older who underwent RP and compare it with the outcome of younger patients. In addition, we evaluate in these patients the influence of RP on the health-related quality of life (HRQOL) with specific attention to continence and potency outcomes. Age should not be a barrier to surgical treatment in this group of healthy patients aged 70 years or older. Based on survival rates, RP should not be excluded in selected elderly patients with a life expectancy of at least 10 years and no or limited morbidity. The rates of urinary continence and potency after RP decrease with advancing age but can be considered more or less acceptable in patients aged 70 years or older. The impact of advanced age on HRQOL after RP should be further examined in order to make better treatment decisions in the elderly with localized PCa.

Keywords Prostate cancer • Radical prostatectomy • Surgery • Elderly • Survival Quality of life

Introduction

With the population aging and the continuing efforts for early detection of PCa, more healthy elderly men over age 70 years will present with localized PCa and will seek treatment [1]. Many questions remain unanswered about the appropriate

H. Van Poppel, M.D., Ph.D.
Department of Urology, University Hospitals Leuven,
Leuven, Belgium
e-mail: hendrik.vanpoppel@uzleuven.be

J.-P. Droz, R.A. Audisio (eds.), *Management of Urological Cancers in Older People*, 105
Management of Cancer in Older People,
DOI 10.1007/978-0-85729-999-4_8, © Springer-Verlag London 2013

treatment of PCa in this age cohort [2]. In the past, RP did not apply to men older than 70 years. As the average life expectancy of men has prolonged, the age limits traditionally used to guide treatment decisions for RP are being questioned. Because PCa frequently has a long natural history, RP is typically recommended for men with a life expectancy of at least 10 years in the guidelines of the European Association of Urology (EAU). However, no upper age limit is suggested.

Many physicians believe that men diagnosed with PCa at ages >70 years will not benefit from an RP because the morbidity of RP in these patients is too high and they are likely to die of causes other than PCa. The European Randomized Study of Screening for Prostate Cancer (ERSPC) and the American randomized Prostate, Lung, Colorectal, and Ovarian (PLCO) Cancer Screening study on PCa mortality suggest that older men with low-risk PCa are unlikely to benefit from PSA screening or PCa active therapy. The update of the randomized Scandinavian Prostate Cancer Group study showed a significant reduction in metastases, cancer-specific survival (CSS), and overall mortality in men aged <65 years but not for older men. Nowadays, there is increasing concern that PSA screening may lead to overdiagnosis and overtreatment of indolent cancers. However, other investigators have suggested a possible beneficial effect of RP in appropriately selected elderly patients (≥70 years) [1–6] even up to the age of 80 years in remarkable healthy men [1, 4, 7]. Refinements in the understanding of the pelvic anatomy, improvements and innovations in surgical technique, and early detection have led to better oncological and functional outcomes following RP. On the other hand, it is possible that RP in some men with localized PCa may result in more harm than good. Considerable controversy exists over the appropriate treatment of the elderly with localized PCa. In recent years, there has been interest in active surveillance to avoid treatment-related side effects and prevent overtreatment.

In this chapter, we will review the survival rates for patients ≥70 years who underwent RP for localized PCa and will also compare it with the outcome of younger patients. In addition, we will evaluate the impact of RP (open, laparoscopic, and robotic-assisted laparoscopic) on the health-related quality of life (HRQOL) with specific attention to continence and potency outcomes in men undergoing RP at the age of 70 or older.

Oncological Outcome

Retropubic RP, laparoscopic RP (LRP), and robotic-assisted RP (RALP) represent effective surgical approaches for the treatment of clinically localized PCa and show no difference with respect to biochemical recurrence-free survival. There are limited data on elderly men undergoing RP. It has been established that as men age, clinicopathological characteristics consistent with aggressive disease become more prevalent which may cause significant PCa mortality within 10 years of diagnosis. Other investigators found that men aged ≥70 years with Gleason scores of 8–10 have the most significant risk of undertreatment. They are often receiving watchful waiting and are potentially losing valuable years of life. A decision analysis suggested that potentially curative therapy (RP or RT) should be seriously considered in healthy men up to 80 years with localized PCa especially for men with high-grade disease [7]. Tewari et al. [8] evaluated the long-term survival probability in 3,159 men (<75 years) with clinically localized PCa. They showed that after adjusting for age and comorbidity in a propensity-scoring model, RP and radiotherapy (RT) gave better survival rates compared with conservative management. Overall survival (OS) rates were 65, 50, and 35 %, respectively. CSS rates were 92, 87, and 79 %, respectively. Within each treatment, OS and CSS were similar in men aged <60, 60–70, and >70 years and were worse for men with a Charlson comorbidity score of >1 than in those with score of 0 or 1 [8].

Table 8.1 gives an overview on studies providing survival rates in men undergoing RP at age 70 years or older. The reported 10-year OS rates are higher than 70 % with exception of the retrospective study of Barry et al. [3] and the population-based Canadian cohort study by Jeldres et al. (2008) [1–6, 9, 10]. The OS of patients ≥70 years after RP ($n=1,591$) in the latter study is only 59.3 % and even worse after external beam radiation therapy (EBRT) ($n=4,592$) with 30.3 % [10]. Few studies examined the relationship between age and CSS after RP. None of them revealed a significant difference in CSS between the age groups [2, 3, 5, 9].

Thompson et al. [1] reported the long-term outcomes after RP in 19 healthy octogenarians (≥80 years) and compared them with those of patients 60–69 years old ($n=6,091$) and 70–79 years old ($n=2,606$). Median follow-up was 10.5 years. In the cohort of octogenarians, 13 (68 %) patients had either stage pT3 disease or Gleason score of 7 or more. No significant difference was found in the 10-year OS after RP comparing the 19 octogenarians with the patients aged 60–69 years and aged 70–79 years (79, 84, 75 %), respectively. The results of this retrospective study indicate that RP is feasible and can be safely performed in well-selected elderly patients and in certain patients aged 80 years or older. Patients should undergo an extensive preoperative medical evaluation and should be informed that after RP the rate of urinary incontinence increases with age [1]. Recently, Pierorazio et al. [4] evaluated the survival in 386 patients aged 70–81 years who underwent RP. The median follow-up was 6.5 (1–22) years. Appropriately selected men aged >70 years had excellent CSS and OS rates of 94 and 82.5 % at 10 years and 90.2 and 68.9 % at 15 years, respectively after RP [4].

Several reports have shown that the oncological outcomes of RP in elderly and younger men are equivalent [2, 5, 9, 11, 12]. Siddiqui et al. [9] observed that younger men even with more favorable clinicopathological features had a similar survival outcome compared to older men following retropubic RP in a retrospective study with 5,509 patients. The five age cohorts were <55 years, 55–59, 60–64, 65–69, and ≥70 years. CSS, systemic progression-free survival (sPFS), and biochemical PFS were similar across age groups. OS was lower in the older age group, consistent with the risk of death from causes other than PCa increasing dramatically in older patients [9]. Malaeb et al. [11] showed that retropubic RP is a feasible treatment option in men aged >70 years with localized PCa and no or mild morbidity. They failed to show a statistically significant difference in the biochemical recurrence

Table 8.1 Survival rates after radical prostatectomy in men aged 70 years or older

Authors, year	n	Age (years)	Recruitment period	10-year overall survival	10-year cancer-specific survival	10-year biochemical progression-free survival
Barry et al. (2001) [3]	180	70–74	1971–1984	65 %		
Thompson et al. (2006) [1]	2,606	70–79	1986–2003	75 %		
	19	>80		79 %		
Siddiqui et al. (2006) [9]	1,527	≥70	1087–1995		99.5 % (low risk)	
					97.5 % (medium risk)	
					94.0 % (high risk)	
Jeldres et al. (2008) [10]	1591	70–89	1989–2000	59 %		
Richstone et al. (2008) [2]	258	≥70	1983–2003	73 %	96 %	74 %
Pfitzenmaier et al. (2009) [5]	100	≥70	1990–2006	71 %	98 %	57 %
Froehner et al. (2010) [6]	329	≥70	1992–2004	77 %		
Pierorazio et al. (2010) [4]	386	70–81	1982–2008	83 %	94 %	60 %

among patients aged >70 years when compared to two younger age groups. The three age groups were patients of 50 years ($n=49$), 50–70 years ($n=601$), and older than 70 years ($n=39$). The 5-year PSA progression-free estimates were 82 % (95 % CI 69–96 %), 82 % (95 % CI 78–86 %), and 65 % (95 % CI 43–86 %), respectively ($P=0.349$). The overall and cause-specific mortalities were not different. A limitation was a relatively small sample size in two of the three age groups. The follow-up might not be long enough. Mean postoperative follow-up was 39 months. Patients aged >70 years did have a higher percentage of T2 (vs. T1) tumors, higher percentage Gleason grade 7–10, and higher mean PSA and were more likely to have seminal vesicle invasion ($P=0.034$) and higher total prostate volume ($P<0.001$) [11]. Similarly, Magheli et al. [12] revealed that increased age is not correlated with inferior biochemical recurrence-free outcomes following RP. On stratified analyses, patients ≤45 years, 46–55, 56–65, and ≥66 years had 5-year biochemical-free survival rates of 93, 89, 89, and 85 %, respectively, and 10-year biochemical-free survival rates of 89, 84, 89, and 78 %, respectively. Despite more favorable pathological features in younger men, no statistically significant differences in biochemical-free survival could be observed among the four age cohorts in this study. Age should not be considered an independent prognosticator for disease recurrence following RP. This was the first study to use propensity score matching to investigate the relationship between patient age and biochemical recurrence outcomes following RP. A major limitation of the study was the relatively short follow-up with a median follow-up of 3 years for the entire cohort [12]. OS and CSS were not reported in the two previous studies [11, 12]. From 1983 to 2003, 258 men aged ≥70 years and 3,777 aged <70 years underwent retropubic RP. Richstone et al. [2] revealed that the patients aged ≥70 years treated with retropubic RP tended to have cancer of higher clinical and pathological stage/grade. Upgrading from biopsy, Gleason sum 2–6 to RP Gleason sum 7–10 was more frequent in older men (≥70 years) than in younger men (<70 years) (45 and 35.2 %) but this was not significant on a multivariate analysis. Upstaging was more frequent in older than in younger men (40.2 and 29.3 %, respectively), and age was associated with upstaging on a multivariate analysis. There was no difference in biochemical progression-free probability (74 and 75 % at 10 years, respectively, $P=0.13$) or CSS (96 % at 10 years, $P=0.33$) between the age groups. Older men had a lower OS than younger men (73 vs. 79 % at 10 years, respectively, $P=0.001$). According to the authors, the preoperative Partin tables and Kattan nomograms remain accurate tools in counselling of older patients considering definitive treatment, in particular retropubic RP [2]. Barlow et al. (2009) investigated in a retrospective study including 1,984 patients the relationship between age at time of surgery and the risk of biochemical failure after RP (open or RALP). Biochemical recurrence was defined as a single PSA level of ≥0.2 ng/mL at least 28 days after RP. It is shown that older patients aged >65 years have more aggressive forms of PCa at the time of RP. The 5-year recurrence-free survival rates were 80.6 % (CI 78.0–82.9 %) for group 1 (40–64 years, $n=1,325$) and 75.6 % (CI 71.5–79.1 %) for group 2 (>65 years, $n=659$). Based on a univariate analysis, older patients who undergo RP appear to have an increased risk of recurrence (hazard ratio HR 1.30, $P=0.012$). However, age does not appear to be an independent predictor of biochemical recurrence when accounting for PSA level, Gleason score, and clinical stage in multivariate analyses (HR 1.04, $P=0.76$) [13].

Pfitzenmaier et al. [5] reported the results of a prospective study evaluating and comparing survival in PCa patients <70 ($n=100$) and ≥70 years ($n=526$) who underwent RP with a median follow-up of 5.3 years. The young and old patients had an organ-confined PCa in 56.3 and 58.0 % ($P=0.826$). They had well and moderately differentiated tumors in 78.7 and 75.0 % of cases and poorly differentiated tumors in 21.3 and 25.0 % ($P=0.198$). Young and old patients had an eastern cooperative oncology group performance status (ECOG) >1 in 2.3 and 7.0 % of cases ($P=0.024$), respectively. A 10-year PSA-free survival for young and old patients was 51.8 and 57.4 % ($P=0.721$), 10-year-disease-specific survival was 92.3 and 97.6 % ($P=0.342$), and 10-year metastasis-free survival was 86.9 and 89.7 % ($P=0.713$). The 10-year OS was 78.1 % for the young and 71.2 % for the old patients ($P=0.565$) and, therefore, by far higher than in the Canadian cohort. The survival outcome in the elderly group is not inferior to that of younger patients on multivariate analysis. Gleason score was not available for all patients and follow-up was relatively short [5]. Selection criteria regarding the health status for RP in the elderly seemed to be more stringent in the study of Pfitzenmaier et al. [5] compared with the Canadian study published by Jeldres et al. [10]. Almost 10 % of the Canadian patients were older than 80 years which was not the case in this study. The Charlson comorbidity index was ≤2 in 69 % of the cases in the Canadian patients, whereas in this study, 93.0 % had an ECOG $\leq$ 1. Pfitzenmaier et al. agree that careful selection must be made before RP is performed in the elderly. RP in the elderly should be limited to the healthy old patient (ECOG $\leq$ 1) with an estimated life expectancy of 10 years and, more probably, 15 years would be even more adequate [5].

Comorbidity has been identified as an independent predictor of survival in men selected for RP in general. Very few data are available on the long-term survival and the prognostic value of comorbidity in men 70 years or older diagnosed with PCa and selected for RP. Early studies found only a weak relationship between comorbidity and survival in men undergoing RP at the age of ≥70 years. A possible explanation can be found in a stricter selection process patients undergo before being scheduled for RP and a high-competing mortality of second malignancies in this age group [6]. In many septa- and octogenarians, comorbidities may undermine the life expectancy estimates and patients who die of non-PCa causes prior to the 10-year threshold are considered as overtreated. Jeldres et al. [10] showed in a population-based study with 6,183 PCa patients aged ≥70 years that 40 % of septa-and octogenarian men who are selected for RP do not have adequate life expectancy (at least 10 years) to warrant active therapy. They questioned the indication to attempt curative therapy in these older patients especially the indication for EBRT (OS 30.3 %). More severe RP selection criteria are needed if the objective is to minimize overtreatment [10]. Froehner et al. [6] showed in a recent study that the Charlson comorbidity score may be used to stratify men selected for RP at age 70 years or older and to estimate long-term survival probability. In this study of 329 consecutive patients aged ≥70 years, RP inappropriately selected patients without adverse tumor-related risk factors or serious morbidity resulted in an excellent 10-year OS rate of 77–100 % (depending on which of the five morbidity classifications were used). The following comorbidity classifications were used: Charlson score, American Society of Anesthesiologists (ASA) physical status classification, New York Heart Association (NYHA), classification of cardiac insufficiency, and classification of angina pectoris of the Canadian Cardiovascular Society (CCS). The Charlson comorbidity score was the best of the tested comorbidity classifications in patients 70 years old or older considered eligible for RP [6].

Quality of Life

Over the last decade, PCa is diagnosed at early stages and treatment is associated with more favorable survival outcomes. Therefore, the basis on which patients select primary therapy has shifted toward the associated complications and "quality of life" (QOL) considerations. The influence of age on QOL with specific attention to potency and continence after treatment of PCa is of interest when counselling patients regarding the expected outcomes following treatment. Many studies have focused on the impact of treatment for PCa on health-related quality of life (HRQOL) outcomes, but little has been published on QOL following RP in men with localized PCa over the age of 70.

The use of validated QOL questionnaires has been encouraged such as the 20-item University of California, Los Angeles Prostate Cancer Index (UCLA-PCI) questionnaire that evaluates urinary, bowel, and sexual domains and the 50-item Expanded Prostate Cancer Index Composite (EPIC) that assesses urinary irritative and incontinence subscales and a hormonal/vitality domain. We review the data available on QOL with specific attention on urinary continence and potency of elderly patients after open RP, LRP, and RALP.

Open Radical Prostatectomy

The use of an EPIC survey in PCa patients of all ages revealed that after treatment with RP (*n* = 234), EBRT (*n* = 135) or (125) I implant (*n* = 74), better urinary continence was noted in those who underwent radiation based therapies. Those who underwent RP had better bowel function and less urinary irritation. Sexual function was impaired with all of these treatment options but it has to be noted that highest scores of impairment of sexual function were seen in those who selected brachytherapy [14]. The general HRQOL is relatively good after RP, EBRT, or brachytherapy for clinically localized PCa, and it does not appear to be affected by treatment. Recently, the Scandinavian Prostate Cancer Group-4 (SPCG-4) randomized study evaluated the long-term QOL outcomes after RP and watchful waiting (WW) performed between 1989 and 1999 with a validated study-specific questionnaire. At that time, the surgeons in this study still prioritized non-nerve-sparing surgery. Men had a median follow-up of 12.2 years (range 7–17) and a median age of 77 years (range 61–88). There was no difference in proportion of patients who reported high self-assessed QOL (35 vs. 34 %, control: 45 %), anxiety (43 vs. 43 %, control: 33 %), and prevalence of erectile dysfunction (84 vs. 80 %, control: 46 %), between the RP and WW group, respectively. Prevalence of urinary leakage at least once daily was more common in the RP group (41 vs. 11 %, control: 3 %). In a longitudinal analysis of men in SPCG-4 who provided information at two follow-up points 9 years apart, 45 % of men of the RP and 60 % of the WW group reported an increase in physical symptoms; 61 and 64 % reported a reduction in QOL, respectively. In the WW group, side effects can be caused by tumor growth or treatment by medical or surgical castration or as a consequence of lower urinary tract symptoms [15].

A few studies that evaluated urinary incontinence and potency in preoperatively potent men of different ages treated with open retropubic RP stratified the functional outcomes by patient age. A limitation of these studies is that continence and potency were not assessed by a validated QOL questionnaire [16–18]. In addition, we review the studies more specifically evaluating QOL in the elderly who underwent RP. In three Japanese studies, patients completed the general and disease-specific HRQOL with the Short Form-36 (SF-36) and the UCLA-PCI questionnaire, respectively, before and 3, 6, 12, and 24 months after surgery [19–21]. The SF-36 covers eight domains, four physical and four emotional. The UCLA-PCI covers urinary, bowel, and sexual problems and the extent of bother from problems in that area.

First, we discuss urinary incontinence because patients rate urinary incontinence after treatment for localized PCa as one of the greatest QOL concerns. The proportion of men ≥70 years who recovered from urinary continence (pad-free) 18 months after retropubic RP in the study published by Kundu et al. [16] was 86 % (371 of 433). This is lower than the outcome in younger men (95 % for men age 40–49, 96 % for men 50–59, 93 % for men 60–69) [16]. Loeb et al. have reported similar rates after 18 months of follow-up [17]. A 2-year longitudinal study measured 112 Japanese men with localized PCa who underwent RP with the SF-36 and the UCLA-PCI questionnaire. Urinary function declined at 3 months and continued to recover at 6, 12, 18, and 24 months but did not return to baseline while urinary bother returned to baseline at 6 months after surgery. Overall, 50.5, 84.4, 87.6, 88.5, and 90.5 % of men were continent (pad-free) at 3, 6, 12, 18, and 24 months, respectively. The authors compared younger (≤65 years, $n=49$) with older men (>65 years, $n=63$). At baseline, there was no significant difference in urinary function between both groups. Both groups reported after RP significantly lower scores than baseline ($P<0.05$ for all time points). Younger men tended to show more rapid recovery in urinary function than older men within 12 months after RP (75.1 vs. 65.8 % and 89.5 vs. 78.6 % at 3 and 6 months). After 18 months, there were no significant differences in urinary function score among the two age groups, and urinary function score in both groups appeared similar by the end of the 2 years [19]. Another study that evaluated the QOL after RP with the SF-36 and UCLA-PCI in 205 elderly men (≥70 years) reported that by 2 years postoperatively, 57 and 81 % of patients had fully returned to baseline urinary function and bother, respectively. In total, 82 % of patients reported continence defined as requiring "no pad". Mean recovery time to baseline urinary function and bother was 8.3 and 4.7 months, respectively [20]. More recently, Namiki et al. [21] evaluated the changes of HRQOL with the SF-36 and UCLA-PCI during the first 2 years after RP ($n = 166$) or EBRT ($n = 118$) in elderly men aged ≥70 years treated for PCa. The RP group is associated with worse scores for urinary function and urinary bother postoperatively, compared with the EBRT group. Only 54 % of the elderly patients (≥70 years) returned to baseline urinary function 2 years after surgery [21] while this proportion was 88 % for younger men (<60 years) in a previous survey using the same methods.

Second, we discuss data on sexual function after RP for patients with localized PCa. Preserving potency is a major concern for those men potent before RP. Kundu et al. [16] revealed that potency rates following bilateral versus unilateral nerve-sparing retropubic RP were better for men <70 years (78 vs. 53 %, $P = 0.001$) compared with those in men aged ≥70 years (52 vs. 56 %, $P = 0.6$) [16]. Loeb et al. have reported similar rates after 18 months of follow-up [17]. Ayyathurai et al. reported the return of erectile function in 1,620 consecutive preoperatively potent men treated with nerve-sparing RP where feasible. Follow-up was minimum 6 months. Of 619 men who had a bilateral and of 178 who had a unilateral nerve-sparing retropubic RP, 72 and 53 %, respectively, were potent. When stratified by age group (≤49, 50–59, 60–69, and ≥70 years), potency rates were 86, 76, 58, and 37 %, respectively. In line with other large studies [16, 17], the authors concluded that potency rates after retropubic RP were better in younger men [18].

A 2-year longitudinal Japanese study ($n = 112$) reported that sexual function score had decreased 3 months after surgery and further continued to improve over the 2 years to a level lower than baseline. The postoperative sexual function scores of the younger men were better than those of the older. Younger men were more likely to have nerve-sparing surgery, which might have influenced the recovery [19]. Another longitudinal outcome study that evaluated the QOL after RP in 205 Japanese elderly men (≥70 years) reported by 2 years postoperatively, a recovery of sexual function and bother to baseline level of 25 and 83 %, respectively. The mean recovery time was 10.9 months for sexual function and 5.3 months for sexual bother [20]. A more recent Japanese longitudinal outcome study reported in elderly patients aged ≥70 years who underwent RP ($n = 166$) or EBRT ($n = 118$) low sexual function after treatment. The score for sexual function decreased over the 2 years in both treatment groups but to a greater extent in the RP group, leading to a comparable score with the EBRT group posttreatment. Similarly, scores of sexual bother were significantly lower at each postoperative time point for the RP group [21]. A limitation of these studies is the relative small sample size which may not be representative of the general elderly population.

Third, the study reported by Kundu et al. [16] showed that, excluding urinary incontinence and impotence, postoperative complications occurred in 9 % of patients (320 of 3,477). The occurrence of postoperative complications was associated with type of surgery (9 % for nerve-sparing surgery and 17 % for non-nerve-sparing surgery) ($P = 0.001$). Overall, the complication rate decreased significantly by era (16.9 % for pre-PSA era vs. 7.4 % for PSA era, $P < 0.0001$). Postoperative complications were associated with age at surgery (4 % for men age 40–49, 7 % of men age 50–59, 9 % for men 60–69, and 14 % for men 70 or older, $P < 0.0001$). The most common complications were anastomotic stricture (2.7 %), inguinal hernia (2.5 %), and thromboembolism (1.3 %) [16]. In the study by Loeb et al. [17], the surgical complication rate ranges from 5 to 7 %. Men aged 70 years or older had a higher rate of surgical complications (9–13 %) [17].

Fourth, the combined results of full urinary continence, sexual potency, and absence of biochemical recurrence represent the "trifecta," the most desired major outcomes following treatment of PCa. To our knowledge, no studies are available that report the trifecta rate after RP for the elderly. Important to note is that the trifecta rate does not consider individual patient preferences and the three outcomes assessed may not have equal importance for each patient.

Laparoscopic Radical Prostatectomy

Nerve-sparing laparoscopic radical prostatectomy (LRP) was an increasingly popular, minimally invasive treatment option that provided satisfactory first year HRQOL outcomes when assessed with the validated EPIC questionnaire.

First, Rogers et al. [22] assessed prospectively urinary continence and potency rates in 369 men who underwent LRP for PCa using the EPIC questionnaire and evaluated the influence of age on HRQOL. The patients were stratified into three age groups; group 1: <50 years ($n=40$), group 2: 50–59 years ($n=176$), and group 3: >60 years ($n=153$). Answers to the EPIC questionnaire were collected before surgery, and then 3, 6, and 12 months after LRP. Older men were less likely to achieve urinary continence (1 pad or less daily) 1 year after LRP (groups 1–3: 100, 91, and 81 %, respectively, $P < 0.01$). Analysis of the older group (>60 years) revealed that 38 of the 72 (53 %) patients were pad-free 1 year after LRP. The mean return to baseline urinary continence based on the EPIC urinary continence subscale at 1 year in group 1–3 was 80, 79, and 74 %, respectively ($P = 0.49$). The authors concluded that the return to baseline urinary continence is similar in all age groups by the end of the first postoperative year [22].

A retrospective study showed that extraperitoneal laparoscopic RP (eL-RP) is feasible and efficacious in elderly patients with localized PCa. Moreover, eL-RP is a minimally invasive procedure showing a lower morbidity and more rapid convalescence in patients >70 years compared with open surgery. Urinary continence was evaluated by the validated short form of the International Continence Society male questionnaire (ICSM). The continence rates in the elderly (>71 years) at 6 months were similar and independent of the surgical approach (67 % for LRP and 70 % for open RP) and lower compared to the continence rate after eL-RP for younger patients (<59 years, 91 %). The observed higher incontinence rate after eL-RP (33 %) in the elderly should be discussed preoperatively. The authors concluded that chronologic age is not a contraindication for offering elderly patients eL-RP for localized PCa. The patients in this group had a higher pathological stage and higher

Gleason score suggesting a biologically more aggressive form of PCa than in the younger patients. In men aged over 70 years, QOL is substantially greater after eL-RP than after open RP. Patients after eL-RP show a comparable recovery in the majority of the QOL subscales independently of their age. Elderly patients seem to be more sensitive to pain perception and need postoperatively significantly more analgesics than the younger men [23].

Second, Rogers et al. [22] revealed that younger men were more likely to be potent and engaging in intercourse with or without phosphodiesterase-5- inhibitors at 1 year after bilateral nerve-sparing LRP (<50 years, 70 %; 50–59 years, 67 %; and >60 years, 46 %, respectively, $P < 0.01$). The mean return to baseline sexual function based on the EPIC sexual function subscale at 1 year in group 1–3 was 68, 65, and 58 %, respectively ($P = 0.56$). The authors concluded that the return to baseline sexual function is similar in all age groups by the end of the first postoperative year. A limitation of the study was the relatively short follow-up of 3–12 months since continence and potency tend to continue to improve during the first 2 years after RP [22].

Poulakis et al. assessed potency by the International Index of Erectile Function (IIEF-5). At 6 months, 10 and 31 % of patients aged >71 and <59 years reached baseline potency, respectively after LRP. There was no significant difference between the percentage of patients >71 years reaching baseline potency at 6 months after LRP or open RP (10 and 11 %, respectively) [23].

Third, Poulakis et al. revealed that complication rates and perioperative morbidity did not differ significantly between older (≥71) and younger men (<59) who underwent LRP. Respiratory insufficiency and delirium were the most common complications in this study and no perioperative deaths occurred. This is probably because elderly patients were highly selected healthy men [23]. It is well known that laparoscopic surgery in the elderly is associated with lower morbidity and shorter convalescence compared with open surgery.

Finally, to our knowledge, there is no study that reports the trifecta rate after LRP in the elderly population.

Robotic-Assisted Laparoscopic Prostatectomy

Robotic-assisted laparoscopic prostatectomy (RALP) is being used increasingly in the surgical management of clinically localized PCa because it is associated with fast recovery, less blood loss, and surgical outcomes comparable to open RP. A recent comparative study of QOL outcomes between LRP and RALP showed statistically similar postoperative urinary function outcomes in both groups and an earlier return of sexual function for RALP patients when compared with LRP patients after bilateral nerve-sparing surgery. A few studies assessed the influence of age on functional outcomes after RALP.

First, Mendiola et al. [24] evaluated in a prospective study age-stratified functional outcomes in 300 patients after RALP for localized PCa. The three age groups included 21, 129, and 150 patients (aged <50, 50–9, and >60 years old, respectively). The authors showed that younger men (<60 years) will likely have an earlier return of continence compared to older men (>60 years) after RALP ($P=0.02$). HRQOL issues were assessed both subjectively by actual patient interview and objectively using the validated SF-36 and UCLA-PCI preoperatively and at 1, 3, 6, and 12 months postoperatively. Using subjective assessment during patient interviews and the strict continence criteria of no pads used per day, continence rates at 3 months after surgery were 67, 55, and 43 % ($P=0.06$) for the three age groups. However, continence results were similar among all age groups after 12 months of follow-up (93, 90, and 92 %, $P=0.80$). These results contradict previously published data from Kundu et al. [16] who observed better continence rates in younger patients after retropubic RP. The improved continence rate in the elderly could be attributed to a possible better apical dissection provided with RALP [24]. Greco et al. [25] assessed continence, return to activity, recovery time, postoperative hospital admission, and complications after RALP in 23 men aged ≥70 years and 150 men aged <70 years. The outcomes in elderly men were comparable to those in younger men, except for a higher pathological Gleason grade, a transient delay in return of full continence, and taking longer to return to driving after surgery. The continence rate, defined as the use of one pad or less per day, was significantly lower in men aged ≥70 years at 6 months after RALP (60 vs. 79 %, $P=0.04$) but was equivalent to those in younger men (<70 years) at 12 months after RALP (83 vs. 89.2 %, $P=0.54$). It should be noted that the difference in continence rate at 6 months was no longer statistically significant (65 vs. 79 %, $P=0.17$) when patients with a previous transurethral resection of the prostate (TURP) were excluded. Only carefully selected elderly men with limited comorbidities were offered RALP, and the elderly patients did not reflect the average elderly patient [25]. Shikanov et al. [26] revealed that there is an acceptable probability of achieving continence after robotic RP in selected elderly patients. Of the patients, 25 % (359) were older than 65 years and 5 % (77) were 70 years old or older. Continence (pad-free) at baseline and 1 year after surgery were evaluated by the UCLA-PCI questionnaire. Age was treated as a continuous variable. Predicted probabilities (95 % CI) of continence at age 65, 70, and 75 years were 0.66 (0.63, 0.69), 0.63 (0.57, 0.68), and 0.59 (0.52, 0.66), respectively, 1 year after robotic RP. On multivariate analysis, age was independently associated with being pad-free (OR 0.97, $P=0.002$). Also in this study, the elderly patients were highly selected healthy patients and results may not be applicable on the average elderly patient of corresponding age [26].

Second, younger men will likely have an earlier return of potency compared to older men (>60 years, $n=150$) and will continue to report superior potency outcomes compared to older men 1 year after surgery. The potency rate after bilateral and unilateral nerve-sparing surgery for men >60 years were 72 and 36 %, respectively. The subjective potency rates for each age group (<50, 50–59, and >60 years old) were 87, 76, and 62 %, respectively, at 12 months [24]. Greco et al. [25] did not report potency results. Shikanov et al. [26] revealed that there is an acceptable probability of achieving potency after robotic RP in selected elderly patients. Potency (erection sufficient for intercourse) at baseline and 1 year after surgery were evaluated by the UCLA-PCI questionnaire. The corresponding probabilities of postoperative 1-year potency after bilateral nerve-sparing surgery were 0.66 (0.62, 0.71), 0.56 (0.49, 0.64), and 0.46 (0.36, 0.56). Age (OR 0.92, $P < 0.0001$) was independently associated with achieving potency [26].

Third, Greco et al. [25] found no significant differences in surgical complications between the younger (<70 years) and older men (≥70 years). Surgical complications included urine leaks (15 vs. 9 %), bladder neck contractures (3.3 vs. 0 %), migrated intravesical clips (3.9 vs. 0 %), deep venous thrombosis (1.7 vs. 0 %), and pulmonary embolism (1.1 vs. 4 %) [25].

Finally, no specific studies that reported trifecta rates after RALP in the elderly were identified.

Discussion

The survival rates after RP in the elderly in the reviewed studies are encouraging (OS: 65–83 %, CSS: 94–96 %, 10-year biochemical PFS: 57–74 %) (Table 8.1). Several authors agree that careful selection must be made before RP is performed in the elderly. Appropriately selected elderly patients with a life expectancy of at least 10 years and no or limited morbidities are considered to be possible candidates for RP.

However, the studies in this chapter have several limitations. Several studies have small sample sizes. There are no universally accepted guidelines for quantifying and reporting urinary incontinence and erectile dysfunction after RP. Although different definitions have been used, urinary incontinence can be quantified and qualified (pads or no pads, leakage or not). Assessment of erectile dysfunction lacks standardization. Partial recovery of potency, adequate rigidity, ability for intercourse, and overall sexual satisfaction are different factors. Age at surgery, preoperative potency, and the use of medication or devices to treat erectile dysfunction should all be reported and associated with reported rates of potency. Next to the UCLA-PCI and EPIC, several other QOL tools have been used such as the International Index of Erectile function (IIEF-5), the International Continence Society male short-form questionnaire (ICS male SF), the Sexual Health Inventory for Men (SHIM), International Consultation on Incontinence Questionnaire (ICIQ), etc. Direct comparison of the QOL studies is frequently not possible because of different definitions of functional outcomes, multiple QOL assessment instruments, different age cut-off points, and variable methods of data analysis.

Using a strict criterion of 0 pads per day, continence rates of 71 % after open RP for patients ≥70 years, using UCLA-PCI [20], 53 % after LRP for patients >60 years, using EPIC [22] and 92 % after RALP for patients >60 years, and using UCLA-PCI [24] were reported in the elderly at 12 months post-surgery. Greco et al. defined urinary continence as requiring one pad or less per day. They found a urinary continence rate of 83 % at 12 months after RALP for patients ≥70 years [25]. Potency rates are better in younger men and after bilateral nerve-sparing surgery. In the elderly, potency rates after bilateral nerve-sparing surgery were reported of 52 and 38 % after open RP for patients ≥70 years using no validated QOL tools[16, 18], 46 % 1 year after LRP for patients >60 years using EPIC [22], and 72 % 1 year after RALP for patients >60 years using UCLA-PCI [24]. Two studies reported that men aged 70 years or older had a higher rate of surgical complications after open RP than younger men (14 vs. 9 % and 9–13 vs. 5–7 %) [16, 17]. The two studies reporting complications after LRP or RALP in the elderly showed no significant differences in surgical complications between younger and older men [23, 25]. To our knowledge, there are no studies describing the "trifecta" rate after RP, LRP, or RALP in the elderly population.

Conclusions

Several investigators have considered RP a viable option for elderly patients based on data of survival outcomes. The rates of urinary continence and potency after RP decrease with advancing age but can be considered more or less acceptable in selected elderly with no or limited morbidities. Healthy elderly patients with localized PCa should not be limited in their treatment options solely on the basis of advanced chronologic age. With advances in technology and techniques, QOL outcomes after RP for men with localized PCa will continue to improve and might further reduce morbidity. Therefore, the influence of advanced age on HRQOL after open RP, LRP, and RALP should be further examined in order to make better treatment decisions in the elderly with localized PCa. Treatment selection is not based only on age, life expectancy, tumor-related prognostic factors, comorbidity, and QOL issues but also on preferences of the individual patient and urologist and the treatment availability. The decision to choose for RP or surveillance is an option that needs to be discussed in detail with the patient.

References

1. Thompson RH, Slezak JM, Webster WS, Lieber MM. Radical prostatectomy for octogenarians: how old is too old? Urology. 2006;68(5):1042–5.
2. Richstone L, Bianco FJ, Shah HH, et al. Radical prostatectomy in men aged>or=70 years: effect of age on upgrading, upstaging, and the accuracy of a preoperative nomogram. BJU Int. 2008;101(5):541–6.
3. Barry MJ, Albertsen PC, Bagshaw MA, et al. Outcomes for men with clinically nonmetastatic prostate carcinoma managed with radical prostatectomy, external beam radiotherapy, or expectant management: a retrospective analysis. Cancer. 2001;91(12):2302–14.
4. Pierorazio PM, Humphreys E, Walsh PC, Partin AW, Han M. Radical prostatectomy in older men: survival outcomes in septuagenarians and octogenarians. BJU Int. 2010;106(6):791–5.
5. Pfitzenmaier J, Pahernik S, Buse S, Haferkamp A, Djakovic N, Hohenfellner M. Survival in prostate cancer patients>or=70 years after radical prostatectomy and comparison to younger patients. World J Urol. 2009;27(5):637–42.

6. Froehner M, Koch R, Litz RJ, Hakenberg OW, Oehlschlaeger S, Wirth MP. Survival analysis in men undergoing radical prostatectomy at an age of 70 years or older. Urol Oncol. 2010;28(6):628–34.
7. Alibhai SM, Naglie G, Nam R, Trachtenberg J, Krahn MD. Do older men benefit from curative therapy of localized prostate cancer? J Clin Oncol. 2003;21(17):3318–27.
8. Tewari A, Raman JD, Chang P, Rao S, Divine G, Menon M. Long-term survival probability in men with clinically localized prostate cancer treated either conservatively or with definitive treatment (radiotherapy or radical prostatectomy). Urology. 2006;68(6):1268–74.
9. Siddiqui SA, Sengupta S, Slezak JM, et al. Impact of patient age at treatment on outcome following radical retropubic prostatectomy for prostate cancer. J Urol. 2006;175(3 Pt 1): 952–7.
10. Jeldres C, Suardi N, Walz J, et al. Poor overall survival in septa- and octogenarian patients after radical prostatectomy and radiotherapy for prostate cancer: a population-based study of 6183 men. Eur Urol. 2008;54(1):107–16.
11. Malaeb BS, Rashid HH, Lotan Y, et al. Prostate cancer disease-free survival after radical retropubic prostatectomy in patients older than 70 years compared to younger cohorts. Urol Oncol. 2007;25(4):291–7.
12. Magheli A, Rais-Bahrami S, Humphreys EB, Peck HJ, Trock BJ, Gonzalgo ML. Impact of patient age on biochemical recurrence rates following radical prostatectomy. J Urol. 2007;178(5):1933–7.
13. Barlow LJ, Badalato GM, Bashir T, Benson MC, McKiernan JM. The relationship between age at time of surgery and risk of biochemical failure after radical prostatectomy. BJU Int. 2010;105(12):1646–9.
14. Frank SJ, Pisters LL, Davis J, Lee AK, Bassett R, Kuban DA. An assessment of quality of life following radical prostatectomy, high dose external beam radiation therapy and brachytherapy iodine implantation as monotherapies for localized prostate cancer. J Urol. 2007;177(6):2151–6.
15. Johansson E, Steineck G, Holmberg L, et al. Long-term quality-of-life outcomes after radical prostatectomy or watchful waiting: the Scandinavian Prostate Cancer Group-4 randomised trial. Lancet Oncol. 2011;12(9):891–9.
16. Kundu SD, Roehl KA, Eggener SE, Antenor JA, Han M, Catalona WJ. Potency, continence and complications in 3,477 consecutive radical retropubic prostatectomies. J Urol. 2004;172(6 Pt 1):2227–31.
17. Loeb S, Roehl KA, Helfand BT, Catalona WJ. Complications of open radical retropubic prostatectomy in potential candidates for active monitoring. Urology. 2008;72(4):887–91.
18. Ayyathurai R, Manoharan M, Nieder AM, Kava B, Soloway MS. Factors affecting erectile function after radical retropubic prostatectomy: results from 1620 consecutive patients. BJU Int. 2008;101(7):833–6.
19. Namiki S, Saito S, Satoh M, et al. Quality of life after radical prostatectomy in Japanese men: 2 year longitudinal study. Jpn J Clin Oncol. 2005;35(9):551–8.
20. Namiki S, Ishidoya S, Tochigi T, Ito A, Arai Y. Quality of life after radical prostatectomy in elderly men. Int J Urol. 2009;16(10):813–9.
21. Namiki S, Ishidoya S, Kawamura S, Tochigi T, Arai Y. Quality of life among elderly men treated for prostate cancer with either radical prostatectomy or external beam radiation therapy. J Cancer Res Clin Oncol. 2010;136(3):379–86.
22. Rogers CG, Su LM, Link RE, Sullivan W, Wagner A, Pavlovich CP. Age stratified functional outcomes after laparoscopic radical prostatectomy. J Urol. 2006;176(6 Pt 1):2448–52.
23. Poulakis V, Witzsch U, de Vries R, Dillenburg W, Becht E. Laparoscopic radical prostatectomy in men older than 70 years of age with localized prostate cancer: comparison of morbidity, reconvalescence, and short-term clinical outcomes between younger and older men. Eur Urol. 2007;51(5):1341–8.
24. Mendiola FP, Zorn KC, Mikhail AA, et al. Urinary and sexual function outcomes among different age groups after robot-assisted laparoscopic prostatectomy. J Endourol. 2008;22(3): 519–24.

25. Greco KA, Meeks JJ, Wu S, Nadler RB. Robot-assisted radical prostatectomy in men aged > or =70 years. BJU Int. 2009;104(10):1492–5.
26. Shikanov S, Desai V, Razmaria A, Zagaja GP, Shalhav AL. Robotic radical prostatectomy for elderly patients: probability of achieving continence and potency 1 year after surgery. J Urol. 2010;183(5):1803–7.

Chapter 9
Radiotherapy in Elderly Prostate Cancer Patients

Pascal Pommier

Abstract Radiotherapy in elderly cancer patient is not a question of "age," but draws the question in that population of the cost/benefit ratio estimation in terms of clinical benefit (overall survival, event-free survival, and quality of life) versus unnecessary treatment-related toxicities and societal costs. In that setting, decision making has to take into account, on the one hand, the aggressiveness of the prostate cancer (i.e., using the D'Amico classification) and, on the other hand, the life expectancy of each individual patient mainly related to the severity of his associated comorbid conditions. Some general recommendations have been proposed by the International Society of Geriatric Oncology and are applicable for radiotherapy decision in elderly patient.

Keywords Radiotherapy • Prostate cancer • D'Amico classification • Elderly patients • Cancer screening • Event-free survival

Introduction

The updated results (median follow-up of 11 years) of the European Randomized Study of Screening for Prostate Cancer demonstrated in a cohort of 162,388 men 55–69 years of age a 21 % relative reduction in the risk of death from prostate cancer (29 % after adjustment for noncompliance) and an absolute reduction in mortality (0.10 deaths per 1,000 person-years) in the screening group [1]. However, several publications have demonstrated that elderly prostate cancer patients are diagnosed with a more advanced disease compared to younger patients that may compromise their life expectancy and quality of life.

P. Pommier, M.D., Ph.D.
Department of Radiation Oncology, Centre Léon Bérard,
Lyon, France
e-mail: pascal.pommier@lyon.unicancer.fr

J.-P. Droz, R.A. Audisio (eds.), *Management of Urological Cancers in Older People*, 121
Management of Cancer in Older People,
DOI 10.1007/978-0-85729-999-4_9, © Springer-Verlag London 2013

More Aggressive Cancer Disease at Diagnosis in Elderly Patients?

Results from the prospective American database "Surveillance, Epidemiology, and End Results" (SEER) revealed that the frequency of metastases at presentation were significantly superior in the oldest population (3, 5, 8, 13, and 17 %, respectively, in patients aged <75, 75–79, 80–84, 85–89, and ≥90 years) [2]. This more advanced stage at the diagnosis is probably one of the major factors explaining in that study a higher incidence of death from PC in the oldest population (3–4, 7, 13, 20, and 30 %, respectively, in patients aged <75, 75–79, 80–84, 85–89, and ≥90 years).

Also based on the SEER data, but selecting 19,639 men more than 66 years old with a localized cancer at the diagnostic who did not receive any active therapy (surgery or radiation within 180 days of diagnosis), Albertsen et al. reported the comparative results for overall survival and cause-specific survival for men below or above 75 years, taking into account the cancer prognostic factors (T1 vs. T2 and for each Gleason score (GS) 5–7 or 8–10) and comorbidities (Charlson comorbidity index 0 vs. 1 vs. ≥2) [3]. In the most favorable cancer prognostic group (T1c, GS 5–7) and in patients with no or few comorbidities (Charlson comorbidity index 0 or 1), 5 and 10 years cause-specific mortality rates were higher in the oldest patients.

A similar observation has been published by Arvold et al. in a large prospective study cohort of low-risk (5,760 patients) and intermediate-risk prostate cancer (3,079 patients) treated either with prostatectomy or brachytherapy [4]. Competing risks multivariable regression was performed to assess the risk of prostate cancer specific mortality after radical prostatectomy or brachytherapy, adjusting for age, year of treatment, cardiovascular comorbidity, and known prostate cancer prognostic factors. The only factor associated with an increased risk of prostate cancer specific mortality ($p=0.03$) was increasing age at treatment in intermediate risk men.

Are Elderly Patients Undertreated?

In a very large cohort issued from the SEER cohort, including 68,797 men aged 65–80 years with cT1-T2 PCa treated with radiotherapy (68 %) or observation (32 %) between the years 1992 and 2005, Abdollah et al. demonstrated that oldest patients (age 75–80 years) were less likely to receive radiotherapy than younger ones (respectively 34.5 % vs. 44.2 %, $p<0.001$) [5]. In addition, radiotherapy patients also had lower comorbidity but harbored higher clinical stage (cT2c: 11.7 % vs. 6.8 %) and higher tumor grade (Gleason score 8–10: 26.7 % vs. 14.8 %, $p<0.001$).

A similar observation has been published by Konety et al. using the multi-institutional CaPSURE database [6]. On multivariate analysis adjusted for sociodemographic factors, diagnostic risk category and the number of comorbidities at diagnosis patients 75 years or older were less likely to be treated with primary therapy than with watchful waiting regardless of the risk category or comorbidity level.

Radiotherapy in Elderly Patients

Competing-Risks Mortality: Does Associated Comorbidities Justify Observation Versus Curative Therapy in Elderly Populations?

One of the main reasons to justify the trend to propose an observation conversely to an active therapy with a curative intent (radiotherapy) in elderly patients is the competing-risks mortality due to more frequently associated comorbidities in these patients. However, this attitude is not fully supported by the literature data.

Indeed, the series reported by Albersten, the 5 and 10 years overall survival for patients with a comorbidity index ≥2 with GS 5–7 was similar in patients aged >75 or 66–74 years old [3].

Fiorica et al. analyzed the predictive factors for overall survival in a cohort of 107 consecutive patients aged ≥75 (median age 79.1 years) receiving radiotherapy alone or associated with a 6-month hormonal therapy [7]. Variables considered were age, stage, comorbidities according to the adult comorbidity evaluation index (ACE-27), and performance status (PS). 23.4 % of patients had no comorbidities, while 46.7 % had mild, 23.4 % moderate, and 6.5 % severe comorbidities, respectively. With a 37.8-month follow-up, a high rate of 5 years overall survival rate was observed (78 %) however significantly higher for patients with no or mild comorbidities ($p < 0.0001$) and a good PS ($p = 0.009$).

The most insightful report has been produced by Abdollah et al. assessing competing-risks mortality after radiotherapy versus observation for localized prostate cancer (PCa), based on the SEER database (see above) [5]. A propensity-score matching was applied to balance the characteristics of the two groups [i.e., age at diagnostic, baseline comorbidity status using the Charlson comorbidity index (CCI) and tumor grade and stage] resulting in a matched cohort of 41,972 patients (36 and 41 % aged respectively 70–74 and 75–80 years). The primary endpoint was cause-specific mortality (CSM), considered more adequate than overall mortality as a great majority of PCa patients will die to causes other than cancer due to the often long natural history of this cancer when localized at the diagnosis. Looking to the whole population, the benefit of radiotherapy versus observation only was significant in patients in the high-risk group cancers (T2C or Gleason Score ≥ 8) (8.8 % vs. 14.4 %; $p < 0.001$), but not in the low to intermediate group cancers. Unfortunately, these two prognostic groups have not been individualized to assess the benefit of radiotherapy especially in the intermediate group. Looking to the impact of comorbidities, the amount of benefit observed with radiotherapy versus observation was similar and significant whatever the CCI score was (respectively 5.7 % vs. 6.5 %, 4.6 % vs. 6.0 %, and 4.2 % vs. 5.0 % for patients with a CCI of 0, 1, and 2). Interestingly, the most elderly patients (75–80 years) were the only ones in multivariate analysis to statistically beneficiate of the CSM reduction due to radiotherapy (5.6 % vs. 7.3 %, $p < 0.001$).

The conclusion of the authors was that "baseline comorbidity and patients age are not as important as PCa characteristics in deciding whether radiotherapy would be beneficial to a patient or not. Indeed, even older patients (ages 75–80) seem to have some benefit when they are treated with radiotherapy instead of observation" [5].

Predictors of prostate cancer-specific mortality (PCSM) in elderly men with intermediate-risk prostate cancer treated with brachytherapy with or without external beam radiation therapy have been assessed by Nanda et al. in a large cohort of 1,978 men of median age 71 (interquartile range, 66–75) years [8]. A multivariable competing risks regression including prevalent cardiovascular disease (CVD), age, year of brachytherapy, PSA level, and tumor category was applied.

In accordance with Abdollah et al. report, in that population, a higher PSA level was significantly associated with an increased risk of PCSM ($p=0.02$). However, conversely to the Abdollah et al. general conclusion, the presence of CVD was significantly associated with a decreased risk of PCSM ($p=0.05$), and in the setting of CVD pretreatment, PSA level was not a significant predictor of PCSM ($p=0.27$).

Life Expectancy to Select "Elderly" Patients Who May Benefit from Radiotherapy?

Life expectancy (LE) beyond 10 years has been adopted by several professional associations' guidelines [9, 10] to offer or not definitive therapy to patients with localized prostate cancer as to avoid unnecessary treatment, treatment-related acute and late toxicity, and societal costs. The accuracy of life tables to predict overall survival has been assessed by Walz et al. in a series of 3,176 patients treated with radiotherapy and who had no clinical evidence of disease relapse [11]. In that series, life table was a statistically significant predictor of overall mortality but with a limited ability to predict life expectancy in patients treated with radiotherapy for prostate. It should therefore be associated with other variables such as age and Charlson comorbidity index.

Is Radiotherapy Effective for Elderly Prostate Cancer Patients Compared to Younger Ones?

Regarding the results of the very large cohort of localized prostate cancer patients issued from the SEER published by Abdollah et al., the effectiveness of external beam radiotherapy (compared to observation), in terms of CSS, has been demonstrated in elderly patients and especially in that series in the oldest ones [5].

Similar results have been published by Fiorica et al. and Geinitz et al. [7, 12]. In the Fiorica series including 107 consecutive patients aged ≥75, no difference was detected for different ages [7]. Geinitz et al. reported their experience using a 3D conformal radiotherapy (median dose 70 Gy) in 80 patients aged >75 years compared to 221 younger patients treated during the same period (no significant differences between patients' characteristics). In that nonrandomized series, older patients had even a biological disease-free survival at 4 years significantly better than younger patients (76 % vs. 61 %, *p*: 0.042) [12].

The efficacy of brachytherapy (exclusive or associated with external beam and/or hormonal therapy) has been assessed by Merrick et al. in 145 men aged more than 75 years (median 76 years) [13]. With a 5.8-year median follow-up, 9-year cause-specific survival, biochemical progression-free survival, and overall survival rates for the entire cohort were 99.3, 97.1, and 64.5 %, respectively. Overall survival and non-cancer deaths were best predicted by tobacco status, and most of the deaths were due to cardiovascular diseases (22 patients) or second malignancies (9 patients).

Is Radiotherapy More Toxic in Elderly Prostate Cancer Patients Compared to Younger Ones?

Based on their nonrandomized large comparative study, Geinitz et al. did not observe any significant differences in acute or late side effects between age groups [12].

In the series reported by Fiorica et al., patients (aged ≥ 75), no difference in acute or late toxicities was detected for different ages [7]. However, patients with higher comorbidities (based on ACE-27 classes) experienced higher acute and late toxicity rate for diarrhea and marginally for urinary toxicity.

The tolerance of radiotherapy in elderly patients (>75 years) has also been assessed in a larger cohort by Liu et al. including 322 elderly patients with at least 24-month follow-up (EBRT in 289 and brachytherapy in 33) compared with a control group of 1,353 patients aged less than 75 years (EBRT in 941 and brachytherapy in 412) [14]. There were no significant differences between the two age groups for EBRT, but a higher rate of late grade 3 gastrointestinal toxicity was reported in elderly patients compared to the younger ones in the brachytherapy series (3 % vs. 0.2 %; *p* = 0.02). However, age group was not a significant predictor for any toxicity when other factors were controlled for.

Combined Hormonal and Radiation Therapy in Elderly Patients

Short-term (at least 6 months) or long term (2–3 years) hormonal therapy associated to radiotherapy has proven a higher efficacy compared to radiotherapy alone (using standard-dose level and fractionation) in prostate cancers classified in the intermediate- and high-risk groups according to D'Amico classification [15–18].

Nguyen et al. performed a subgroup analysis in a phase III trial to assess the potential additional benefit of 6 months of androgen suppression therapy (AST) in addition to 70 Gy external beam radiotherapy (RT) in oldest men (defined as above the median age) [19]. In patients with mild or no comorbidity, combination of RT + AST was associated with a significantly lower risk of death on multivariable analysis, but conversely, RT + AST was associated with a higher risk of death among men with moderate or severe comorbidity.

The same medical team also demonstrated that hormonal therapy may be detrimental in patients with history of coronary disease, congestive heart failure, or myocardial infarction [20].

New Technologies in Radiotherapy: Better Cost/Benefit for Elderly Patients?

Intensity-Modulated Radiotherapy (IMRT)

IMRT may be considered as an advanced radiotherapy technique that permits to obtain a higher conformal target volume irradiation compared with the now "standard" 3D conformal radiotherapy (3D-CRT). The difference is mainly marked for concave target volume and is, therefore, well adapted in prostate cancer radiotherapy with the rectal wall that is included in the posterior concave shape of the prostate.

This theoretical benefit on rectal toxicity has been assessed and demonstrated by Bekelman et al. specifically in older men (more than 65 years; 45 % more than 75) in the SEER observational cohort, including nonmetastatic prostate cancer treated either with IMRT (5,845) or 3D-CRT (6,753) [21].

Hypofractionation

Hypofractionation has recently been showed in a randomized trial to be an alternative to conventional high-dose fractionation in high-risk cancer patients with similar acute and late toxicity rates and a significantly 3-year freedom from biochemical failure (FFBF) rates were 87 and 79 % in favor of the hypofractionation arm [22, 23]. That trial mainly enrolled elderly patients with a median age of 75 years (range 54–82), and this fractionation may be applied to this population. However, no specific analysis based on age has been reported.

Recommendations

The International Society of Geriatric Oncology (SIOG) has published in 2010 recommendations that should provide the highest standard of care for older men with localized and advanced prostate cancer based on a systematic bibliographic search

Table 9.1 Expert panel recommendations for localized prostate cancer (SIOG)

Group		
1	"Fit" or "healthy" older men	Should receive the same standard treatment as younger patients. More specifically, they should receive curative therapy in cases of high-risk localized prostate cancer
2	"Vulnerable" (i.e., reversible impairment)	Should receive standard treatment after resolution of any geriatric problems through geriatric interventions
3	"Frail" (i.e., irreversible impairment)	Should receive an adapted treatment
4	"Too sick" with "terminal illness"	Should receive only symptomatic palliative treatment

[24]. The consensus was that "older men with prostate cancer should be managed according to their individual health status, which is mainly driven by the severity of associated comorbid conditions, and not according to chronological age."

The minimal screening for decision making should include an evaluation of comorbidities, dependence status and nutritional status, and a geriatric intervention in case of "vulnerability" or "fragility" as to classify patients into four prognostic groups regarding life expectancy, regardless of the "real" age of the patient.

The recommendation of the SIOG for active therapy based on this classification is reported in Table 9.1.

In addition, several additional recommendations have been proposed for decision making taking into account cancer-related prognostics using the D'Amico classification: "High risk group (D'Amico) with life with a chance of surviving for >10 years are likely to benefit from curative treatment ; Older men in the 'low-risk' and possibly in the 'intermediate-risk' groups [../..] are likely to benefit from an active surveillance approach." Regarding hormonal therapy in localized prostate cancer, "the benefits and harms of ADT [../..] should be carefully balanced in older men. Attention is drawn to an increased risk of diabetes, cardiovascular complications, and osteoporosis and bone fractures."

References

1. Schröder FH, Hugosson J, Roobol MJ, Tammela TL, Ciatto S, Nelen V, Kwiatkowski M, Lujan M, Lilja H, Zappa M, Denis LJ, Recker F, Páez A, Määttänen L, Bangma CH, Aus G, Carlsson S, Villers A, Rebillard X, van der Kwast T, Kujala PM, Blijenberg BG, Stenman UH, Huber A, Taari K, Hakama M, Moss SM, de Koning HJ, Auvinen A, ERSPC Investigators. Prostate-cancer mortality at 11 years of follow-up. N Engl J Med. 2012;366(11):981–90.
2. Scosyrev E, Messing EM, Mohile S, Golijanin D, Wu G. Prostate cancer in the elderly: frequency of advanced disease at presentation and disease-specific mortality. Cancer. 2012;118(12):3062–70.
3. Albertsen PC, Moore DF, Shih W, Lin Y, Li H, Lu-Yao GL. Impact of comorbidity on survival among men with localized prostate cancer. J Clin Oncol. 2011;29(10):1335–41.

4. Arvold ND, Chen MH, Moul JW, Moran BJ, Dosoretz DE, Bañez LL, Katin MJ, Braccioforte MH, D'Amico AV. Risk of death from prostate cancer after radical prostatectomy or brachytherapy in men with low or intermediate risk disease. J Urol. 2011;186(1):91–6.

5. Abdollah F, Sun M, Schmitges J, Thuret R, Tian Z, Shariat SF, Briganti A, Jeldres C, Perrotte P, Montorsi F, Karakiewicz PI. Competing-risks mortality after radiotherapy vs. observation for localized prostate cancer: a population-based study. Int J Radiat Oncol Biol Phys. 2012;84(1): 95–103.

6. Konety BR, Cowan JE, Carroll PR, CaPSURE Investigators. Patterns of primary and secondary therapy for prostate cancer in elderly men: analysis of data from CaPSURE. J Urol. 2008;179(5):1797–803.

7. Fiorica F, Berretta M, Colosimo C, Berretta S, Ristagno M, Palmucci T, Palmucci S, Lleshi A, Ursino S, Fisichella R, Spartà D, Stefanelli A, Cappellani A, Tirelli U, Cartei F. Safety and efficacy of radiotherapy treatment in elderly patients with localized prostate cancer: a retrospective analysis. Arch Gerontol Geriatr. 2010;51(3):277–82.

8. Nanda A, Chen MH, Moran BJ, Braccioforte MH, Dosoretz D, Salenius S, Katin M, Ross R, D'Amico AV. Predictors of prostate cancer-specific mortality in elderly men with intermediate-risk prostate cancer treated with brachytherapy with or without external beam radiation therapy. Int J Radiat Oncol Biol Phys. 2010;77(1):147–52.

9. Heidenreich A, Aus G, Bolla M, Joniau S, Matveev VB, Schmid HP, Zattoni F, European Association of Urology. EAU guidelines on prostate cancer. Eur Urol. 2008;53(1):68–80.

10. Thompson I, Thrasher JB, Aus G, Burnett AL, Canby-Hagino ED, Cookson MS, D'Amico AV, Dmochowski RR, Eton DT, Forman JD, Goldenberg SL, Hernandez J, Higano CS, Kraus SR, Moul JW, Tangen CM, AUA Prostate Cancer Clinical Guideline Update Panel. Guideline for the management of clinically localized prostate cancer: 2007 update. J Urol. 2007;177(6):2106–31.

11. Walz J, Gallina A, Perrotte P, Jeldres C, Trinh QD, Hutterer GC, Traumann M, Ramirez A, Shariat SF, McCormack M, Perreault JP, Bénard F, Valiquette L, Saad F, Karakiewicz PI. Clinicians are poor raters of life-expectancy before radical prostatectomy or definitive radiotherapy for localized prostate cancer. BJU Int. 2007;100(6):1254–8.

12. Geinitz H, Zimmermann FB, Thamm R, Schumertl A, Busch R, Molls M. 3D conformal radiation therapy for prostate cancer in elderly patients. Radiother Oncol. 2005;76(1):27–34.

13. Merrick GS, Wallner KE, Galbreath RW, Butler WM, Brammer SG, Allen ZA, Adamovich E. Prostate brachytherapy in men>or =75 years of age. Int J Radiat Oncol Biol Phys. 2008;72(2):415–20.

14. Liu M, Pickles T, Keyes M, Moravan V, Agranovich A, Morris J. Tolerance of elderly patients (>75 years) to prostate external beam radiotherapy or brachytherapy. Eur J Cancer. 2005;3:S233–4.

15. D'Amico AV, Whittington R, Malkowicz SB, Schultz D, Blank K, Broderick GA, Tomaszewski JE, Renshaw AA, Kaplan I, Beard CJ, Wein A. Biochemical outcome after radical prostatectomy, external beam radiation therapy, or interstitial radiation therapy for clinically localized prostate cancer. JAMA. 1998;280(11):969–74.

16. Bolla M, Collette L, Blank L, Warde P, Dubois JB, Mirimanoff RO, Storme G, Bernier J, Kuten A, Sternberg C, Mattelaer J, Lopez Torecilla J, Pfeffer JR, Lino Cutajar C, Zurlo A, Pierart M. Long-term results with immediate androgen suppression and external irradiation in patients with locally advanced prostate cancer (an EORTC study): a phase III randomised trial. Lancet. 2002;360(9327):103–6.

17. D'Amico AV, Chen MH, Renshaw AA, Loffredo M, Kantoff PW. Androgen suppression and radiation vs radiation alone for prostate cancer: a randomized trial. JAMA. 2008;299(3): 289–95.

18. D'Amico AV, Chen MH, Crook J, Armstrong JG, Malone S, Steigler A, Dunne M, Kantoff PW, Denham JW. Duration of short-course androgen suppression therapy and the risk of death as a result of prostate cancer. J Clin Oncol. 2011;29(35):4682–7.

19. Nguyen PL, Chen MH, Renshaw AA, Loffredo M, Kantoff PW, D'Amico AV. Survival following radiation and androgen suppression therapy for prostate cancer in healthy older men: implications for screening recommendations. Int J Radiat Oncol Biol Phys. 2010;76(2):337–41.

20. Nguyen PL, Chen MH, Beckman JA, Beard CJ, Martin NE, Choueiri TK, Hu JC, Hoffman KE, Dosoretz DE, Moran BJ, Salenius SA, Braccioforte MH, Kantoff PW, D'Amico AV, Ennis RD. Influence of androgen deprivation therapy on all-cause mortality in men with high-risk prostate cancer and a history of congestive heart failure or myocardial infarction. Int J Radiat Oncol Biol Phys. 2012;82(4):1411–6.
21. Bekelman JE, Mitra N, Efstathiou J, Liao K, Sunderland R, Yeboa DN, Armstrong K. Outcomes after intensity-modulated versus conformal radiotherapy in older men with non metastatic prostate cancer. Int J Radiat Oncol Biol Phys. 2011;81(4):325–34.
22. Arcangeli G, Fowler J, Gomellini S, Arcangeli S, Saracino B, Petrongari MG, Benassi M, Strigari L. Acute and late toxicity in a randomized trial of conventional versus hypofractionated three-dimensional conformal radiotherapy for prostate cancer. Int J Radiat Oncol Biol Phys. 2011;79(4):1013–21.
23. Arcangeli G, Saracino B, Gomellini S, Petrongari MG, Arcangeli S, Sentinelli S, Marzi S, Landoni V, Fowler J, Strigari L. A prospective phase III randomized trial of hypofractionation versus conventional fractionation in patients with high-risk prostate cancer. Int J Radiat Oncol Biol Phys. 2010;78(1):11–8.
24. Droz JP, Balducci L, Bolla M, Emberton M, Fitzpatrick JM, Joniau S, Kattan MW, Monfardini S, Moul JW, Naeim A, van Poppel H, Saad F, Sternberg CN. Management of prostate cancer in older men: recommendations of a working group of the International Society of Geriatric Oncology. BJU Int. 2010;106(4):462–9.

Chapter 10
Selective Minimally Invasive Therapy in Older Patients for Localized Prostate Cancer: A Way to Mitigate Harm and Retain Benefit?

Louise Dickinson, Hashim Uddin Ahmed, and Mark Emberton

Abstract The benefits of screening and treatment of localized prostate cancer are increasingly in question. Some of this uncertainty can be attributed to the treatment-related morbidity and impact on quality of life that exists from current standard treatment options, e.g., external beam radiotherapy and radical prostatectomy. A potential strategy that offers cancer control with reduced treatment-related harm is known as "focal therapy," which targets treatment to the tumor rather than the whole organ. This chapter explores the rationale for this new treatment concept, its application within the elderly population, and the diagnostic investigations and therapeutic technologies available to us for localization of disease and targeting of treatment. We also explore the results of recent clinical trials in this area and possible future directions in this new treatment strategy.

Keywords Focal therapy • Localized prostate cancer • Multiparametric MRI • Ultrasound • Transperineal template biopsies • Index lesion • Ablative therapies

Introduction

The benefit versus harm question in the screening and treatment of localized prostate cancer has never been more actively in debate. The US Preventive Services Task Force attributed a grade D to PSA screening in 2011 deeming it of "moderate or high certainty that the service has no net benefit or that the harm outweighs the benefits," having already recommended against any benefit of screening in men

L. Dickinson, M.B.B.S., B.Sc.(Hons), MRCS (✉) • H.U. Ahmed, MRCS(Ed), BM, BCh (Oxon), B.A.(Hons) • M. Emberton, M.D., FRCS (Urol)
Department of Urology, University College Hospitals NHS Foundation Trust, London, UK
e-mail: misslouisedickinson@gmail.com; hashim.ahmed@ucl.ac.uk; markemberton1@btinternet.com

J.-P. Droz, R.A. Audisio (eds.), *Management of Urological Cancers in Older People*, 131
Management of Cancer in Older People,
DOI 10.1007/978-0-85729-999-4_10, © Springer-Verlag London 2013

aged 75 years and older in their previous statement in 2008 [1]. During 2009, the results of the European Randomized Study of Screening for Prostate Cancer (ERSPC) were published, demonstrating a 20 % reduction in prostate cancer mortality in the screened population compared to the control arm [2]. However, 1,410 men needed to be screened and 48 diagnosed and treated in order that one prostate cancer-related death was avoided over a 9-year interval. These results reinforce those of the earlier Scandinavian randomized controlled trial, which compared surgery and watchful waiting, and showed an absolute risk reduction in preventing cancer mortality within 8 years of only 5 % (from 14 to 9 %) [3]. The benefits of screening and treatment become even more equivocal in the older population, when diminishing life expectancy, and an increase in other comorbidities largely outweigh the risks of prostate cancer specific mortality.

Furthermore, conclusions on the benefits are difficult to draw upon for the subgroup of older men from large randomized controlled studies, as those over 75 years were excluded.

Since the PSA era began, there has been a shift in disease profile, with an increased detection of low-volume and low-risk disease. The apparent poor benefit-to-risk ratio for the treatment of prostate cancer therefore partly relates to overtreatment of low-risk disease that would be unlikely to result in death if left untreated. Even the benefits of treating intermediate disease are equivocal, based on early reports from the recently completed Prostate Cancer Intervention Versus Observation Trial (PIVOT), although the full report is awaiting publication. The alternative approach to treatment, active surveillance, requires a high burden of PSA blood tests and biopsy procedures (with their associated risks), and the psychological morbidity of living with untreated disease until curative treatment is sought. A significant proportion of men elect to have treatment, despite an absence of evidence of biochemical or histopathological progression, reiterating the detrimental psychological impact from this management strategy. The second problem relates to the significant treatment-related morbidity and the impact on quality of life that exists from current standard treatment options (e.g., external beam radiotherapy, radical prostatectomy). Men undergoing radical prostatectomy can expect anything between 2 and 60 % risk of incontinence and up to 90 % risk of impotence. Approximately 20 % of patients receiving external beam radiotherapy experience significant urinary or rectal symptoms, and potency rates are comparable to radical surgery. Recent refinements in surgical technique and minimally invasive access (laparoscopic or robot-assisted) have offered potential improvements in quality of life outcomes, genitourinary function, and shorter hospital stays. However, improved outcomes from robotic-assisted or laparoscopic techniques have larger been anecdotal to date, with very little published objective evidence of significant differences compared to conventional open surgery. Arguably some of the lack of conclusive evidence can be attributed to the current learning curves associated with the introduction of a new surgical technique. However, any significant overall benefit to patients has yet to be determined. Advances in radiotherapy applications have also led to more conformal treatments, with less damage to the surrounding anatomical structures (nerves, vessels, bladder wall, sphincters, rectum), and potentially fewer side effects.

A solution to reducing treatment-related harm might occur if the therapies offered were well tolerated, with a minimal recovery period, and overall fewer side effects, while still effectively treating the areas of cancer within the prostate. A number of minimally invasive therapies are now in use that seek to achieve these aims. For example, cryotherapy and high-intensity focused ultrasound (HIFU) have become established alternative primary treatments for localized prostate cancer within clinical practice over the last few years. They have also been used for salvage treatment of radiorecurrent disease, albeit with a higher risk of significant genitourinary and bowel (e.g., rectourethral fistula) complications. Other newer primary treatment modalities such as photodynamic therapy (PDT) and laser therapies are currently under evaluation within clinical trials. These minimally invasive therapies can be given in the day-case setting, and do not require intra-abdominal surgical access with the advantage that recovery and return to usual daily activities are quicker. These factors are of particular importance within the elderly population in who added risks from reduced mobility, such as hospital-acquired infections and thromboembolic events, accumulate with prolonged hospital stays.

An additional advantage to these ablative therapies is the feasibility of reducing treatment coverage to a smaller area of the prostate, as an alternative to treating the whole gland. Such a selective approach could allow treatment to conform more closely to the area (or areas) of cancer, with preservation of surrounding normal prostatic tissue. This concept has been termed "focal therapy" and encompasses a range of therapeutic protocols that offer a tissue-sparing approach with the aim of reducing the treatment insult to the surrounding anatomical structures and, consequently, potentially leading to lower rates of genitourinary side effects. There has been growing interest in the potential role of focal therapy as a treatment for localized prostate cancer. Clinicians with expertise in the field have met in recent years to discuss terminology and standards for treating patients focally and to recommend protocols for future focal therapy trials within international consensus meetings [4, 5]. One of these expert groups defined focal therapy as "a type of treatment that aims to eradicate known cancer within the prostate and at the same time preserve uninvolved prostatic tissue with the aim of preserving genitourinary function" [4].

Trial data is now available from early phase I/II trials of focal therapy for the primary treatment of localized prostate cancer using different minimally invasive technologies. They have demonstrated promising results for obtaining early oncological outcome together with preservation of genitourinary function. Phase III randomized controlled trials are now under way. Trial results will be further discussed later in this chapter in reference to each minimally invasive technology.

The Place of Minimally Invasive Therapies Within Current Treatment Recommendations for Older Patients

While the results of the recent large randomized trials (such as ERSPC) suggest that we are overdiagnosing and overtreating localized prostate cancer, how do these results help us to advise management in the older population with localized prostate cancer, and how might minimally invasive treatments be utilized? In contrast to the concerns on overtreatment, several papers have highlighted that older men are generally under-treated on the basis of their chronological age, with little regard to general health status and fitness. Elderly men are more likely to be offered "watchful waiting" or immediate hormone ablation therapy as a means of obtaining cancer control, rather than curative radical treatment. Radical surgery tends to be offered only to those men under 70 years, in view of the accumulation of risks with age, and number of coexisting comorbidities. For those offered external beam radiotherapy, the treatment required is prolonged and time intensive. Whole-gland treatment with a minimally invasive therapy could offer an attractive alternative in this subgroup, offering a quicker post-operative recovery period, and usually a single hospital visit for treatment.

The International Society of Geriatric Oncology (SIOG) recently published recommendations for the management of prostate cancer specifically in older men [6]. In relation to localized prostate cancer, they firstly advised treatment decisions based on a full health assessment taking into account comorbidities and patient preference, in addition to (and not instead of) chronological age. Secondly, they advised an active surveillance approach to men with D'Amico low- and intermediate-risk disease but suggested that carefully selected ("fit" and "vulnerable") men with high-risk disease are likely to benefit from curative treatment. Finally, caution was advised in the use of hormone ablation therapy, with careful balancing of the benefits and harms on a patient-by-patient basis. The minimally invasive techniques of cryotherapy, brachytherapy, and HIFU were referenced by this group. HIFU and cryotherapy were considered as potential alternatives for curative treatment to surgery or radiotherapy, pending further results from longer-term studies, although the place of brachytherapy was questioned in this age group due to the restriction to low-risk disease for eligibility.

What Place Could "Selective" (or Focal) Treatment Take in the Elderly?

A more "selective," or focal, approach to treatment could be considered as an alternative to two patient cohorts in the elderly population. Firstly, as an alternative to active surveillance in men with low-risk disease, who are medically fit, and in whom the benefits of treatment outweigh life expectancy. Secondly, men with intermediate to high-risk disease, who are denied radical treatment due to chronological age or comorbidities, or alternatively, decline radical treatments or hormone ablation therapy due to treatment burden and concerns over the side effects.

Cancer Cure Versus Cancer Control? (Fig. 10.1)

Radical treatments aim to remove or ablate the whole prostate gland together with a necessary tissue margin for destruction of all known cancer. The advantages of this

Fig. 10.1 Illustrations of the two potential treatment protocols within focal therapy, i.e., cancer cure (treatment of all identifiable disease) versus cancer control (treatment of the index lesion)

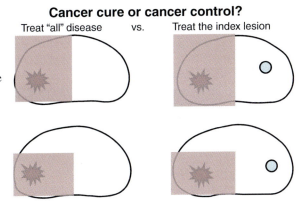

Cancer cure or cancer control?

Treat "all" disease   vs.   Treat the index lesion

are self-explanatory in that all cancer is intended for treatment and cancer cure is sought. However, this approach comes at a price, as the margins required have an impact on the surrounding neurovascular bundles and the other anatomical structures around the prostate. Focal treatment may offer a means of obtaining cancer control, with a lower impact on genitourinary function, through preservation of at least one neurovascular bundle. Focal treatment could follow two different approaches; firstly, all identified cancer could be treated, with an appropriate tissue margin. This strategy would incorporate that group of patients with unifocal and unilateral disease, a disease profile occurring in 20–40 % of men. The second approach allows treatment in further cohort of men that have a dominant or "index" lesion. Treatment could be targeted to this lesion, while deliberately leaving any contralateral low-volume, low-risk disease untreated and closely monitored over time. This strategy assumes the biology of other solid organ cancers, i.e., that the largest "index" lesion confers the main prognostic risk. The index lesion in prostate cancer accounts for up to approximately 80 % of the total tumor volume [7]. The other nondominant lesions account for 0.1–0.4 cc of tumor on average and tend to be of low grade. Lesions above 0.5 cc are the ones that tend to harbor Gleason scores of 7 or greater and are responsible for extracapsular extension if present. Thus, ablation of only the index lesion, or its hemi-gland, could reduce prostate-specific mortality risk with less treatment-related harm than "standard" therapies. This approach is likely to suit the older population, whereby achieving cancer control rather than cancer cure, together with a reduced side-effect risk, may allow preservation of quality of life without significant impact on life expectancy from prostate cancer.

Preservation of Genitourinary Function and Overall Quality of Life

The protracted natural history of prostate cancer means that prostate-related mortality benefit from treatment is difficult to determine and greater reliance is placed on surrogate biochemical markers of oncological success, e.g., serial PSA levels. The effects of prostate cancer treatments on general and prostate-specific quality of life, and adverse events, tend to have a greater impact on men in the shorter term. The complications related to these treatments are known to influence a range of life aspects, including general well-being, interpersonal relationships, sexual function, and social status.

Erectile function, although multifactorial in etiology, declines as part of the "normal" aging process with a significantly greater prevalence of dysfunction in men over 70 years compared to those in their 50s or 60s [8]. Baseline erectile function is an important measure to establish in order to know the true impact of a prostate cancer therapy. Unfortunately, relatively few studies report on this. The range of reported erectile function rates is large. A review of the epidemiology of erectile function showed a prevalence of 5–20 % of moderate to severe erectile dysfunction across all age groups. However, this prevalence ranged from 2 to 30 % in the <50-year-old age group to 38–57 % in men of 70–79 years [9]. Salomon et al. reported dysfunction ranging from mild to severe on IIEF score in 48 % of 1,330 men with localized prostate cancer awaiting radical prostatectomy [10]. Whether there is a decline in continence function as part of normal aging is less certain, but out of 3,810 men within the ERSPC study, up to 9 % of men had urinary leakage several times a week.

Many men place at least as much importance on preservation of function, even if diminished, as cancer cure, in particular when presented with the information on the natural history of the disease and their own personal risk profile. As the advising doctors, we should be sympathetic to the needs of the patients to maintain quality of life, and how this should balance against cancer risk. Focal treatment may allow modification of prognosis through cancer control, with minimal to no compromise on function. Conversely, the arguments for more invasive and extensive treatments become difficult to justify, while the benefits of treatment to life expectancy are so uncertain.

Planning Focal Treatments

One of the impediments to focal treatments in the past has been the absence of diagnostic tests that can "map" cancer lesions for targeting of treatments. As a result, the whole prostate has needed to be treated. The current standard diagnostic test, transrectal ultrasound (TRUS)-guided biopsy, involves "blind" (nonimage targeted) sampling of prostate tissue from a predefined area of the prostate. This technique allows a diagnosis (positive or negative for cancer) and, when positive, a representation of the maximal grade and volume of disease that assume that the biopsies sampled the highest risk cancer. However, TRUS biopsy is known to either misdiagnose or underdiagnose men in around 30 % of cases, through missing or under-sampling of clinically significant lesions. Furthermore, this technique cannot be relied on to accurately side and locate clinically significant lesions in order to

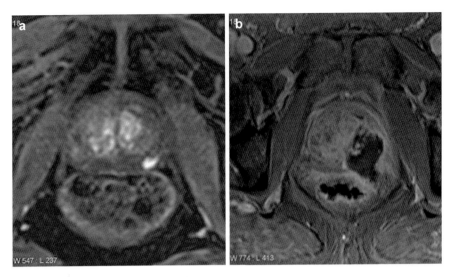

Fig. 10.2 (**a**) Multiparametric MRI showing a discrete left peripheral zone tumor on the dynamic contrast-enhanced sequence. Targeted transperineal prostate biopsies to this area confirmed a Gleason 4 + 3 prostate cancer with no disease identified elsewhere on standard sampling of the prostate. (**b**) Early (1 week) postoperative MRI following focal HIFU treatment demonstrating a lack of gadolinium uptake in the lower left quadrant indicating tissue necrosis at the site of the previous tumor

plan tissue-sparing treatments. Other diagnostic approaches are therefore required. New imaging and biopsy techniques are now available that can accurately localize and characterize prostate cancer burden.

Imaging Techniques

Multiparametric MRI (Fig. 10.2)

MRI has traditionally been included within the prostate cancer diagnostic pathway in order to stage disease for treatment planning. In this context, MRI has comprised of two sequences, T1- and T2-weighted, that allow intra- and extra-prostatic tumor burden to be grossly assessed. However, a major limitation of this "conventional" MR imaging is that differentiation between tumor and biopsy hemorrhage artifact is difficult, and precise information on tumor burden, localization, and characterization is impossible to achieve. Until now, MRI has therefore not had a place within the diagnostic pathway. However, advances in MR platforms and technique have allowed evolution of more sophisticated imaging, by combining additional sequences (MR spectroscopy, diffusion-weighted, dynamic contrast-enhanced) as "multiparametric" (mp) MRI. In this form, a shift in the use of MRI for cancer diagnosis has become possible. Accuracy rates of 90 % for ruling out clinically significant prostate cancers of at least 0.5 cc have been achieved by a number of groups, when preoperative mpMRI findings were compared against radical prostatectomy as the reference standard [11].

Some groups are now using mpMRI pre-biopsy in men with suspected prostate cancer (raised PSA or abnormal digital rectal examination) for detection of disease and risk stratification of any identified lesions. By introducing MRI at the pre-biopsy stage, the problems of biopsy hemorrhagic artifact are overcome, with improved imaging interpretation. Furthermore, biopsy sampling strategies can be tailored according to the results of the mpMRI, including the addition of image-targeted cores to the lesion. Improved detection rates for clinically significant disease have been achieved with targeted biopsies, compared to standard (nonimage directed) sampling [12]. There is also evidence that mpMRI can provide information on Gleason grade and D'Amico risk classification [13] albeit with poor sensitivity for detecting low-volume and low-grade disease. However, in considering targeted treatment to those lesions of clinical significance, mpMRI may contribute an ideal platform for identifying candidates for selective therapy, while omitting detection of clinically insignificant disease that does not warrant treatment.

Ultrasound

There are now a number of new ultrasound techniques in use, both within the clinical setting and under evaluation within trials. All are seeking to provide a technique that can accurately detect prostate cancer. There are significant advantages to ultrasound above other imaging techniques. Firstly, it can be performed in the outpatient clinic setting by both radiologists and urologists. It is cost- and resource effective, requiring less time than CT or MRI, and without ionizing radiation. Furthermore, it provides the visual platform for performing biopsies. Some cancer lesions show as discrete hypoechoic areas on gray-scale ultrasound, the conventional technique used in TRUS guidance of biopsies. However, the sensitivity and specificity are not sufficiently high for accurate cancer detection, with less than a third of cancers showing up on gray-scale ultrasound. Other newer ultrasound techniques are beginning to demonstrate a higher diagnostic yield.

Doppler ultrasound assesses regional blood flow and its relative velocity. However, its poor detection of slow-moving blood flow within the microvasculature of cancer lesions is a significant limitation, even despite the use of power Doppler, a technique that increases sensitivity. Contrast-enhanced ultrasound (CEUS) has since been developed, which uses contrast agents containing microbubbles. These are smaller than red blood cells and therefore capable of perfusing microvessels. CEUS-guided biopsies have demonstrated double the rate of prostate cancer detection compared to standard TRUS biopsies [14], and CEUS has also demonstrated detection of higher Gleason grade disease compared with gray-scale ultrasound and power Doppler [15]. Another ultrasound technique is HistoScanning™, which uses a computerized quantification method for analyzing TRUS data and detecting and localizing the acoustic signatures produced by tissue of altered morphology, i.e., tumors, compared with normal tissue. Pre-trained algorithms are applied that interrogate raw backscatter 3D ultrasound data and translate them into visual, interpretable signals, indicating the presence or absence of disease. The results of an open-phase study were recently published, showing a sensitivity of 93 % of HistoScanning™ for the detection of lesions >0.2 cc in volume, against radical prostatectomy as the reference standard [16]. There were limitations in the limited design, in that all patients were known to have cancer, and results were unblinded to some users. However, a subsequent blinded multicenter study is currently under way. Finally elastography is a technique that assesses the differences in elastic properties, or stiffness, between normal and cancerous tissue when pressure is applied. Prostate cancer detection rates were found to be roughly equivalent with elastography-targeted biopsies, compared to a standard 10-core systematic biopsy, but with significantly fewer biopsies required [17].

Overall, these newer ultrasound techniques are demonstrating promise in the detection and localization of prostate cancer. However, they are still a little way from showing sufficient accuracy to be able to define the index lesion or plan selective treatments. There may be scope for a "multiparametric" technique, with a combination of a number of ultrasound techniques in order to enhance overall sensitivity. Ultrasound experts have already begun an assessment of this concept within the clinical setting, and further definitive results are awaited.

Biopsy Strategies (Fig. 10.3)

While we continue to evaluate imaging techniques for the accurate localization of disease and planning focal treatments, histological confirmation remains the most reliable method. However, the current standardized 10- to 12-core sampling biopsy technique is insufficient for these purposes. Despite a systematic approach to sampling each area of the prostate, clinically significant lesions can still be missed (anterior and apical areas in particular as these are difficult to reach), or misclassified as insignificant if not directly sampled. An increase in biopsy core number has not demonstrated a significant increase in detection rates, when the TRUS-guided technique is used.

Transperineal prostate biopsies, an alternative sampling strategy, involve sampling of the prostate via a brachytherapy gird placed on the perineum, usually under general anesthetic. Advantages to this technique are that the anterior and apical areas of the prostate are more easily sampled. In addition, sepsis rates are far lower than following TRUS biopsies as they are taken via the skin, rather than via the rectum. Reported urinary retention rates are variable (3–30 %) and higher than following TRUS biopsy (0.5–1 %), although perioperative use of an alpha-blocker and careful sampling to avoid inadvertent "overshooting" of the biopsy needle into the bladder wall can diminish this risk. Transperineal template biopsies, with samples taken every 5 mm, have demonstrated improved detection rates of cancer compared to TRUS biopsy [18] and can provide an accurate "map" of disease location for

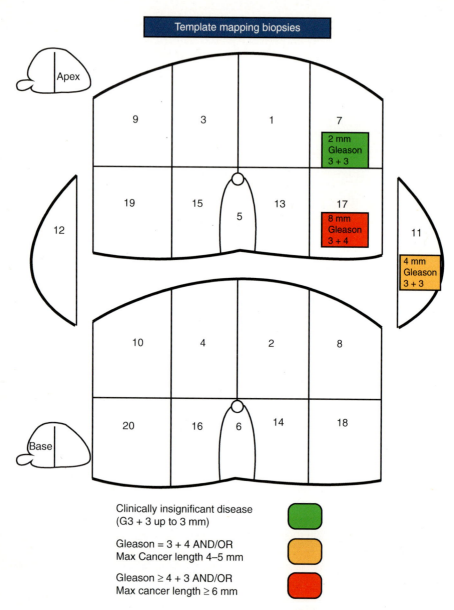

Fig. 10.3 An example visual transperineal template mapping biopsy report, using two definitions of clinically significant disease (See also Ahmed et al. [27]). This patient could receive a left hemi-ablation treatment of the biopsy identified disease

focal treatment planning. However, this technique requires a high saturation of biopsies, causing additional procedural burden to the patient, and a significant amount of histopathology processing and reporting effort. With improved imaging, a future strategy that targets biopsies only to visualize lesions with fewer cores and sparing of "normal" tissue appears potentially feasible. If mpMRI is demonstrated as the more sensitive imaging technique, registration of the MRI image onto an ultrasound platform would allow accurate targeting and avoid the costly and time-consuming requirement for "in-bore" biopsy within the MR scanner. Such MR-US registration techniques are currently under development.

Summary

Focal therapy is now a feasible concept, with advances in imaging techniques and biopsy strategies enabling detection and localization of clinically significant disease, and the index lesion, for treatment planning. However, further work is needed to refine these techniques. Furthermore, accurate techniques are needed to register, or fuse, the information acquired from mpMRI onto an ultrasound platform for targeting of biopsies and delivery of ultrasound-based focal therapies.

Minimally Invasive Technologies in Current Clinical Practice

There are several minimally invasive technologies currently in use (cryotherapy, HIFU, brachytherapy) within clinical practice for treatment of localized prostate cancer, in both the primary and salvage setting. Others, such as photodynamic therapy, are under evaluation within clinical trials. A common theme to all of these therapies is there has been a shift in approach from whole-gland treatment to focal ablation of the target cancer area. The conduct and clinical outcomes of each minimally invasive technique is explored in the next section.

Cryotherapy

Cryotherapy involves freezing of prostate tissue via cryoneedles placed in the perineum using transrectal ultrasound guidance. The freezing process causes cytolysis both directly and indirectly through ice-crystal formation, ischemic necrosis, and activation of immune responses and apoptosis. It has been granted approval as a treatment option for localized prostate cancer by the Centers for Medicare and Medicaid Services (CMS) (since 1999) and the Food and Drug Administration.

There have been a number of advances in technique and conduct since cryotherapy was first introduced as an alternative to radical prostatectomy in the 1960s. First-generation cryosurgery involved "blind" transurethral placement via a perineal incision. The lack of monitoring of needle placement position and the real-time freezing effect, plus the absence of a urethral warmer, led to a significant rate of morbidity (urethra-cutaneous fistulae, urethral sloughing, and incontinence). Following a gap in its clinical use, a more refined technique was introduced by Onik and team several years later. Second-generation cryosurgery introduced visual feedback with ultrasound guidance and use of the percutaneous route for probe placement. The probes were reduced in size from a large 8-mm probe to several smaller 3-mm ones, allowing more precise tissue coverage. As a result, morbidity rates, and cancer ablation, improved. Later device updates included a change from liquid nitrogen to argon gas, the use of even smaller probes via a fixed template as an alternative to free-hand placement, urethral warmers to reduce urethral sloughing rates, thermosensors for local tissue temperature feedback, and intraoperative injection of saline into Denonvilliers' fascia to separate the rectum from the prostate.

Summary of Clinical Results

There are now a number of clinical series within the literature on the outcomes of whole-gland cryotherapy for primary treatment of localized prostate cancer. In addition, a large, independently audited, IRB-approved web-based Cryo On-Line Database (COLD) now exists, for registry data collection from cryotherapy procedures. Biochemical disease-free survival rates have been variable in reported series, although a number of different biochemical definitions have been applied (e.g., using a range of PSA nadirs between <1 and <0.2 ng/ml), and postoperative biopsy for histological determination of disease control not always performed. Neo-adjuvant or adjuvant hormone ablation therapy use has also varied. However, all have demonstrated feasibility of cancer control with favorable urinary toxicity outcomes to other radical treatment options, and with low fistula rates (0–2 %). However, impact on potency has been consistently significant with preservation of function in as few as 5–10 % of men within some series.

As a result, the cryotherapists explored the notion of nerve-sparing cryotherapy in an attempt to improve treatment-related genitourinary function. In a pilot study in 2002, treatment was confined to a hemi-gland in 11 men with unilateral cancer identified on TRUS biopsy (at least 6-core) [19]. The contralateral neurovascular bundle was spared. Of the nine patients completing follow-up, all had a stable PSA level over a mean 36 months (range 6–72 months). One-year postoperative biopsies were benign in the six men that received them, and potency was preserved in seven out of nine men. Thereafter, the notion of a "male lumpectomy" was proposed, reflecting on the similarities with breast oncology, whereby a reduction in the detrimental psychological and physical impacts was achieved by targeting the cancer lesion rather than the organ and applying a tissue-sparing approach to therapy.

Further clinical reports of focal cryotherapy within relatively small numbers of patients supported a significant improvement in potency to approximately 80 %, by using a tissue-sparing technique. Over the years, the number of patients receiving focal cryotherapy has increased significantly. Reported data from the COLD registry have shown that over 1,000 patients had received focal treatment in 2011, with an increase from 2.1 % of all recorded cryotherapy cases in 1999 to 38.2 % of cases in 2007 [20]. Patients receiving tissue-sparing treatment tended to be younger, with a lower clinical grade and stage, and in the lower risk category. The same paper reported on the outcomes of 1,160 patients receiving primary focal cryoablation within the COLD registry. They showed a biochemical disease-free survival (using ASTRO criteria) rate of 75.7 % at 36 months follow-up. Only 14.1 % of men received postoperative biopsy, triggered by a rising PSA and suspicion of residual disease, with a reported positive biopsy rate of 26.3 % but overall assumed rate of only 3.7 % (43/1,160) from the treated cases. This was similar to an overall reported positive biopsy rate of 3 % following whole-gland treatment (125/4,099 patients). Only one rectourethral fistula was reported after focal treatment, and full continence was achieved in 98.4 % of men (compared to 96.9 % following whole-gland cryo-surgery). Sexual function sufficient for intercourse was maintained in 58.1 % of men with focal therapy, compared with 32.3 % after whole-gland therapy.

Summary

The cryotherapists were therefore the first to demonstrate that a change in strategy from treatment of the whole organ to treatment targeted to the cancer itself could result in improved genitourinary function, without significant impact on short to medium-term cancer control. The COLD registry has allowed the collection and reporting of results from a large cohort of patients with benefits for assessing outcomes, but with the limitations that clinical practice and follow-up has not been standardized.

High-Intensity Focused Ultrasound

High-intensity focused ultrasound (HIFU) is another well-established ablative therapy that has been in clinical use for the treatment of prostate cancer since the 1990s. The largest reported series of primary HIFU treatment originate from Japan, UK, France, and Germany, but the availability of long-term outcome data is still limited. As a result, recommendations on its use vary between medical associations, with some approving its use in the primary or salvage setting, and others recommending its use only within controlled clinical trials.

HIFU uses the same properties as diagnostic ultrasound, whereby cyclical sound pressures at varying frequencies are passed through a piezoelectric material. The spectrum of frequencies differs for diagnostic (1–20 kHz) and therapeutic (0.8–3.5 MHz) purposes. HIFU uses short wavelengths in combination with high frequencies to deliver the energy density required for a focused heating effect, achieving temperatures of around 80–90 °C. Alternating cycles of pressure from the propagation of ultrasound waves through tissue result in compression and rarefaction, causing cell death from cavitation. A second mechanism of cell death is from direct thermal damage that occurs from temperatures above 56 °C, as long as this temperature is sustained for at least 1 s.

The ultrasound beam is focused onto the prostate via a transducer within a transrectal probe, creating a treatment volume of 1–3 mm in transverse length × 8–15 mm along the longitudinal axis. Although the surrounding tissue is largely unharmed, there is some "near-field" deposition of energy to the tissue interfaces that sit between the transducer and the target tissue. However, the ultrasound wave frequency rapidly diminishes with proximity to the transducer; therefore, the heating effect outside the target area is kept to a minimum. Clinicians should clearly be aware of this effect when planning and conducting HIFU treatments, as excessive near-field heating risks injury to the perirectal tissue and the possibility of a rectourethral fistula.

There are currently two commercially available HIFU devices, the Ablatherm® (Edap-Technomed, France) and Sonablate® 500 (Focus Surgery, USA). Both devices deliver HIFU treatment via a transrectal transducer with real-time visual feedback on ultrasound imaging. Safety mechanisms to prevent damage to the rectum include cooling via continuous irrigation of degassed water and monitoring of rectal energy deposition levels. Treatment using the Ablatherm® device is delivered on a treatment "module" with the patient placed in the lateral position. Ablation to each hemi-gland is delivered using a preset protocol, with ellipsoidal blocks of ablation that cover the full anterior-posterior distance. A bladder neck incision or transurethral prostate resection is usually performed, either a few weeks prior to treatment or in the same session, in order to reduce the size of the gland for effective coverage and to reduce the risk of postoperative stricture formation. The Sonablate® 500 device comprises of separate imaging and therapeutic transducers. Treatment is delivered in anterior to posterior zones, using different focal lengths (3, 4, or 4.5 cm) planned by the surgeon dependent on the size of the prostate and position of the tumor. Rather than a protocol-driven treatment, the surgeon adjusts the delivered power levels dependent on real-time visual feedback of treatment response, represented by "steam," or gray-scale changes known as "Uchida changes."

Limitations to HIFU treatment include gland size as the focal length is limited; the anterior aspect cannot generally be reached in glands over approximately 50 cc in volume (usually smaller for treatment with the Ablatherm® device). Dense deposits of calcification cause poor penetration of the ultrasound to distal target areas. Patients with prior rectal surgery or anorectal disease may not be able to tolerate insertion of the transrectal probe. A significant benefit of HIFU, like several other ablative therapies, is that treatment can be repeated if required.

Summary of Clinical Results

Eight-year outcomes following primary HIFU treatment for T1c-T3, N0, and M0 disease were recently published by Uchida's group in Japan, using several generation Sonablate® devices [21]. A total of 517 men were treated, with a median follow-up period of 24 months and an average 1.2 treatments, and a 66 % neo-adjuvant hormone ablation therapy rate. There were no prostate cancer-related deaths. Biochemical disease-free survival rates (using Phoenix criteria of PSA nadir + 2 ng/

ml) at 5 years were 84, 64, and 45 % in low-, intermediate-, and high-risk groups, respectively. Of 483 men undergoing 6-month follow-up biopsy, 401 (83 %) showed no evidence of residual cancer. Grade 3 or 4 urethral strictures were seen in 16.6 % of men, grade I incontinence in 0.8 %, and prolonged catheterization (more than 14 days) in 13.2 % of men. The fistula rate was 0.9 %. Preservation of erectile function was achieved in 71.1 %. Another large multicenter series, this time of 803 men (T1-2, N0, M0) treated with the Ablatherm® device, was published by Crouzet et al. The 5- and 7-year biochemical disease-free rates (Phoenix criteria) were 83–75, 72–63, and 68–62 % for low-, intermediate-, and high-D'Amico-risk patients, respectively. Control 6-month postoperative biopsies were performed in 73.3 % of patients, with a negative histology rate of 77.9 %. Adverse events and genitourinary outcomes were not reported.

These series, and other published smaller series, have demonstrated that satisfactory cancer control can be achieved with HIFU, with disease-free rates correlating with preoperative risk status. Furthermore, the treatment can be delivered in the day-case setting and is repeatable. Genitourinary function appears to be comparable to other radical treatments, with a favorable incontinence and fistula rate. Reported stricture rates have been significant but appear to have decreased with progressive learning curves and changes in clinical conduct (e.g., a move from perioperative urethral to suprapubic catheterization) and improved technologies. However, as with the cryosurgeons, it appeared feasible and necessary to explore the concept of focal treatment using HIFU in an aim to improve functional outcomes.

The first prospective phase I/II trial of focal therapy using HIFU was published by Ahmed et al. in 2011 [22]. Twenty men received a hemi-gland treatment of all identifiable disease (Gleason ≤ 7) from transperineal template mapping biopsy. Postoperative cancer control was assessed with protocol-mandated biopsies of the treated area at 6 months, and demonstrated an absence of clinically significant disease (defined as > Gleason 3 and/or maximum cancer core length >3 mm) in all men (19 of 19 men biopsied). In addition, 95 % of the 20 men preserved erectile dysfunction and pad-free continence over a 12-month follow-up period. The results of a second short-term (12-month) focal HIFU trial by the same group have recently been published Ahmed et al. in 2012 [28] An encouraging trifecta rate - defined as preservation of erectile function (with or without PDE-inhibitor use, pad-free, leak-free continence, and absence of clinically significant disease - was achieved in 89% in a cohort of 41 men receiving unilateral or bilateral focal treatment of all identifiable disease (Gleason ≤ 7) on transperineal template mapping biopsy. A third trial has recently completed follow-up and is awaiting publication (clinicaltrials.gov NCT00988130). Furthermore, a larger prospective phase II multicenter trial of focal HIFU treatment is now under way in the UK (clinicaltrials.gov NCT01194648). Transperineal template (5-mm sampling) prostate biopsy is being used to assess eligibility at entry and will also be performed at final 36-month follow-up to assess cancer outcomes. This trial will provide further information on the medium-term outcomes following focal therapy and, in particular, will provide an opportunity to interrogate the behavior of any contralateral untreated clinically insignificant lesions from follow-up biopsy.

Summary

Longer-term results of whole-gland primary HIFU are now becoming available, demonstrating good cancer control and comparable genitourinary function to other radical therapies. As with other surgical procedures, advancements in HIFU technique and knowledge have led to greater expertise and are likely to have improved outcomes. A move toward focal treatment has demonstrated significantly improved rates of preserved genitourinary function, without compromise to cancer control, albeit within only short-term follow-up so far.

Photodynamic Therapy

Photodynamic therapy (PDT) uses a photosensitizer agent activated by light to cause localized tissue necrosis. It has been used in the treatment of tumors of the head and neck and pancreas, as well as being evaluated within clinical trials for the treatment of prostate cancer. The photosensitizer is administered orally, topically, or intravenously, in its inactive form. When light of a certain wavelength is delivered to the target organ, activation of the photosensitizer occurs, with conversion of its inactive form to an unstable energized state and the formation of reactive oxygen species and localized cell death. Light is delivered via optical fibers placed into the prostate using ultrasound guidance and a brachytherapy grid. The procedure takes place under general anesthetic, with the patient in the lithotomy position. A urethral catheter is usually inserted at the time and removed within 24 h.

There are two main forms of photosensitizers – those that are activated in the vasculature and those that are activated in the tissue itself. Tissue-activated photosensitizers, e.g., aminolevulinic acid (ALA), take several days to accumulate in the target organ, and therefore the drug and light are given in separate sessions. They also require several weeks to clear from the body. Careful protection is required during that time from sunlight, or even indoor light, in order to avoid sunburn-type damage to the eyes and skin, where the drug can also accumulate. Vascular-activated photodynamic therapy (VTP) uses a photosensitizer, e.g., the palladium bacteropheophorbide photosensitizers Padoporfin and Padeliporfin (Steba Biotech, the Netherlands), that is activated within the vasculature within minutes of administration, with rapid clearance. The photosensitizer and light source can be administered as a same-day treatment, with no requirements for prolonged protection from light.

Canine studies have been used in the preclinical investigation of PDT photosensitizers and conduct of therapy. As a result of these studies, procedural optimization and light dosing could be determined prior to use within the clinical setting. For example, transurethral light delivery was found to lead to higher levels of urethral necrosis and urinary retention; therefore transperineal delivery was adopted. In addition, canine models were used to demonstrate the effective use of early (7 day) MRI scans to assess treatment, with good correlation found between the volume-lacking gadolinium uptake on MRI and the volume of tissue necrosis on whole-mount prostatectomy specimens. Current clinical trials also use preoperative MRI scans to plan the PDT treatment protocol, including the number of light fibers required, and their placement within the prostate.

Summary of Clinical Results

The earliest clinical report of photodynamic therapy for the treatment of prostate cancer was from a letter published in the *Lancet* in 1990 [23]. Two patients were treated with tissue-activated PDT 6 weeks after two separate prostatic resections. Follow-up 3-month prostate biopsies were benign, and there were no adverse events reported. One patient died from an unrelated condition, and postmortem evaluation of his prostate showed no histological evidence of residual cancer. Subsequent clinical trials using tissue-activated PDT were performed as a salvage therapy for radiorecurrent disease. Initial low light doses were increased, or the therapy repeated, when patchy effects of treatment were seen on postoperative CT. The treatment was well tolerated in these early studies. One group reported a rectourethral fistula following a postoperative rectal biopsy, and limited incidences of stress incontinence and acute urinary retention. The first clinical trials of tissue-activated photosensitizers in primary cases also demonstrated that PDT was well tolerated with little more than transient irritative bladder symptoms in most men. However, cancer control outcomes were variable.

Subsequently, a lipophilic vascular-activated photosensitizer, Padoporfin (WST-09, Tookad®; Steba Biotech, The Hague, the Netherlands) was developed, which required a carrier (Cremophor) to be administered by intravenous infusion. It was also first evaluated within a phase I/II trial as a salvage treatment for radiorecurrent disease, and a dose escalation regimen was used with correlation against treatment volume on early postoperative MRI scans. Tissue response correlated with dose. There were no episodes of adverse skin photosensitivity. Padoporfin has since been evaluated as a primary therapy within a dose escalation trial, and the results of this trial are awaiting publication. However, it became apparent that several men had hypotensive episodes or other evidence of cardiac toxic effects, thought to be secondary to the Cremophor carrier. As a result, a water-soluble version of the drug has been developed, Padeloporfin (WST-11 Tookad® Soluble). Early phase I/II clinical trials have demonstrated improved safety and tolerability levels. A European multicenter phase III trial is currently under way that randomizes men with localized low-risk prostate cancer to active surveillance or PDT (with WST-11).

Summary

In a similar manner to the other minimally invasive therapies described, PDT has been used for both whole-gland and focal treatments. It was initially thought that PDT might spare peripheral nerves and that this would be reflected in erectile function rates. However, this has not yet been proven as the case. More recent photosensitizer vascular-activated agents allow treatment to be given in the day-case setting, with minimal risk of photosensitivity reactions. The development of a new water-soluble photosensitizer (WST-11) appears to have significantly reduced the risk of cardiac toxicity described with older agents. The potential of PDT for offering cancer control and preserved function with a focal approach is currently being explored within a large European multicenter randomized controlled trial.

Future Minimally Invasive Therapies for Focal Therapy

Two approaches are being taken in the development of other minimally invasive therapies that could treat in a focal manner. Firstly, more established techniques, e.g., brachytherapy, that are already used in the treatment of prostate or other solid organ cancers are now being considered as potential focal therapies. Secondly, new focal treatments are being developed and explored within phase I/II trials. The emphasis in development of most of the latter group of therapies is in the use of imaging to effectively guide and monitor the effects of treatment.

Low-dose-rate brachytherapy, the technique of inserting radioactive pellets into the prostate, is already offered as a first-line treatment for localized low-risk disease. It is an attractive alternative to external beam radiotherapy as it can be performed in a single sitting as a day-case procedure. Treatment planning is performed using TRUS, either preoperatively or intraoperatively, to calculate the number and placement of seeds required to cover the prostate as an isodose, with reduced density to the urethra. Only recently has it been proposed as a potential form of delivering focal treatment. Two early focal brachytherapy trials are now under way, one involving treatment to a hemi-gland (clinicaltrials.gov NCT01354951) and the other a "more focal" approach. Preliminary results are awaited. A recent international consensus meeting was held to discuss the feasibility of low-dose-rate brachytherapy as a focal treatment [5]. The group reached consensus on appropriate patient selection, principles and technical considerations of brachytherapy treatment conduct, and potential measures for monitoring outcomes. In addition, the group agreed on an appropriate protocol proposal for a randomized phase II trial, comparing focal and whole-gland brachytherapy arms. Another novel radiotherapy technique, CyberKnife, is a method for delivering hypofractionated stereotactic radiotherapy via a robotic arm. It allows a dose gradient, with maximal treatment density to the tumor target, and a steep downward gradient to the surrounding normal tissue. It is currently being used to treat the whole gland and is demonstrating very promising results compared to conventional external beam radiotherapy for reduced bowel, urinary, and sexual side effects. Early discussions are under way to assess the feasibility of delivering treatment in a more focal manner.

Other novel focal therapies utilize real-time MR imaging to accurately locate lesions for accurate targeting of treatment and for monitoring of treatment response. Microwave treatment has been used in the treatment of radiorecurrent prostate cancer in five men [24]. MR thermometry demonstrated good correlation between the visualized heating effect and the areas of tissue necrosis. Another group have reported on phase I trials of MR targeted photothermal laser ablation in 12 patients with low-risk prostate cancer [25]. Six-month postoperative TRUS biopsy demonstrated a 50 % overall cancer-free outcome and early (7-day) postoperative gadolinium contrast-enhanced MRI verified the position of the treated area with hypoperfused tissue volume. Another group have subsequently performed real-time MR imaging-guided laser ablation in two patients [26] with successful ablation of the target area and correlation of the temperature changes seen on imaging.

Post-op Monitoring

A challenge for minimally invasive therapies is in the use of appropriate follow-up investigations to gauge success. There is currently no agreed standardized definition for biochemical success. As a result, a number of definitions from radical therapies, such as ASTRO and Phoenix criteria, have been adopted. The Stuttgart criteria (PSA nadir + 1.2 ng/ml) were recently proposed for monitoring postoperative response following whole-gland HIFU. However, this definition has yet to be validated using prospective data. The problem becomes even greater in the case of focal therapy, as PSA levels never decrease to a negligible nadir due to continued PSA production by preserved normal prostatic tissue. Histological verification of treatment effect has been assessed with follow-up TRUS biopsies in many minimally invasive published studies, although biopsy protocols tend to differ. Increasingly, imaging, usually in the form of gadolinium-enhanced MRI, is being used to assess outcome, particularly within focal therapy trials. Imaging may become the most reliable form of both short- and long-term follow-up following focal treatment, as response to treatment and the presence of residual or new disease can potentially be visualized and monitored over time. However, one of the crucial tasks of future focal therapy trials is to prospectively evaluate the accuracy of imaging techniques to identify, or exclude, residual disease warranting further treatment.

Conclusions

We have presented data on a number of currently available minimally invasive technologies, which potentially offer alternative treatment options to the elderly population as either whole-gland or focal therapies. The main objective for treatment, particularly within the elderly population, is to reduce the risk of prostate cancer-related death while causing minimal impact on quality of life, and the prime obligation for urologists and oncologists is in assessing the risk to benefit ratio of treatment and appropriate patient selection. We have described some of the recent advances in diagnostics that will allow us to improve our detection and localization of disease for the purposes of planning focal treatments. These investigations are additionally likely to provide an important means of appropriately risk-stratifying patients prior to electing for active surveillance or whole-gland therapies.

This chapter has focused primarily on the use of minimally invasive technologies for primary treatment of localized prostate cancer. However, all of these therapies have also demonstrated encouraging outcomes within the whole-gland salvage setting. Furthermore, it may be that tissue-sparing salvage treatment of focal recurrent disease would allow hormone ablation therapy to be deferred (and its significant side effects) and may have implications for life expectancy. Current and future focal therapy trials will provide further valuable information on the success, or otherwise, of focal therapy in the primary and salvage settings.

Finding appropriate definitions of success should be one of the priorities of future clinical trials evaluating whole-gland and minimally invasive therapies. Once established, improved standardization of outcomes will allow more robust comparison between published data, and more conclusions can be drawn regarding the place of these therapies within standard practice.

References

1. Chou R, Croswell JM, Dana T, et al. Screening for prostate cancer: a review of the evidence for the U.S. Preventive services task force. Ann Intern Med. 2011;155:762–71.
2. Schroder FH, Hugosson J, Roobol MJ, et al. Screening and prostate-cancer mortaility in a randomized European study. N Engl J Med. 2009;360:1320–8.
3. Bill-Axelsen A, Holmberg L, Mirrja Ruuth, et al. Watchful waiting and prostate cancer. N Engl J Med. 2005;352:1977–84.
4. De la Rosette J, Ahmed HU, Barentsz J, et al. Focal therapy in prostate cancer – report from a consensus panel. J Endourol. 2010;24:775–80.
5. Langley S, Ahmed HU, Al-Qaisieh B, et al. Report of a consensus meeting on focal low dose rate brachytherapy for prostate cancer. BJU Int. 2012;109 Suppl 1:7–16.
6. Droz JP, Balducci L, Bolla M, et al. Background for the proposal of SIOG guidelines for the management of prostate cancer in senior adults. Crit Rev Oncol Hematol. 2010;73:68–91.
7. Bott SRJ, Ahmed HU, Hindley RG, et al. The index lesion and focal therapy: an analysis of the pathological characteristics of prostate cancer. BJU Int. 2010;106:1607–11.
8. Korfage I, Roobol M, de Koning HJ, et al. Does 'normal' aging imply urinary, bowel, and erectile dysfunction? A general population survey. Urology. 2008;72:3–9.
9. Kubin M, Wagner G, Fugl-Meyer AR. Epidemiology of erectile dysfunction. Int J Impot Res. 2003;15:63–71.
10. Salomon G, Isbarn H, Budaeus L, et al. Importance of baseline potency rate assessment of men diagnosed with clinically localized prostate cancer prior to radical prostatectomy. J Sex Med. 2009;6:498–504.
11. Villers A, Puech P, Mouton D, et al. Dynamic contrast enhanced, pelvic phased array magnetic resonance imaging of localized prostate cancer for predicting tumor volume: correlation with radical prostatectomy findings. J Urol. 2006;176:2432–7.
12. Hambrock T, Somford DM, Hoeks C, et al. Magnetic resonance imaging guided prostate biopsy in men with repeat negative biopsies and increased prostate specific antigen. J Urol. 2010;183:520–7.
13. Rastinehad AR, Baccala AA, Chung PH, et al. D'Amico risk stratification correlates with degree of suspicion of prostate cancer on multiparametric magnetic resonance imaging. J Urol. 2011;185:815–20.

14. Halpern EJ, Ramey JR, Strup SE, et al. Detection of prostate carcinoma with contrast-enhanced sonography using intermittent harmonic imaging. Cancer. 2005;104:2373–83.

15. Xie SW, Li HL, Du J, et al. Contrast-enhanced ultrasonography with contrast-tuned imaging technology for the detection of prostate cancer: comparison with conventional ultrasonography. BJU Int. 2012;109:1620–6. doi:10.1111/j.1464-410X.2011.10577.x.

16. Simmons LA, Autier P, Zát'ura F, et al. Detection, localisation and characterisation of prostate cancer by Prostate HistoScanning(™). BJU Int. 2011. doi:10.1111/j.1464-410X.2011.10734.x [Epub ahead of print].

17. Aigner F, Pallwein L, Junker D, et al. Value of real-time elastography targeted biopsy for prostate cancer detection in men with prostate specific antigen 1.25 ng/ml or greater and 4.00 ng/ml or less. J Urol. 2010;184:913–7.

18. Barqawi AB, Rove KO, Gholizadeh S, et al. The role of 3-dimensional mapping biopsy in decision making for treatment of apparent early stage prostate cancer. J Urol. 2011;186:80–5.

19. Onik G, Narayna P, Vaughan D, et al. Focal 'nerve-sparing' cryosurgery for treatment of primary prostate cancer: a new approach to preserving potency. Urology. 2002;60:109–14.

20. Ward JF, Jones JS. Focal cryotherapy for localized prostate cancer: a report from the national Cryo On-Line Database (COLD) Registry. BJU Int. 2012;109:1648–54. doi:10.1111/j.1464-410X.2011.10578.x [Epub ahead of print].

21. Uchida T, Shoji S, Nakano M, et al. Transrectal high-intensity focused ultrasound for the treatment of localized prostate cancer: eight-year experience. Int J Urol. 2009;16:881–6.

22. Ahmed HU, Freeman A, Kirkham A, et al. Focal therapy for localized prostate cancer: a phase I/II trial. J Urol. 2011;185:1246–54.

23. Windahl T, Andersson SO, Logfren L. Photodynamic therapy of localised prostate cancer. Lancet. 1990;336:1139.

24. Chen JC, Moriarty JA, Andrew Derbyshire J. Prostate cancer: MR imaging and thermometry during microwave thermal ablation – initial experience. Radiology. 2000;214:290–7.

25. Lindner U, Weersink RA, Haider MA, et al. Image guided photothermal focal therapy for localized prostate cancer: phase 1 trial. J Urol. 2009;182:1371–7.

26. Raz O, Haider MA, Davidson SRH, et al. Real-time magnetic resonance imaging-guided focal laser therapy in patients with low-risk prostate cancer. Eur Urol. 2010;58:173–7.

27. Ahmed HU, Hu Y, Carter T, et al. Characterizing clinically significant prostate cancer using template prostate mapping biopsy. J Urol. 2011;186:458–64.

28. Ahmed HU, Hindley RG, Dickinson L, et al. Focal therapy for localised unifocal and multifocal prostate cancer: a prospective development study. Lancet Oncol. 2012;13:622–32.

Chapter 11
Active Surveillance and Watchful Waiting in Indolent Elderly Prostate Cancer Patients

Nicolas Mottet and Helen Boyle

Abstract PSA screening, even after the age of 70, has led to the diagnosis of prostate cancers considered to be indolent. They represent a subgroup of low-risk, low-volume tumors. Active surveillance is a curative attitude based on initial surveillance and active, still curative, treatment when more aggressive tumor characteristics become evident. It is based on repeated biopsies and PSA tests. Available data are very promising, even though the available follow-up is still quite short. The 10-year specific survival is higher than 97 %. By contrast, watchful waiting is a palliative attitude where treatment is delayed until symptomatic progression occurs. This later attitude has been shown to be non inferior for overall survival compared to radical prostatectomy in non-screen-detected men above the age of 65 with a median 13 years of follow-up or screen-detected patients with a 10-year follow-up. It leads to more local symptoms, most of them being unrelated to cancer progression. It could become the standard of care for low-risk patients except for those with the longest life expectancy where active surveillance should be considered first. Both attitudes require patient's full comprehension of the issues at stake and his acceptance. It also implies regular clinical follow-up.

Keywords Prostate cancer • Gleason score • Low-risk disease • Active surveillance Watchful waiting • Insignificant cancer

N. Mottet, M.D., Ph.D. (✉)
Department of Urology, University Hospital of St. Etienne,
St. Etienne, France
e-mail: nicolas.mottet@chu-st-etienne.fr

H. Boyle, M.D.
Department of Medicine, Center Léon-Bérard,
Lyon, France
e-mail: helen.boyle@lyon.unicancer.fr

J.-P. Droz, R.A. Audisio (eds.), *Management of Urological Cancers in Older People*,
Management of Cancer in Older People,
DOI 10.1007/978-0-85729-999-4_11, © Springer-Verlag London 2013

The standard of thinking in oncology is often that once diagnosed, a cancer needs a systematic immediate active treatment. It is clear nowadays that using this attitude in low-risk prostate cancer (PCa) will lead to major overtreatment: most patients being treated without any benefit but with significant long-term side effects. This observation has lead to the development of two different attitudes: active surveillance and watchful waiting. But the physician's attitude remains often too active and aggressive in low-risk patients, especially in the elderly. Our aim is to summarize the current evidence supporting these two different attitudes.

The concepts of active surveillance and watchful waiting are fundamentally different. The aim of active surveillance is to delay the treatment of a potentially curable prostate cancer that is growing very slowly (nonsignificant lesion) until it presents aggressive features but is still at a potentially curable stage. This concept is possible only for a subgroup of low-risk clinically T1c or T2a lesions. Unlike active surveillance, the watchful waiting attitude is a palliative attitude where treatment is postponed until symptoms occur, without any curative attempt. In practice it is a "challenge": the disease and its related symptoms will evolve slower compared to the patient's general condition worsens, and an effective palliative treatment will always be available. This attitude can be applied to both localized lesions and advanced T3 or N1 disease and can even sometimes be discussed for metastatic lesions. We will focus on D'Amico's low-risk lesions only (T1c-2a, Gleason < 7, PSA < 10 ng/ml).

Active Surveillance

Cohort studies of patients with screen-detected and untreated prostate cancer (stage T1c) have shown that overall survival is comparable to that of the general population in a subgroup characterized primarily by a Gleason score equal or below 7 [1], with a 10-year-specific survival rate between 90 and 95 %. The only published randomized trial comparing radical prostatectomy with no treatment was reported by Bill-Axelson et al. [2]. It favored active treatment, but patients were not screen detected. For screen-detected patients, the still unpublished PIVOT trial did not show any overall survival difference at 10 years, neither for the entire cohort nor for low-risk patients [3]. In both studies, the control group was offered watchful waiting only. Therefore, active surveillance, based on a stricter follow-up policy, might represent the best option for many elderly patients having a very long life expectancy.

Importance of the Gleason

Whatever the therapeutic approach, all studies show the prognostic importance of tumor differentiation. A significant relationship between tumor volume, pT stage, and prognosis is recognized. It is possible to isolate a subset of PCa as potentially insignificant [4] by combining these three criteria: intracapsular lesion (pT < pT3), Gleason score less than 7, and tumor volume less than 0.2–0.5 cc. The growth rate is so slow (with a volume doubling time over 5 years) that they will not have any impact in patient's overall survival. Recently, the tumor volume considered clinically insignificant has been revised upward, following data from the ERSCP cohort, and could reach up to 1.3 cc [5].

If screening can diagnose earlier stages, it leads to more frequent discovery of insignificant lesions, with the resulting increased risk of overtreatment. This was confirmed by the Rotterdam team [6] reporting 49 % insignificant lesions in the screening arm of the ERSPC study. Numbers up to 67 % have recently been suggested [7], underscoring the potential importance of this issue.

Characterization of Insignificant Lesions on Biopsy

Insignificant lesions were characterized on surgical specimens but must be defined with the prostate still in place: the possibility of delayed treatment in potentially curable disease requires accurate initial characterization.

It is recognized that a single positive core is insufficient to characterize a tumor as insignificant [8]. In 1992, Terris proposed the combination of a PSA below 10 ng/ml, a Gleason score below 7, and the presence of a single positive core with a minimal length of 10 mm, containing less than 3-mm cancer [9] to define an insignificant lesion. In 1994, Epstein et al. proposed similar predictive criteria based on prostatectomy specimens: biopsy Gleason score less than 7, less than half of the cores being positive (with at least six cores taken), less than half of each core with cancer, and a PSA density (PSAD) less than or equal to 0.15 ng/ml/g [10]. But this was a retrospective analysis and it was based on six biopsies performed on prostatectomy specimens; therefore, the usefulness of these criteria is limited [10]. If their specificity is generally excellent, the sensitivity is poor.

There is also a clear Gleason undergrading between the 6-core sampling and the prostate specimen (underestimation in up to 40 % of cases) [7]. Increasing the number of cores to 10 or more improves concordance between biopsy Gleason score and prostatectomy Gleason score [11].

A correlation between tumor volume and the number of positive cores has been suggested by Ochiai et al. in a cohort of 207 prostatectomies: 42, 16.4, and 5.5 % of insignificant lesions were found, respectively, when a single, two, or three or more positive cores were obtained [12].

The reliability of current imaging modalities to define tumor volume is still debatable although some promising work is underway [13], especially for the detection of anterior lesions [14]. Current biological data such as PCA3 are too preliminary to be used, despite the initial interest [15].

Rebiopsy: A Must?

Indirect means, such as saturation biopsies, have been proposed to better define the tumor volume and Gleason score. Suggested in 2005 by Epstein et al. [4], it was confirmed by Boccon-Gibod et al. [16]. If the Gleason undergrading is improved by the rebiopsy strategy, it is usually an upgrade from 6 (3 + 3) to 7 (3 + 4) and not 4 + 3, even if possible. Furthermore biopsying might lead to finding multiple positive cores (more than 50 %), which is predictive of an extracapsular lesion.

Prostate biopsies are performed routinely, and with up to 15 cores, minor complications are not uncommon, but serious complications are rare. A significant increase in the number of cores will probably increase this incidence [16].

Predictors of Insignificant Cancer

Cheng et al. [17] performed a multivariate analysis looking for factors that could predict a tumor volume of less than 0.5 cc, from 336 surgical specimens. The number of positive cores and the length of the tumor on each core were independent factors. One of the rare series available where more than six cores were taken at biopsy is that of Ochiai et al. [12]. Two hundred and seven patients were diagnosed with prostate cancer on biopsies with at least 10 cores and treated by radical prostatectomy. Forty five (21.7 %) had a tumor described as insignificant. Predictive factors of insignificant cancer, in a multivariate analysis, in patients with only a single positive biopsy were Gleason score 7 (3 + 4) or less, less than 2 mm of cancer, and a prostate volume larger than 50 g. When more than two cores were positive, only a Gleason score less than 7 was predictive of insignificant cancer.

Repeated biopsies in potential candidates for active surveillance are thus probably the most important factor to determine which tumors are really insignificant. Nomograms have been proposed, mainly by Steyerberg et al. [6]. Steyerberg et al. has been validated on an independent cohort, but unfortunately it requires to know the prevalence of insignificant cancer in the studied population.

Current Cohorts

Several cohorts of active surveillance have been reported, the most advanced being based on 450 patients [18]. An active surveillance strategy was proposed if all the following criteria were present: T1c–T2a, PSA less than or equal to 10 ng/ml, and Gleason score less than 7. For patients with a life expectancy of more than 15 years, the Epstein criteria [13] were added: less than three positive cores and tumor in less than half of each positive core. The follow-up was based on a digital rectal examination and a PSA test every 3 months for 2 years and every 6 months afterward and systematic biopsies at 1 year and then every 3 years up to the age of 80. Active treatment was offered at patient's request or in the presence of grade 4 on repeat biopsies or for a PSA doubling time (based on at least eight samples) of less than 3 years. At 10 years, overall survival was 85 %, specific survival was 97.2 %. After a median follow-up of 6.8 years, 66 % of the entire cohort has not yet been treated. The most

Table 11.1 Criteria for active surveillance in the main cohorts

	$N =$	Median age	Criteria
Dall'Era et al. [20]	376	62	Gleason $\leq 3+3$, PSAd ≤ 0.15 ng/dl, $5 \leq$ T2, ≤ 33 % biopsies+, ≤ 50 % core
Van den Bergh et al. [19]	616	66	Gleason $\leq 3+3$, PSA ≤ 10 ng/ml, PSAd $\leq 0,2$ ng/dl, T$\leq$T2, ≤ 2 biopsies+
Van As et al. [13]	326	67	Gleason $\leq 3+4$, PSA ≤ 15 ng/ml, T$\leq$T2a, ≤ 50 % biopsies+
Soloway et al. [26]	230	64	Gleason ≤ 6, PSA ≤ 10 ng/dl, T$\leq$T2, ≤ 2 biopsies+, ≤ 20 % core +
Klotz et al. [18]	453	70	Gleason ≤ 6, PSA ≤ 10 ng/dl, (until 1999: Gleason $\leq 3+4$, PSa ≤ 15 ng/ml)
Tosoian et al. [27]	633	66	Gleason $\leq 3+3$, PSAd ≤ 0.15 ng/dl, T1, ≤ 2 biopsies+, ≤ 50 % core
Adamy et al. [28]	238	64	Gleason $\leq 3+3$, PSA ≤ 10 ng/ml, T$\leq$T2a, ≤ 3 biopsies+, ≤ 50 % length

Table 11.2 Current results from the main series of active surveillance

	Median follow-up (months)	Progression grade/ volume (%)	Progression PSA/PSA DT (%)	Treatment at patient's request (%)	Overall survival	Specific survival	Progression-free survival
Dall'Era et al. [20]	47	35	5	8	97	100	54
Van den Bergh et al. [19]	52	/	13	18	91	100	68
Van As et al. [13]	22	13	18	2	98	100	73
Soloway et al. [26]	32	10	/	/	100	100	86
Klotz et al. [18]	82	9	14	3	68	97	70
Tosoian et al. [27]	32	14	/	9	98	100	54
Adamy et al. [28]	22	13	14	11	/	/	/

common criteria leading to treatment was a PSA doubling time (PSA DT) of less than 3 years (15 % of patients) or a direct request of patients (12 %) reflecting their anxiety. But among the 24 patients who underwent radical prostatectomy, 58 % were pT3, and 8 % were pN+. These two points represent the limitations of inclusion and surveillance criteria used by the team. Other studies have been reported from the ERSCP [19], the UCSF [20], or the MSKCC [21]. They all confirm the importance of repeated biopsies, but they are all limited by their mean follow-up of less than 4 years. The main studies are shown in Tables 11.1 and 11.2. Anxiety is the second leading cause of treatment in some studies. It is interesting to note that in the work reported by Steineck et al., there was no significant difference between the treated and the non-treated patients when considering quality of life and well-being subjective criteria, assessed by self-administered questionnaires [22].

Criteria for Transition to an Active Treatment

There is currently no single marker of tumor progression. Therefore, the consistent attitude is to monitor all the parameters, leading to characterize a tumor as insignificant: digital rectal examination, PSA, and repeated biopsies containing at least 10 cores (Gleason score, number of positive cores, and tumor length). The appearance of grade 4 on the repeated biopsies is a key point for switching to active treatment. It is unclear whether this increase in grade is secondary to lesion progression, or whether it simply reflects better tumor sampling [23]. The PSA value is an imperfect trigger, the benign component of the prostate playing probably a major role in the PSA level, considering the low volume of these lesions. The kinetics of total serum PSA has been proposed to overcome this difficulty. The PSA DT is one method to analyze this kinetics [24]. It has been used in the ERSPC cohort: a PSA DT of less than 3 years led to active treatment. The importance of this factor is being questioned, especially given its low correlation with grade progression on repeated biopsies [25].

The results of active surveillance could be further improved by the use of simple noninvasive treatments such as 5-α reductase inhibitors as suggested by the REDEEMER study. More importantly, the discussion of active surveillance for a probably nonsignificant cancer might be a good opportunity to suggest changes in diet and lifestyle, allowing a reduction in cardiovascular morbidity. It is important to remember that cardiovascular death is the leading cause of death in patients with insignificant PCa [23]. This simple approach should be widely used in health educational programs, as opposed to taking 5-α reductase inhibitors, which remains an experimental option.

To conclude, the current results of active surveillance protocols are acceptable at 10 years. They are perfectible in terms of patients' selection and follow-up modalities. But based on the available results, they represent at least a major treatment option in patients above 70 years of age, fulfilling all the above-mentioned criteria. The real question in this population is the inclusion criteria. They might be too strict in senior adults where a watchful waiting attitude might be as effective and less aggressive in all low-risk situations, except for those with a really long expected survival, based on comorbidity.

Watchful Waiting

For localized lesions (i.e., T1–2), the data are primarily based on the SEER data [1]. A cohort of 14,516 men with untreated T1–T2 PCa was followed for a median time of 8.3 years. The average age was 78 years, 42 % of patients had stage T2, and 70 %

had no significant comorbidity (Charlson 0). At the end of the study, there were only a few prostate cancer-related deaths, and most patients were either alive or dead from another disease. The main predictor of survival at 10 years, apart from age, was biopsy Gleason score greater than 7. These data confirm observations from previous cohorts on non-screen-detected PCa but with better survival in this cohort. The lead time bias might explain this difference.

Similarly the risk of delayed treatment and its modality are again directly related to the patient's age and the biopsy Gleason score. For moderately differentiated lesions (Gleason scores 5–7), 23 % of men between 66 and 74 had a secondary potentially curative treatment compared to only 6 % after 75 years. These results are very different depending on whether the diagnosis was made by PSA screening or because of symptoms: only 13 % of the non-screen-detected men underwent an attempted curative treatment, compared to 23 % in the screen-detected patients. The difference does not exist beyond 75 years. For these moderately differentiated lesions, 60–70 % of patients received hormonal therapy.

These data have been recently confirmed by the preliminary report of the PIVOT trial. This randomized trial compared the survival of patients treated with a radical prostatectomy or randomized to a watchful waiting policy. Of the 731 randomized patients, 40 % had a low-risk lesion, 50 % had a T1c. The mean and median PSA were 10 and 7 ng/ml, respectively. Seventy percent of patients had a Gleason score less than 7. After a median follow-up of 10 years, neither overall mortality (HR: 0.88, $p=0.22$) nor specific mortality (HR: 0.63, $p=0.09$) differed for the entire cohort and for patients with low-risk disease [3].

The data are very different for lesions with a Gleason above 7: the number of curative, hormonal, or secondary palliative treatment are almost identical for patients 66–74 years screen detected or not, and absolutely identical beyond 75 years in both groups, highlighting again the aggressiveness of these lesions where more than 80 % of patients received hormonal therapy at some point. Besides these survival data, serious complications such as spinal cord compression treated with surgery or radiotherapy were rare: 0.9 % for Gleason 5–7 and 6.9 % for Gleason greater than 8.

Voiding troubles are often considered as a local complication. A major difference must be made between a locally advanced huge disease on DRE and a prostate mainly enlarged by a benign condition. For voiding symptoms if the medical treatment becomes ineffective, a transurethral resection is usually very effective, and the prostate volume by itself, apart from very large prostates, has no real impact on its efficacy.

Conclusions

For symptomatic patients, neither attitude has any role, but a clear difference between enlarged prostate mainly through benign condition and large T2 lesions (no longer classified as low risk) has to be made. For asymptomatic patients with very long life expectancy (clearly beyond 10 years) and harboring a low-risk disease, active surveillance should probably be the standard of care, as long as the individual probability of life is more than 10 years. The current criteria for deciding on active surveillance, except a Gleason score below 7, still need to be clarified in the population of senior adults and could probably be safely extended (especially regarding the number of positive biopsies accepted to consider an active surveillance attitude). Otherwise watchful waiting might be the attitude of choice. For low-risk patients bothered by voiding symptoms, a standard treatment of these symptoms should be proposed, usually ignoring the insignificant-associated cancer. Such attitudes can only be engaged if they are fully accepted by the patient, his family, and his treating physician. This requires long and detailed discussions balancing the pros and cons. A systematic active treatment in such low-risk situations would for sure be over-treatment for most if not all patients.

References

1. Lu Yao GL, Albertsen PC, Moore DF, et al. Outcomes of localized prostate cancer following conservative management. JAMA. 2009;302:1202–9.
2. Bill-Axelson A, Holmberg L, Ruutu M, et al. Radical prostatectomy versus watchful waiting in early prostate cancer. N Engl J Med. 2011;364:1708–17.
3. Wilt TJ. The VA/NCI/AHRQ CSP#407: prostate cancer intervention versus observation trial (PIVOT). J Urol. 2011; 185. LBA.
4. Epstein JE, Sanderson H, Ballentine Carter H, et al. Utility of saturation biopsy to predict insignificant cancer at radical prostatectomy. Urology. 2005;66:356–60.
5. Wolters I, Roobol MJ, van Leeuwen PJ, et al. A critical analysis of the tumor volume threshold for clinically insignificant prostate cancer using a data set of a randomized screening trial. J Urol. 2011;185:121–5.
6. Steyerberg EW, Roobol MJ, Kattan MW, et al. Prediction of indolent prostate cancer: validation and updating of a prognostic nomogram. J Urol. 2007;177:107–12.
7. Welch HG, Black WC. Overdiagnosis in cancer. J Natl Cancer Inst. 2010;102:605–13.
8. Boccon-Gibod LM, Dumonceau O, Toublanc M, et al. Micro-focal prostate cancer: a comparison of biopsy and radical prostatectomy specimen features. Eur Urol. 2005;48:895–9.
9. Terris MK, Mcneal JE, Stamey TA. Detection of clinically significant prostate cancer by transrectal ultrasound-guided systematic biopsies. J Urol. 1992;148:829–32.
10. Epstein JI, Walsh PC, Carmichael M, et al. Pathologic and clinical findings to predict tumor extent of nonpalpable (stage T1c) prostate cancer. JAMA. 1994;272:368–74.
11. Elabbady AA, Khedr MM. Extended 12-core prostate biopsy increases both the detection of prostate cancer and the accuracy of Gleason score. Eur Urol. 2006;49:49–53.
12. Ochiai A, Troncoso P, Chen ME, et al. The relationship between tumor volume and the number of positive cores in men undergoing multisite extended biopsy: implication for expectant management. J Urol. 2005;174:2164–8.
13. van As NJ, de Souza NM, Riches SF, et al. A study of diffusion-weighted magnetic resonance imaging in men with untreated localised prostate cancer on active surveillance. Eur Urol. 2009;56:981–8.
14. Lawrentschuk N, Haider MA, Daljeet N, et al. Prostatic evasive anterior tumours': the role of magnetic resonance imaging. BJU Int. 2010;105:1231–6.
15. Ploussard G, Durand X, Xylinas E, et al. Prostate cancer antigen 3 score accurately predicts tumour volume and might help in selecting prostate cancer patients for active surveillance. Eur Urol. 2011;59:422–9.

16. Boccon Gibod LM, de Longchamps B, Toublanc M, et al. Prostate saturation biopsy in the reevaluation of microfocal prostate cancer. J Urol. 2006;176:961–4.
17. Cheng L, Poulos CK, Pan C-X, et al. Preoperative prediction of small volume cancer (less than 0.5 ml) in radical prostatectomy specimens. J Urol. 2005;174:898–902.
18. Klotz L, Zhang L, Lam A, et al. Clinical results of long-term follow-up of a large, active surveillance cohort with localized prostate cancer. J Clin Oncol. 2010;28:126–31.
19. Van den Bergh RC, Roemeling S, Roobol MJ, et al. Outcomes of men with screen-detected prostate cancer eligible for active surveillance who were managed expectantly. Eur Urol. 2009;55:1–8.
20. Dall'Era MA, Konety BR, Cowan JE, et al. Active surveillance for the management of prostate cancer in a contemporary cohort. Cancer. 2008;112:2664–70.
21. Eggener SE, Mueller A, Berglund RK, et al. A multi-institutional evaluation of active surveillance for low risk prostate cancer. J Urol. 2009;181:1635–41.
22. Steineck G, Helgesen F, Adolfsson J, et al. Quality of life after radical prostatectomy or watchful waiting. N Engl J Med. 2002;347:790–6.
23. Cooperber MR, Caroll PR, Klotz L. Active surveillance for prostate cancer: progress and promise. J Clin Oncol. 2011;29:3669–76.
24. Khatami A, Aus G, Damber JE, et al. PSA doubling time predicts the outcome after active surveillance in screening-detected prostate cancer: results from the European randomized study of screening for prostate cancer, Sweden section. Int J Cancer. 2007;120:170–4.
25. Ross AE, Loeb S, Landis P, et al. Prostate-specific antigen kinetics during follow-up are an unreliable trigger for intervention in a prostate cancer surveillance program. J Clin Oncol. 2010;28:2810–6.
26. Soloway MS, Soloway CT, Eldefrawy A, Acosta K, Kava B, Manoharan M. Careful selection and close monitoring of low-risk prostate cancer patients on active surveillance minimizes the need for treatment. Eur Urol. 2010;58:831–5.
27. Tosoian JJ, Trock BJ, Landis P, et al. Active surveillance program for prostate cancer: an update of the Johns Hopkins experience. J Clin Oncol. 2011;29:2185–90.
28. Adamy A, Yee DS, Matsushita K, et al. Role of prostate specific antigen and immediate confirmatory biopsy in predicting progression during active surveillance for low risk prostate cancer. J Urol. 2011;185:477–82.

Chapter 12
Decision Making in Elderly Localized Prostate Cancer

Nicolas Mottet, Helen Boyle, and Jean-Pierre Droz

Abstract Decision making in senior adults suffering from a prostate cancer is a balance between tumor aggressiveness and patient's survival probability. The latter is the main survival prognostic factor and might be approached through several scores, such as the Charlson. Screening tools such as the G8 might be helpful to consider referring patients for a more precise geriatric evaluation. The main determinant of tumor aggressiveness is the biopsy Gleason score. Only those with a Gleason equal or above 8 have a significant risk of dying in the next 10 years, especially in non-screen-detected lesions. An active surveillance strategy or a watchful-waiting attitude should be systematically proposed, especially for low- or intermediate-risk lesions, based on comorbidities. Active treatment modalities such as surgery, external beam or brachytherapy can be offered in selected intermediate- or high-risk lesions, provided that a clear survival benefit and minimal accepted side effects are obtained.

Keywords Prostate cancer • Specific mortality • Natural history • Radical prostatectomy • Radiotherapy • Watchful waiting

N, Mottet, M.D., Ph.D. (✉)
Department of Urology, University Hospital of St. Etienne,
St. Etienne, France
e-mail: nicolas.mottet@chu-st-etienne.fr

H. Boyle, M.D.
Department of Medicine, Center Léon-Bérard,
Lyon, France
e-mail: helen.boyle@lyon.unicancer.fr

J.-P. Droz, M.D., Ph.D.
Department of Medical Oncology, Lyon-RTH Laënnec School of Medicine,
Centre Léon-Bérard, Lyon, France
e-mail: jpdroz@orange.fr

J.-P. Droz, R.A. Audisio (eds.), *Management of Urological Cancers in Older People*, 163
Management of Cancer in Older People,
DOI 10.1007/978-0-85729-999-4_12, © Springer-Verlag London 2013

Prostate cancer occurs predominantly in senior adults. According to the Surveillance, Epidemiology, and End Results (SEER) registry in the USA, the median age at diagnosis in the years 2000–2007 was 68 years. Respectively, 60 and 25.7 % of new cases were diagnosed, and over 90 and 71.2 % of prostate cancer-specific deaths occurred in men ≥65 and ≥75 years of age [1]. The overall growth and aging of the world's population is expected to increase the burden of prostate cancer since the proportion of men aged ≥70 years is expected to increase from 0.8 % in 2000 to 17.2 % by 2050 [2]. The introduction of PSA screening has dramatically changed the presentation of the disease, with patients now diagnosed at a younger age and with lower grade/organ-confined disease. However, given the long natural history of prostate cancer, many patients who were not of senior age at the time of diagnosis are likely to be managed for PSA relapse and disease progression in their old age. These epidemiological statistics illustrate the need for information and guidelines specifically targeting senior adults with prostate cancer. The International Society of Geriatric Oncology (SIOG) has specifically addressed the issue of decision making for the management of elderly patients with prostate cancer [3]. The National Cancer Center Network (NCCN) has developed Senior Adult Oncology Guidelines based on classical approaches of geriatric oncology and likely applicable to prostate cancer patients [4, 5].

Clinical Presentation

The decision-making process will be discussed after a clear diagnostic based on biopsies. The reason for having the biopsy done has been discussed extensively elsewhere. Three questions have to be answered for this decision-making process: firstly, what would be the individual probability of survival for this individual without a prostate cancer? This question has usually been answered before even considering PSA and biopsy. But it must be reassessed after a confirmed diagnosis. Secondly, what is the aggressiveness of his disease? Finally, what are the benefits and drawback to be expected from any form of treatment?

Health Status Evaluation in Elderly Prostate Cancer Patients

The experts who developed the SIOG guidelines [3] limited patient assessment to dependence, nutrition, and comorbidities. All three domains are likely to be detected by screening tools, and, for comorbidities, evaluation may allow immediate management. Some screening tools are available and might help clinicians to discriminate those who require an in-depth geriatric assessment. This has been discussed elsewhere. Tools such as basic daily living activities scale (ADL) (bathing, dressing, toileting, transfer, continence, and feeding) [6] or instrumental ADL (IADL) [7] (financial management, medication management, use of transportation, and use of

Table 12.1 Health status evaluation and decision making

Health status evaluation/groups	Fit	Vulnerable	Frail	Terminal illness
Comorbidity CISR-G (23)	Grades 0/1/2	At least one grade 3	Several grade 3 or one grade 4	Multiple
	And	Or	Or	And/or
Dependence				
ADL (21)	No abnormality	No abnormality	At least one or more	Dependence
IADL (22)	No abnormality	≥1 abnormality	ADL abnormality	
	And	Or	Or	And/or
Malnutrition	Weight loss < 5 %	Weight loss 5–10 %	Weight loss > 10 %	Malnutrition
Geriatric intervention	None	One domain	Multiple domains	Multiple domains
Cancer treatment	Standard	Standard after geriatric intervention	Adapted treatment	Palliative treatment

the telephone) are useful. Comorbidities are evaluated through many scales, such as the CIRS-G (Cumulative Illness Rating System – Geriatrics) [8].

Nutritional status is estimated very simply from the variation of weight during the past 3 months. A comprehensive geriatric assessment (CGA) is recommended in frail patients and in some vulnerable patients identified by screening tools such as the recently described G8 tool [9].

Elderly patients are divided in four health status groups: fit, vulnerable, frail, and patients too sick for intervention. Fit patients have no serious comorbidity, are functionally independent (no dependence in IADL and ADL), and have no malnutrition. Their health status is considered sufficiently good for them to tolerate any form of standard cancer treatment, provided a significant benefit. Vulnerable patients are dependent in one or more IADL (but not in ADL), or they present one uncontrolled comorbid condition or a risk of malnutrition. These patients may benefit from additional geriatric intervention and may receive standard cancer treatment after resolution of geriatric problems. Frail patients are dependent in one or more ADL, have two or more uncontrolled comorbid conditions, or show major malnutrition. Patients in this group should benefit from a geriatric intervention and can be given specific adapted cancer treatment. Patients who are considered too sick for intervention have a very poor health status resulting from a combination of different impairments. These patients are only eligible for end-of-life palliation (Table 12.1). Geriatric evaluation is therefore mandatorily incorporated in the decision-making process and must be at the initial stage. This has been even more highlighted by the recent SEER database cohort where comorbidity was by far the leading cause of death in untreated PCa patients, regardless of Gleason score at 10 years, for men above 65 years [10]. The influence of comorbidity on survival has been studied by Tewari et al. [11] who have shown that the risk of non-prostate cancer mortality is three times higher in patients with severe comorbidity (Charlson score ≥ 2) than in those with mild comorbidity (Charlson score 0–1). In a recent Swedish nationwide cohort of 6,849 men aged 70 years or older [12], with a Gleason score < 8 and serum PSA values < 20 ng/ml, the PCa death rate at 10 years was 3.6 % in the group receiving surveillance and watchful waiting, 2.4 % after prostatectomy, and 3.3 % after EBRT. When adjusting for risk category, Charlson score, and socioeconomic status, there was a significantly lower risk of specific death after surgery or EBRT compared to surveillance. The rate of non-prostate cancer death was 19 % in the surveillance group versus 8.5 % with prostatectomy and 14.2 % with EBRT, highlighting the impact of initial selection for the different treatment modalities. In a multivariate analysis, Charlson score above 2 and lower socioeconomic status were associated with decreased nonspecific survival.

What Is the Aggressiveness of This PCa?

Staging Procedures

Accurate tumor staging, in particular the determination of whether or not the tumor is confined to the prostate gland, is essential for treatment decision making. It is based on the TNM staging developed by the American Joint Committee on Cancer and International Union against Cancer which is the most widely used system worldwide and is now available online [13].

The methods for local and regional staging include DRE, serum PSA level determination, and, in some specific situations, computerized tomography (CT) scan and magnetic resonance imaging (MRI). Potential nodal involvement is based on nodal size and is never specific. Suspicious is based on a size above 1 cm in the shorter axis. The gold standard for node evaluation is histological examination during lymph node dissection, a situation which is exceptional in the elderly population. The presence of distant metastases is assessed by CT scan, MRI, and bone scan. The later images are not disease specific, especially in elderly patients with extensive osteoarthritis. Improved imaging modalities have been proposed such as FNa bone scan [14]. If curative treatment is considered, a complete work-up is needed. MRI appears to be superior to CT scan for local staging, but not for assessing nodal extension. However, MRI could be of interest as no nephrotoxic vascular injection is required, and it could replace bone scan, allowing a complete workout with a single exam [15].

PCa Prognostic Factors

The optimal management of patients with prostate cancer requires accurate assessment of the risk of unfavorable outcome. The most widely used prognostic factors are clinical T stage, pretreatment serum PSA level, and Gleason score on prostate biopsy. These factors are the basis of a widely used risk stratification tool developed by D'Amico et al. to evaluate the probability of biochemical relapse 5 years after curative therapy [16]. In patients of the low-risk group (<25 % probability of PSA failure at 5 years), tumor stage is T1c–T2, serum PSA level < 10 ng/ml, and Gleason score ≤ 6. Recently, the NCCN guidelines have identified a subgroup of patients with stage T1c, Gleason score ≤ 6, PSA < 10 ng/ml, less than 3 positive cores, each with less than 50 % of cancer component, and PSA density < 0.15 ng/ml/g [4]. These patients are at very low risk of long-term relapse, and no immediate active treatment is recommended. In the D'Amico classification, patients in the high-risk group (>50 % probability of PSA failure at 5 years) have a tumor stage ≥ T2c, a serum PSA level > 20 ng/ml, or a Gleason score ≥ 8, whereas other patients are classified in the intermediate-risk group (25–50 % probability of PSA failure at 5 years). This classification has been widely published and validated. Results of a retrospective cohort study from the SEER database have confirmed that the Gleason score is the main driver for 10-year survival in clinically localized PCa regardless of age at diagnosis [17]. The 10-year specific survival for patients with a Gleason score below or equal to 7 is 90 % for T1c/T2 disease between 75 and 79 years of age and around 85 % after 80 years. It falls below 80 % for those with a Gleason score above 7. Non-prostate cancer survival at 10 years is 40 % for patients aged between 75 and 79 years and around 20 % after 80 years. These specific survival results are clearly better than those observed in non-screened patients [18].

Prediction of pathological stage, as initially suggested using Partin's tables, was based on DRE, PSA level, and biopsy Gleason score [19]. However, these factors only predict pathological probability, not patient survival, and clearly underestimate node involvement. Prediction of outcome from surrogate markers, mainly PSA relapse-free survival, has been proposed in various scores and nomograms. Most are based on either pre-therapeutic data. Some of these scores have been validated by several institutions and therefore might represent useful tools for assessing individual patients [20].

In case of relapse after an initial local treatment, the most significant specific survival predictive factor is the PSA kinetics, mainly the PSA doubling time (PSA-DT) [21, 22]. The usual threshold is 12 months, and the lower the PSA-DT, the worse the prognosis. But the calculation of the doubling time is still a matter of debate; it requires several values at several months (years) distance. Assessment of the predictive value of PSA-DT in 381 senior patients undergoing radiation therapy for clinically localized prostate cancer [23] has shown a direct relationship between 10-year specific survival and the D'Amico risk group (ranging from 100 to 55 %). Conversely, the estimated 10-year non-prostate cancer death was respectively 27, 17, and 12 % in patients at high, intermediate, and low risk. Nearly identical estimates of death from prostate cancer or from other causes were observed in PSA-relapsing men with a PSA-DT ≤ 12 months. Despite their old age, the cause of death in these patients with short PSA-DT was nearly exclusively prostate cancer.

Treatment of Localized Disease

Radical Prostatectomy

The results of a Scandinavian randomized trial of 695 men (mean age, 65 years) with localized prostate cancer demonstrate that, compared with conservative management, radical prostatectomy (RP) reduces prostate cancer mortality and the risk of metastases, but there is no, or little, further increase in benefit at 10 or more years after surgery [24]. Furthermore, a subgroup analysis revealed that the survival benefit was limited to patients below 65 years of age. However, the risk of death and of postoperative complications following RP is more a function of severity of comorbidities than chronological age [25], especially in elderly patients [26]. The recently presented PIVOT trial on screen-detected lesions highlights the lack of survival benefit after a 10-year follow-up period for the entire cohort [27]. Regarding subgroup analysis, only intermediate- and mainly high-risk disease have an improved overall and specific survival. But no patient above 70 years was included.

Lymph node dissection is optional in low-risk patients but mandatory in those with intermediate or high risk. Neoadjuvant hormonal treatment has no place in the neoadjuvant setting [28] and remains controversial in the adjuvant situation [29]. Positivity of surgical margins is associated with an increased risk of relapse. However, its impact on specific and overall mortality is still unclear [30]. In patients at high risk of relapse, three trials have shown a benefit of adjuvant over salvage radiotherapy in terms of PSA relapse-free survival [31–33]. However, only one of these trials has tested metastasis-free survival and survival benefits [31], while another is negative regarding survival [32].

Urinary incontinence is a common complication of RP, with reported incidence rates between 3 and 74 % [25], and older age has been consistently identified as a risk factor [34]. The analysis of 11,522 prostatectomized men from the SEER-Medicare database confirmed that long-term incontinence was significantly related to increasing age (24 % after 75 years vs. 17–18 % before, $p < 0.001$) but also to the severity of comorbidities (from 18 % for Charlson 0–21 % for Charlson ≥ 2, $p = 0.03$) [25]. In clinical practice, it is important to consider that older patients who have a good mobility score and are physically active are likely to suffer a level of incontinence similar to that of younger patients. Conversely, older patients who live a sedentary lifestyle are at higher risk of developing persistent incontinence after surgery. Impotence is the second significant side effect of RP, especially when a non-nerve-sparing procedure is used or in older patients. However, the data available are even more imprecise. Finally, age itself is still discussed as a possible prognostic factor for recurrence [35], possibly related to PSA level, Gleason score, and T status [36].

Altogether, it appears reasonable to conclude that senior adult patients who are candidates for radical prostatectomy should (a) have poor-risk prostate cancer (i.e., a high risk of prostate cancer-specific death); (b) be in good health, either in the fit or the vulnerable groups (i.e., high probability of survival at 5–10 years); and (c) have a low risk of incontinence (good pelvic floor tonicity).

External Beam Radiation Therapy (EBRT)

There is one randomized trial comparing old-fashioned EBRT and watchful waiting which is unable to show any survival benefit at 15 years [37]. But the old-fashioned low-dose radiation modality might partly explain the lack of benefit. Three-dimensional conformal radiotherapy (3D-CRT) is the gold standard of treatment, and intensity-modulated radiotherapy (IMRT), an optimized form of 3D-CRT, has become an increasingly interesting option. No patient should receive a dose below 70 Gy which, even for low-risk patients, has been associated with decreased relapse-free survival [38]. For patients with locally advanced or high-risk disease, EBRT alone is no longer the standard of care and must be combined with ADT, based on the results of randomized clinical trials showing a clear overall survival benefit at 10 years using either a neoadjuvant concomitant [39] or a concomitant adjuvant treatment [32]. The duration of ADT must be prolonged up to 3 years [40]. A population-based study of 31,643 nonmetastatic prostate cancer patients aged 65–85 years and treated with EBRT and/or brachytherapy has shown improved 5-year and 8-year survival rates in patients with stage T3/T4 disease receiving adjuvant ADT, but no survival advantage for men with T1/T2 disease [41]. These findings are consistent with clinical practice guidelines. However, the survival advantage associated with combining EBRT and ADT in high-risk prostate cancer patients may apply only to those with no or minimal comorbidities (i.e., fit patients) [42]. A retrospective analysis of 527 patients with nonmetastatic prostate cancer has shown the absence of relationship between age (four groups, <60, 60–69, 70–74, and ≥75 years) and risk of acute or late genitourinary or gastrointestinal toxicity after EBRT [43]. With modern irradiation techniques and increased dose, long-term toxicity is usually low, with less than 5 % expected severe toxicities, the dominant morbidity being the late genitourinary toxicity [44]. After more than 2 years of follow-up, the impotence rate is around 50 %. The outcome, in terms of cancer control and treatment-related late comorbidity, of senior patients undergoing EBRT is similar to that of younger patients. However, a discordant trial suggests that age itself might be an independent predictor of time to death from prostate cancer, with patients above 75 years of age having a decreased specific survival compared to younger patients [45].

Brachytherapy

Brachytherapy is indicated in patients with clinical stage T1b–T2a-b tumors, N0, M0, Gleason score ≤ 6, and PSA level ≤ 10 ng/ml, with a prostate volume < 50 cc and low International Prostate Symptom Score (IPSS) [46, 47]. This technique appears to be suitable for the treatment of older prostate cancer patients. Nevertheless, the survival benefit in senior adult patients with low-risk localized disease is not established. Complications of brachytherapy appear to be slightly less severe than those associated with EBRT or RP, but evidence from the SEER database suggests that urinary, bowel, and erectile complications significantly increase with both age and severity of comorbidities [48]. Results from a multivariate analysis have shown that the Charlson comorbidity index is a stronger predictor of brachytherapy complications than chronological age. However, the place of brachytherapy in senior adults is questionable as indications for brachytherapy are almost the same as for watch and wait management.

Comparison of Surgery, EBRT, and Brachytherapy

No randomized trial has compared the three treatment modalities. The same team has repeatedly reported a retrospective cohort analysis, with nearly similar rates of biochemical relapse-free survival at 8 years for RP and EBRT (72 and 70 %, respectively, $p=0.010$). The slightly higher rate reported with EBRT was attributed to the higher number of high-risk patients in this group and to insufficient dose (<72 Gy). Age (<65 vs. ≥65 years) was not an independent predictor of treatment relapse ($p=0.78$) [49]. In a recent study of 10,472 localized prostate cancer patients, no overall survival difference between surgery, EBRT, and brachytherapy has been reported [50]. After adjusting for age, comorbidities, stage, and biopsy Gleason score, a specific survival benefit has been observed for RP. This nonrandomized retrospective trial has not been published yet, and results must be interpreted with caution.

Regarding quality of life (QOL) or overall side effects, results from the Prostate Cancer Outcome Study have demonstrated that urinary incontinence is significantly more common with surgery (14–16 %) than with EBRT (4 %), while bowel urgency and painful hemorrhoids are significantly worse with EBRT (29 and 20 %, respectively) than with surgery (19 and 10 %, respectively) [51]. Similar differences between surgery and EBRT have been observed by different investigators, with less urinary stress incontinence after radiation therapy and better bowel and urinary functions after surgery. Sexual function is always impaired, though to a lesser extent when using brachytherapy. Quality of life has also been shown to vary with the number of physical symptoms, and it is statistically significantly better in the treated group than in nontreated patients [52].

Alternative Local Treatments: HIFU and Cryotherapy

Minimally invasive high-intensity focused ultrasound (HIFU) has emerged as a potential therapeutic option in patients with clinically localized, low-, or intermediate-risk prostate cancer and prostate volume<50 ml [53]. However, this treatment remains experimental [47]. Longer follow-up and comparison with established therapies are required to confirm HIFU efficacy before it can be recommended as a standard of care, and a comparison to surveillance is more than needed if the primary target are the low-risk patients.

The ideal candidates for cryosurgery are patients at low or intermediate risk [47], with a prostate volume ≤ 40 ml. A randomized trial comparing EBRT and cryosurgery in 244 patients with clinically localized low and intermediate prostate cancer has been published recently [54]. After a median follow-up of 100 months, no difference in disease progression at 36 months, overall, or disease-specific survival has been reported. However, patient numbers were too small to draw significant clinical conclusions.

Androgen Deprivation Therapy Alone

Following recent results obtained with EBRT and ADT, the place of the combination modality should be clarified, compared to ADT alone. Three prospective randomized clinical trials conducted in locally advanced N0 M0 patients have recently been presented [55–57], two of which already published. Both have evidenced a clear benefit in disease-specific survival and metastasis-free survival. Of note, no increased cardiac death rate has been reported in patients treated with the combination compared to EBRT alone.

In patients unfit to undergo aggressive local treatment or who refuse intervention, the question of immediate ADT, as is frequently used in the USA, is raised. This question has been recently examined by the EORTC trial 30891 [58]. After a median follow-up of 7.8 years, it was shown that an immediate ADT provides a small but statistically significant benefit in overall survival, but not in disease-specific survival. Most deaths are related to prostate cancer or cardiovascular disease. The many side effects of the therapy and the marginal survival benefit to be expected highlight the need for a straightforward, in-depth discussion with every patient before treatment initiation. Only for a subgroup of patients above 70 years of age, with PSA > 50 ng/ml and PSA-DT < 1 year, might really benefit from this approach.

Relapse and Survival: Is There a Relationship?

It must be highlighted that most available data on treatment efficacy are related to biological relapse-free survival, except for RP and recently EBRT where survival data are available. Biological relapse is still discussed as a surrogate endpoint for overall or specific survival [59].

Watch and Wait Policy

Two strategies are available for patients not receiving immediate treatment: "watchful waiting" (also "watch and wait" policy) and "active surveillance." These strategies have very different objectives. The rationale for watchful waiting is based on the assumption that many patients who die while having prostate cancer do not die of the cancer. On the opposite, suitable candidates for active surveillance are patients who have very low-risk tumors (low Gleason score, PSA level, and clinical stage), who might be cured by immediate active treatment. Treatment is postponed until signs of progression occur while the patient is still potentially curable [60]. Both attitudes have been extensively discussed elsewhere and should be systematically offered, especially in senior adults with low and intermediate risk. The decision between watchful waiting and active surveillance in senior adult patients should not be based solely on chronological age but rather on the estimated individual risk of dying of prostate cancer or of other causes.

Finally, Which Treatment for Which Patient?

Evidence suggests that, in both the USA [61] and Europe [62], only a minority of senior adults with localized prostate cancer receive curative therapy. The 2012 EAU guidelines recommend that "as a standard, an assessment of the patient's life expectancy, overall health status and tumor characteristics is necessary before any treatment decision can be made." It is also stated that "life expectancy, rather than patient age, should be the factor considered in treatment selection" [47]. These assumptions are perfectly in-line with the finding of the major role of <Gleason [17] and comorbidity [10] in terms of survival in localized PCa.

Alibhai et al. have evaluated treatment efficacy in men older than 65 years with localized prostate cancer by using a decision model integrating patient age, comorbidity, Gleason score, patient preferences, and treatment efficacy data [63]. Their results show that prostatectomy and EBRT significantly improve life expectancy and quality-adjusted life expectancy in older men with mild comorbidity and moderately or poorly differentiated prostate cancer. They conclude that "curative therapy should be seriously considered in men up to age 80 years who have high-grade disease." A population-based cohort study of men aged 75–84 years with clinically localized prostate cancer has shown that aggressive treatment (RP or EBRT) was more likely to induce urinary, bowel, and erectile dysfunction than conservative management [64]. The adjusted disease-specific mortality ratio was 0.43, favoring an aggressive treatment. However, the absolute 5-year disease-specific survival difference between groups was small (98 % vs. 92 %) since most deaths were from other causes. When offering patients older than 75 years aggressive treatments associated with uncertain survival benefits, a balance between expected survival and possible adverse treatment effects should be presented. As with the Swedish cohort of men older than 70 years [12], an observational study of 44,630 US patients aged 65–80 years with localized, well-, or moderately differentiated prostate cancer has suggested a significant overall survival advantage for patients receiving curative treatment, including men aged 75–80 years [65]. The survival benefit was again attributed to a reduction in non-prostate cancer mortality. Results of a Canadian population-based cohort of 6,183 men aged older than 70 years have demonstrated that 40 % of the patients selected for RP did not have sufficient life expectancy to warrant attempting curative therapy, and 70 % of those who received radiation therapy died before the 10-year cutoff point [66]. These findings highlight the need for more stringent selection criteria for radiation therapy and prostatectomy, including accurate health status assessment. This suggests that treatment decisions in senior adults should balance the risk of dying of prostate cancer with the risk of dying from another cause (i.e., severity and number of comorbidities that contribute to the patient's health status in general).

Finally, given that half of the patients with newly diagnosed prostate cancer are older than 70 years (corresponding to the group of elderly patients), specific studies must be performed to refine the decision making in this group. The objective is to eventually increase their chance of survival and their quality of life.

References

1. Altekruse SF, Kosary CL, Krapcho M, et al. SEER cancer statistics review, 1975–2007, National Cancer Institute. Bethesda. Available at: http://seer.cancer.gov/csr/1975_2007/, based on November 2009 SEER data submission, posted to the SEER web site; Accessed on January 2012..
2. U.S. Census Bureau, International Data Base. Available at: http://www.census.gov. Accessed on January 2012.
3. Droz JP, Balducci L, Bolla M, et al. Management of prostate cancer in older men: recommendations of a working group of the International Society of Geriatric Oncology. BJU Int. 2010;106:462–9.
4. NCCN guidelines on prostate cancer. Available at: http://www.nccn.org/professionals/physician_gls/PDF/prostate.pdf. Accessed on January 2012.
5. NCCN guidelines in senior adult oncology. Available at: http://www.nccn.org/professionals/physician_gls/PDF/senior.pdf. Accessed on January 2012.
6. Katz S, Ford AB, Moskowitz RW, Jackson BA, Jaffe MW. Studies of illness I the aged. The index of ADL: a standardized measure of biological and psychosocial function. JAMA. 1963;185:914–9.
7. Lawton MP, Brody EM. Assessment of older people: self-maintaining and instrumental activities of daily living. Gerontologist. 1969;9:179–86.
8. Linn BS, Linn MW, Gurel L. Cumulative illness rating scale. J Am Geriatr Soc. 1968;16:622–6.
9. Soubeyran P, Bellera C, Goyard J, et al. Validation of the G8 screening tool in geriatric oncology: the ONCODAGE project. J Clin Oncol. 2011;29(Suppl):9001.
10. Albertsen PC, Moore DF, Shih W, et al. Impact of comorbidity on survival among men with localized prostate cancer. J Clin Oncol. 2011;29:1335–41.
11. Tewari A, Johnson CC, Divine G, et al. Long-term survival probability in men with clinically localized prostate cancer: a case–control, propensity modeling study stratified by race, age, treatment and comorbidities. J Urol. 2004;171:1513–9.
12. Stattin P, Holmberg E, Johansson JE, Holmberg L, Adolfsson J, Hugosson J. Outcomes in localized prostate cancer: national prostate cancer register of Sweden follow-up study. J Natl Cancer Inst. 2010;102:950–8.
13. TNM Online. Available at: http://www3.interscience.wiley.com/cgibin/mrwhome/104554799/HOME. Accessed on January 2012.
14. Even Sapir E, Metser U, Mishina E, Lievshitz G, Lerman H, Leibovitch I. The detection of bone metastases in patients with high-risk prostate cancer: 99mTc-MDP planar bone scintigraphy,

single- and multi-field-of-view SPECT, 18F-fluoride PET, and 18F-fluoride PET/CT. J Nucl Med. 2006;47:287–97.

15. Gutzeit A, Doert A, Froehlich JM, et al. Comparison of diffusion-weighted whole body MRI and skeletal scintigraphy for the detection of bone metastases in patients with prostate or breast carcinoma. Skeletal Radiol. 2010;39:333–43.

16. D'Amico AV, Moul J, Carroll PR, Sun L, Lubeck D, Chen MH. Cancer-specific mortality after surgery or radiation for patients with clinically localized prostate cancer managed during the prostate-specific antigen era. J Clin Oncol. 2003;21:2163–72.

17. Lu-Yao GL, Albertsen PC, Moore DF, et al. Outcomes of localized prostate cancer following conservative management. JAMA. 2009;302:1202–9.

18. Albertsen PC, Hanley JA, Fine J. 20-year outcomes following conservative management of clinically localized prostate cancer. JAMA. 2005;293:2095–101.

19. Partin AW, Kattan MW, Subong EN, Walsh PC, Wojno KJ, Oesterling JE, et al. Combination of prostate-specific antigen, clinical stage, and Gleason score to predict pathological stage of localized prostate cancer. A multi-institutional update. JAMA. 1997;277:1445–51.

20. Shariat SF, Karakiewicz PI, Roehrborn CG, Kattan MW. An updated catalog of prostate cancer predictive tools. Cancer. 2008;113:3075–99.

21. D'Amico AV, Moul JW, Carroll PR, Sun L, Lubeck D, Chen MH. Surrogate end point for prostate cancer-specific mortality after radical prostatectomy or radiation therapy. J Natl Cancer Inst. 2003;95:1376–83.

22. Freedland SJ, Humphreys EB, Mangold LA, et al. Death in patients with recurrent prostate cancer after radical prostatectomy: prostate-specific antigen doubling time subgroups and their associated contributions to all-cause mortality. J Clin Oncol. 2007;25:1765–71.

23. D'Amico AV, Cote K, Loffredo M, Renshaw AA, Schultz D. Determinants of prostate cancer-specific survival after radiation therapy for patients with clinically localized prostate cancer. J Clin Oncol. 2002;20:4567–73.

24. Bill-Axelson A, Holmberg L, Filen F, et al. Radical prostatectomy versus watchful waiting in localized prostate cancer: the Scandinavian prostate cancer group-4 randomized trial. J Natl Cancer Inst. 2008;100:1144–54.

25. Begg CB, Riedel ER, Bach PB, et al. Variations in morbidity after radical prostatectomy. N Engl J Med. 2002;346:1138–44.

26. Sanchez-Salas R, Prapotnich D, Rozet F, et al. Laparoscopic radical prostatectomy is feasible and effective in 'fit' senior men with localized prostate cancer. BJU Int. 2010;106:1530–6.

27. Wilt TJ. The VA/NCI/AHRQ CSP#407: prostate cancer intervention versus observation trial (PIVOT). J Urol. 2011;185. LBA.

28. Shelley MD, Kumar S, Wilt T, Staffurth J, Coles B, Mason MD. A systematic review and meta-analysis of randomised trials of neo-adjuvant hormone therapy for localised and locally advanced prostate carcinoma. Cancer Treat Rev. 2009;35:9–17.

29. Wong YN, Freedland S, Egleston B, Hudes G, Schwartz JS, Armstrong K. Role of androgen deprivation therapy for node-positive prostate cancer. J Clin Oncol. 2009;27:100–5.

30. Boorjian SA, Karnes RJ, Crispen PL, et al. The impact of positive surgical margins on mortality following radical prostatectomy during the prostate specific antigen era. J Urol. 2010;183:1003–9.

31. Thompson IM, Tangen CM, Paradelo J, et al. Adjuvant radiotherapy for pathological T3N0M0 prostate cancer significantly reduces risk of metastases and improves survival: long-term followup of a randomized clinical trial. J Urol. 2009;181:956–62.

32. Bolla M, van Poppel H, Collette L, et al. Postoperative radiotherapy after radical prostatectomy: a randomised controlled trial (EORTC trial 22911). Lancet. 2005;366:572–8.

33. Wiegel T, Bottke D, Steiner U, et al. Phase III postoperative adjuvant radiotherapy after radical prostatectomy compared with radical prostatectomy alone in pT3 prostate cancer with postoperative undetectable prostate-specific antigen: ARO 96-02/AUO AP 09/95. J Clin Oncol. 2009;27:2924–30.

34. Stanford JL, Feng Z, Hamilton AS, et al. Urinary and sexual function after radical prostatectomy for clinically localized prostate cancer: the Prostate Cancer Outcomes Study. JAMA. 2000;283:354–60.

35. Xu DD, Sun SD, Wang F, et al. Effect of age and pathologic Gleason score on PSA recurrence: analysis of 2911 patients undergoing radical prostatectomy. Urology. 2009;74:654–8.
36. Barlow LJ, Badalato GM, Bashir T, Benson MC, McKiernan JM. The relationship between age at time of surgery and risk of biochemical failure after radical prostatectomy. BJU Int. 2010;105:1646–9.
37. Widmark A, Tomic R, Modig H, et al. Int J radiat Oncol Biol Phys. 2011;81(5). LBA. Available at: http://www.redjournal.org/content/astro_abstracts.
38. Kupelian P, Kuban D, Thames H, et al. Improved biochemical relapse-free survival with increased external radiation doses in patients with localized prostate cancer: the combined experience of nine institutions in patients treated in 1994 and 1995. Int J Radiat Oncol Biol Phys. 2005;61:415–9.
39. Roach III M, Bae K, Speight J, et al. Short-term neoadjuvant androgen deprivation therapy and external beam radiotherapy for locally advanced prostate cancer: long-term results of RTOG 8610. J Clin Oncol. 2008;26:585–91.
40. Bolla M, de Reijke TM, Van Tienhoven G, et al. Duration of androgen suppression in the treatment of prostate cancer. N Engl J Med. 2009;360:2516–27.
41. Zeliadt SB, Potosky AL, Penson DF, Etzioni R. Survival benefit associated with adjuvant androgen deprivation therapy combined with radiotherapy for high- and low-risk patients with nonmetastatic prostate cancer. Int J Radiat Oncol Biol Phys. 2006;66:395–402.
42. D'Amico AV, Chen MH, Renshaw AA, Loffredo M, Kantoff PW. Androgen suppression and radiation vs radiation alone for prostate cancer: a randomized trial. JAMA. 2008;299:289–95.
43. Jani AB, Parikh SD, Vijayakumar S, Gratzle J. Analysis of influence of age on acute and chronic radiotherapy toxicity in treatment of prostate cancer. Urology. 2005;65:1157–62.
44. Zelefsky MJ, Levin EJ, Hunt M, et al. Incidence of late rectal and urinary toxicities after three-dimensional conformal radiotherapy and intensity-modulated radiotherapy for localized prostate cancer. Int J Radiat Oncol Biol Phys. 2008;70(4):1124–9.
45. D'Amico AV, Cote K, Loffredo M, Renshaw AA, Chen MH. Advanced age at diagnosis is an independent predictor of time to death from prostate carcinoma for patients undergoing external beam radiation therapy for clinically localized prostate carcinoma. Cancer. 2003;97:56–62.
46. Heidenreich A, Aus G, Bolla M, et al. EAU guidelines on prostate cancer. Eur Urol. 2008;53:68–80.
47. European Association of Urology. Online guidelines on prostate cancer. Available at: http://www.uroweb.org/gls/pdf/Prostate%20Cancer%202010%20June%2017th.pdf. Accessed on February 2012.
48. Chen AB, D'Amico AV, Neville BA, Earle CC. Patient and treatment factors associated with complications after prostate brachytherapy. J Clin Oncol. 2006;24:5298–304.
49. Kupelian PA, Elshaikh M, Reddy CA, Zippe C, Klein EA. Comparison of the efficacy of local therapies for localized prostate cancer in the prostate-specific antigen era: a large single-institution experience with radical prostatectomy and external-beam radiotherapy. J Clin Oncol. 2002;20:3376–85.
50. Stephenson RA. Comparison of overall survival in localized prostate cancer with prostatectomy. EBRT and brachytherapy. J Urol. 2010;183:113.
51. Potosky AL, Davis WW, Hoffman RM, Stanford JL, Stephenson RA, Penson DF, et al. Five-year outcomes after prostatectomy or radiotherapy for prostate cancer: the prostate cancer outcomes study. J Natl Cancer Inst. 2004;96:1358–67.
52. Johansson E, Bill-Axelson A, Holmberg L, Onelov E, Johansson JE, Steineck G. Time, symptom burden, androgen deprivation, and self-assessed quality of life after radical prostatectomy or watchful waiting: the Randomized Scandinavian Prostate Cancer Group Study Number 4 (SPCG-4) clinical trial. Eur Urol. 2009;55:422–30.
53. Crouzet S, Rebillard X, Chevallier D, et al. Multicentric oncologic outcomes of high-intensity focused ultrasound for localized prostate cancer in 803 patients. Eur Urol. 2010;58:559–66.
54. Donnelly BJ, Saliken JC, Brasher PM, et al. A randomized trial of external beam radiotherapy versus cryoablation in patients with localized prostate cancer. Cancer. 2010;116:323–30.

55. Warde P, Mason MD, Ding K, et al. Intergroup randomized phase III study of androgen deprivation plus radiation therapy in locally advanced prostate cancer. Lancet. 2011;378: 2104–11.
56. Mottet N, Peneau M, Mazeron J, Molinie V, Richaud P. Impact of radiotherapy combined with androgen deprivation (ADT) versus ADT alone for local control in clinically locally advanced prostate cancer. J Clin Oncol. 2010;28:15s.
57. Widmark A, Klepp O, Solberg A, et al. Endocrine treatment, with or without radiotherapy, in locally advanced prostate cancer (SPCG-7/SFUO-3): an open randomised phase III trial. Lancet. 2009;373:301–8.
58. Studer UE, Whelan P, Albrecht W, et al. Immediate or deferred androgen deprivation for patients with prostate cancer not suitable for local treatment with curative intent: European Organisation for Research and Treatment of Cancer (EORTC) Trial 30891. J Clin Oncol. 2006;24:1868–76.
59. Collette L, Burzykowski T, Schroder FH. Prostate-specific antigen (PSA) alone is not an appropriate surrogate marker of long-term therapeutic benefit in prostate cancer trials. Eur J Cancer. 2006;42:1344–50.
60. Cooperber MR, Caroll PR, Klotz L. Active surveillance for prostate cancer: progress and promise. J Clin Oncol. 2011;29:3669–76.
61. Bubolz T, Wasson JH, Lu-Yao G, Barry MJ. Treatments for prostate cancer in older men: 1984–1997. Urology. 2001;58:977–82.
62. Houterman S, Janssen-Heijnen ML, Hendrikx AJ, van den Berg HA, Coebergh JW. Impact of comorbidity on treatment and prognosis of prostate cancer patients: a population-based study. Crit Rev Oncol Hematol. 2006;58:60–7.
63. Alibhai SM, Naglie G, Nam R, Trachtenberg J, Krahn MD. Do older men benefit from curative therapy of localized prostate cancer? J Clin Oncol. 2003;21:3318–27.
64. Hoffman RM, Barry MJ, Stanford JL, Hamilton AS, Hunt WC, Collins MM. Health outcomes in older men with localized prostate cancer: results from the Prostate Cancer Outcomes Study. Am J Med. 2006;119:418–25.
65. Wong YN, Mitra N, Hudes G, et al. Survival associated with treatment vs observation of localized prostate cancer in elderly men. JAMA. 2006;296:2683–93.
66. Jeldres C, Suardi N, Walz J, et al. Poor overall survival in septa- and octogenarian patients after radical prostatectomy and radiotherapy for prostate cancer: a population-based study of 6183 men. Eur Urol. 2008;54:107–16.

Part IV
Prostate Cancer: Metastatic Disease

Chapter 13
Clinical Management of Elderly Patients with Metastatic Prostate Cancer Chemotherapy

Guru Sonpavde and Cora N. Sternberg

Abstract Docetaxel and cabazitaxel chemotherapy have modestly extended survival as first- or second-line chemotherapy for patients with metastatic castration-resistant prostate cancer. Mitoxantrone chemotherapy may continue to play a palliative role in selected patients. In general, elderly age alone does not preclude chemotherapy or other therapies in patients that qualify based on a satisfactory biologic age, i.e., with no serious uncontrolled comorbidities, ECOG performance status 0–2, adequate organ and cognitive function, and satisfactory nutritional status and social support. Despite trends for increasing toxicities, selected elderly patients appear to generally tolerate chemotherapy and derive benefits similar to their younger counterparts. However, given the increased prevalence of comorbidities, functional impairments, and organ dysfunctions in the elderly, careful selection of patients coupled with dose modifications and prophylactic measures to avoid toxicities is necessary. Trials are also investigating the role of docetaxel for earlier stages of prostate cancer and comparing docetaxel with cabazitaxel as first-line chemotherapy. In the context of an increasing pipeline of novel approved agents (abiraterone acetate, sipuleucel-T) and emerging agents (radium-223, MDV-3100), optimal survival will probably be realized by the sequential utilization of several different classes of agents.

G. Sonpavde, M.D. (✉)
Section of Medical Oncology, Department of Medicine, Genitourinary medical oncology,
UAB Comprehensive Cancer Center,
Birmingham, Alabama, USA
e-mail: gsonpavde@gmail.com

C.N. Sternberg, M.D., FACP
Department of Medical Oncology, San Camillo and Forlanini Hospitals,
Rome, Italy
e-mail: cstern@mclink.it

J.-P. Droz, R.A. Audisio (eds.), *Management of Urological Cancers in Older People*,
Management of Cancer in Older People,
DOI 10.1007/978-0-85729-999-4_13, © Springer-Verlag London 2013

Keywords Metastatic • Castration-resistant prostate cancer • Abiraterone • MDV3100 • Docetaxel • Cabazitaxel • Mitoxantrone • Chemotherapy

Introduction

Even in the era of biologic agents, systemic chemotherapy continues to play an important role in the therapy of men with metastatic castration-resistant prostate cancer (CRPC). The continuing relevance of chemotherapy was recently demonstrated by the extension of survival by a novel taxane, cabazitaxel, in a docetaxel-pretreated population [1]. Given the advanced age of these patients in general, these data also indicate the relevance of chemotherapy in selected elderly patients. However, given the toxicity profile of cytotoxic agents, data supporting the elderly and fragile population warrants careful examination.

Functional Assessment and Definition of the "Elderly"

No consensus exists regarding a definitive age threshold to define elderly patients, with 65, 70, and 75 years commonly employed. Performance status alone may not adequately capture the functional status of elderly patients (Fig. 13.1). Additionally, it is unclear whether a poor functional status secondary to advanced tumor should be managed differently (potentially more aggressively) as opposed to poor functional status from advanced age or comorbidities (potentially less aggressively). Age leads to physiologic reduction in organ function, and the reduction of renal and hepatic function in particular may impact the pharmacokinetic and pharmacodynamic properties of drugs leading to poorer clearance and increased toxicities. Moreover, the reduction of bone marrow reserve may increase the risk of severe myelosuppression. Malignancies in the elderly are associated with adverse functional consequences, i.e., vulnerability and frailty [2]. The caveat is that while the healthy and frail patients are relatively easy to identify, the clinically healthy but functionally susceptible, i.e., vulnerable, appear to be difficult to identify.

Nevertheless, it may be conceptually relevant and clinically useful to functionally classify the elderly into healthy, vulnerable, and frail patients as suggested by the comprehensive geriatric assessment (CGA) scale (Fig. 13.2) [3]. CGA constitutes a comprehensive evaluation of an older individual's functional status, comorbidities, cognition, psychological state, social support, and nutritional status, and a review of medications. According to National Comprehensive Cancer Network (NCCN), CGA should be adopted for vulnerable older cancer patients. However, its adoption has been retarded by a lack of resources and problematic interpretation of results. The geriatric assessment includes an assessment of activities of daily living (ADLs) and instrumental activities of daily living (IADLs). ADLs represent basic self-care, i.e., the ability to bathe, dress, toilet, feed oneself, maintain continence, and transfer from a bed or chair without assistance. IADL skills are higher level

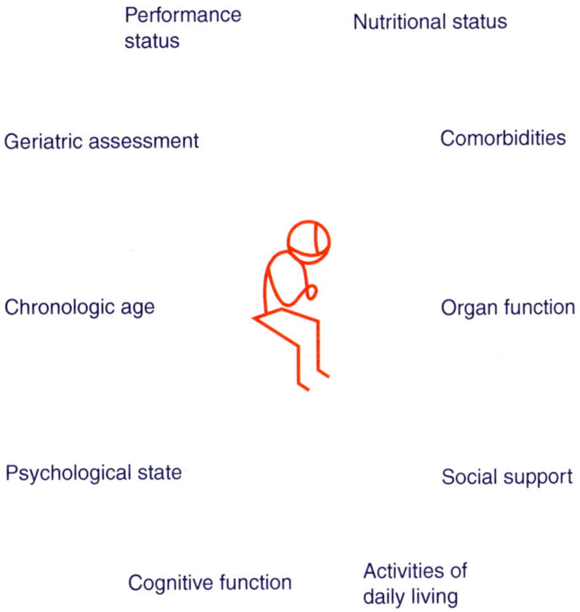

Fig. 13.1 Pre-chemotherapy clinical evaluation of elderly men with metastatic CRPC

Performance status

Nutritional status

Geriatric assessment

Comorbidities

Chronologic age

Organ function

Psychological state

Social support

Cognitive function

Activities of daily living

skills required to maintain independence including using the telephone, transportation, shopping, housework, and managing finances and medications.

One clinical tool for recognizing frailty combines several components of a comprehensive geriatric assessment, including age > 85 years, dependence in ≥1 activities of daily living, ≥3 comorbidities, and the presence of a geriatric syndrome [4]. Another assessment tool is the Vulnerable Elders Survey (VES)-13, with vulnerability defined as a score of ≥3 [5]. The component variables in the VES-13 score are age (1 point for age 75–84 years and 3 points for age 85 years or older), self-rated health status (1 point for fair or poor), difficulty with physical activities (1 point for difficulty with each of six physical activities, with a maximum of 2 points), and difficulties with functional activities (maximum of 4 points for presence of any functional limitation). Recently, a brief geriatric assessment tool consisting of functional status, comorbidity, cognitive function, psychological state, social support, and nutritional status appeared suitable for inclusion in clinical trials [6]. This tool took a median of 22 min to complete and may facilitate routine geriatric assessment in patients with advanced malignancies.

Comorbidity Assessment

The consistent emergence of comorbidities as an independent prognostic factor suggests that the comorbidity index may be ready for prime time and for formal incorporation in trials and clinical decision making. Comorbidities are likely to have the

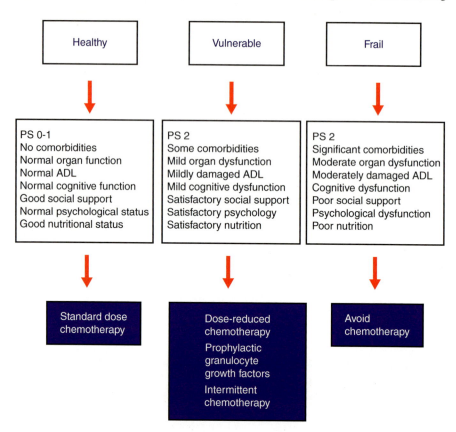

Fig. 13.2 Decision making regarding chemotherapy for elderly patients ≥75 years with metastatic CRPC

greatest negative impact in those expected to survive longer, i.e., those with a more favorable malignancy-related prognosis [7]. The Charlson comorbidity index (CCI) is easy to calculate and is widely used in both benign and malignant conditions [8]. However, the CCI was developed in an inpatient population admitted for various medical conditions and not specifically in those with malignancies. Thereafter, the CCI has been identified to be prognostic in multiple advanced malignancies, although prospective validation is warranted. There are 22 variables that are necessary to calculate the CCI in addition to age including the presence or absence of AIDS (acquired immunodeficiency syndrome), cerebrovascular disease, chronic pulmonary disease, congestive heart failure, connective tissue disease, dementia, hemiplegia, leukemia, lymphoma, myocardial infarction, peripheral vascular disease, and peptic ulcer disease. Additionally, the following diseases are graded: diabetes mellitus (with or without end organ damage), liver disease (none, mild, moderate, severe), renal disease (none, mild, moderate, severe), and malignant solid tumor (none, nonmetastatic, metastatic).

The Adult Comorbidity Evaluation (ACE)-27 has been specifically validated as an independent prognostic factor for patients with a range of solid malignancies, although it requires an independent reviewer and is not patient self-assessed [9]. It is noteworthy that discrimination with ACE-27 was highest for early prostate cancer. ACE-27 grades diseases into 1–3 levels of severity, and an overall comorbidity score (none, mild, moderate, severe) is assigned based on the highest-ranked single disease. Patients are deemed to have severe comorbidities if ≥2 moderately severe organ decompensations are detected. Both the CCI and ACE-27 can be derived by calculators available online or by handheld devices. Furthermore, other comorbidity indices exist in addition to the CCI and ACE-27 that are beyond the scope of description in this chapter. More extensive and prospective malignancy-specific validation of comorbidity indices is warranted to identify a tangible role in clinical decision making.

Docetaxel-Based Chemotherapy

The TAX327 and SWOG-9916 trials accrued both symptomatic and relatively asymptomatic patients and demonstrated survival benefits regardless of risk groups based on pain, visceral metastasis, anemia, and bone scan progression [10, 11].

Activity of Docetaxel

Docetaxel-based chemotherapy replaced mitoxantrone-prednisone (MP) as a standard in 2004 for the management of metastatic CRPC based on the pivotal TAX327 and SWOG-9916 trials (Table 13.1) [11, 12]. Although the median age was 68–70 years in these trials, men up to ~90 years were enrolled (Table 13.1). In the phase III TAX-327 study, 1,006 men were recruited and randomized to weekly (30 mg/m^2 every week for 5 of 6 weeks) or every 3-week (75 mg/m^2) schedules of docetaxel or the historical standard, mitoxantrone (12 mg/m^2 every 3 weeks), with all patients receiving prednisone 5 mg twice daily orally [3]. Therapy was administered until progressive disease and up to a maximum of 10 cycles for the groups given docetaxel or mitoxantrone every 3 weeks and up to 5 cycles (of 6 weeks each) in the weekly docetaxel group. Dose reductions and/or delays were required for grade 4 neutropenia for ≥7 days, infection, neutropenic fever, absolute neutrophil count <1,500/mm^3 for those on 3-week schedules (<1,000/mm^3 for those receiving weekly docetaxel), or platelet count <50,000/mm^3 on a treatment day. Treatment with granulocyte colony-stimulating factor was allowed for patients with febrile neutropenia.

Eligible patients were required to exhibit progressive disease defined as increasing serum PSA on three consecutive measurements at least 1 week apart or by clinical or radiographic criteria. The Karnofsky performance status score was required

Table 13.1 Reported randomized phase III chemotherapy trials for metastatic CRPC

Author (reference)	N	Median age (range) in years	Setting	Control group	Experimental group	Improved survival
Tannock et al. [18]	161	69 (63–75)	First line	P	MP	No, improved QOL
Kantoff et al. [30]	242	72 (65–75)	First line	H	MH	No, improved PFS
Tannock et al. [10]	1,006	68 (36–92)	First line	MP	DP	Yes
Petrylak et al. [11]	770	70 (43–88)	First line	MP	EMP-Docetaxel	Yes
Sternberg et al. [32]	950	70 (42–88)	Second line	P	Satraplatin-P	No, improved PFS
de Bono et al. [1]	755	68 (62–73)	Second line	MP	Cabazitaxel-P	Yes

Index: *N* number of patients, *P* prednisone, *MP* mitoxantrone/prednisone, *QOL* quality of life, *H* hydrocortisone, *MH* mitoxantrone/hydrocortisone, *PFS* progression free survival, *DP* 3-weekly docetaxel/prednisone, *EMP* estramustine phosphate

to be at least 60 %. Patients with brain or leptomeningeal metastases and peripheral neuropathy $\geq$ grade 2 were excluded. Prior radiotherapy was limited to no more than 25 % of the bone marrow. Additionally, adequate hematologic (neutrophil count $\geq$1,500/mm^3, a hemoglobin $\geq$10.0 g/dL, a platelet count $\geq$100,000/mm^3), hepatic (bilirubin level < the upper limit of the normal [ULN] and serum ALT, AST 1.5 times ULN), and renal function (creatinine $\leq$ 1.5 $\times$ ULN).

Progressive disease was defined as pain progression (defined as an increase in the PPI score (present pain intensity) of $\geq$1 point from the nadir, an increase in the analgesic score of $\geq$25 %, or a requirement for palliative radiotherapy); PSA progression was defined as an increase from the nadir of either $\geq$25 % for men with no PSA response or $\geq$50 % for all others or objective progression of measurable disease. Pain response was defined as a reduction in the PPI score of $\geq$2 points from baseline without an increase in the analgesic score or as a reduction of $\geq$50 % in the analgesic score without an increase in the PPI score, either of which was maintained for $\geq$3 weeks.

The median age of enrolled patients was 68 years and ~20 % were $\geq$75 years old. Approximately 45 % had pain. The median survival was 19.2 months in the 3-week docetaxel group, 17.8 months with weekly docetaxel, and 16.3 months with mitoxantrone. The 3-year survivals were 17.9, 16.7, and 13.7 %, respectively [12]. Only 3-week docetaxel plus prednisone attained statistical superiority when compared to MP. The survival benefit of docetaxel plus prednisone given every 3 weeks was consistent across subgroups defined according to the presence or absence of pain, Karnofsky performance status score ($\leq$70 vs. $\geq$80), and age (<65 vs. $\geq$65 years). More patients in the 3-week docetaxel arm experienced a significant reduction in pain compared to mitoxantrone (35 vs. 22 %, $P = 0.01$). Nearly a quarter of patients in each docetaxel arm (22 % with 3-week and 23 % with weekly) exhibited a significant improvement in quality of life (QOL) compared with mitoxantrone (13 %). PSA response rate was better in each docetaxel arm: 45 % with every-3-week administration and 48 % with weekly administration versus 32 %

with mitoxantrone. Men with minimal symptoms had prolonged survival (median, 25.6 months) compared with symptomatic patients (median, 17.1 months; $P=0.009$), but they were more likely to have initial deterioration of QOL with weekly docetaxel [13]. PSA and pain response, but not QOL response, were independently associated with survival.

In the Southwest Oncology Group (SWOG)-9916 phase III trial, 770 patients with metastatic CRPC were randomized to combination docetaxel-EMP or MP [11]. A SWOG performance status score of 0–2 was necessary although a performance status of 3 was allowed if the score was due to bone pain. Patients were ineligible if they had received prior radioisotope, radiotherapy to 30 %, or more of the bone marrow; were currently on anticoagulant therapy (excluding aspirin); and had active thrombophlebitis, hypercoagulability, or a history of pulmonary embolus.

Patients in the docetaxel-EMP group received docetaxel 60 mg/m^2 every 3 weeks plus 5 consecutive days of EMP 280 mg given orally for 3 times a day. Patients in the MP group received mitoxantrone 12 mg/m^2 every 3 weeks plus continuous prednisone at a dose of 5 mg twice a day. Patients who did not experience grade 3/4 toxicity in the first cycle of therapy underwent dose escalation of docetaxel to 70 mg/m^2 and mitoxantrone to 14 mg/m^2. The protocol was amended to include daily coumadin (2 mg) and aspirin (325 mg) in the docetaxel-EMP group. Treatment continued until disease progression or unacceptable adverse effects occurred or until a maximum of 12 cycles of docetaxel-EMP or 144 mg/m^2 of mitoxantrone had been administered. Progression was defined as objective or PSA progression (≥ 25 % and ≥ 5 ng/mL increase in the serum PSA over the last preregistration or nadir measurement, with confirmation of the increase at least 4 weeks later) or death.

The median age of enrolled men was 70 years, with a range of ~47–88 years. The median survival was significantly improved by the docetaxel-EMP combination (17.5 vs. 15.6 months, $P=0.02$), the relative risk of death was reduced by 20 %, and the PSA response rate was significantly better (50 vs. 27 %, $P<0.001$). The median time to progression was 6.3 months for docetaxel-EMP and 3.2 months for MP ($P<0.001$).

Toxicity Profile of Docetaxel

In the TAX327 trial, Grade 3/4 neutropenia occurred in 32 % of patients treated with every-3-week docetaxel, 22 % treated with mitoxantrone, and only 1.5 % treated with weekly docetaxel. However, febrile neutropenia and infection were uncommon in all groups (0–3 %), and there were no septic deaths. There was a higher incidence of grade 3–4 cardiac dysfunction among patients who received mitoxantrone compared to both docetaxel groups (7 vs. 1–2 %). Docetaxel induced more fatigue, alopecia, diarrhea, nail changes, sensory neuropathy, anorexia, changes in taste, stomatitis, dyspnea, tearing, peripheral edema, and epistaxis. Most adverse events associated with docetaxel were low grade and not life threatening, with loss of sensation in the fingers and toes being particularly annoying to some patients. Most patients received the prescribed doses on schedule, with 8–12 % requiring a dose reduction and 21–34 % requiring at least one chemotherapy infusion to be delayed.

In the SWOG-9916 trial, docetaxel-EMP was more toxic with more grade 3/4 gastrointestinal (20 vs. 5 %), hematologic (neutropenic fever, 5 vs. 2 %), cardiovascular (15 vs. 7 %), metabolic (6 vs. 1 %), and neurologic events (7 vs. 2 %). A similar number of men had therapy-related deaths (n = 8 and n = 4, with docetaxel-EMP and MP, respectively).

Necessity of Estramustine and Prednisone

Weekly docetaxel may be considered in more frail patients, given the palliative benefits and lower myelosuppression, although the value of this strategy compared to dose-reduced docetaxel every 3 weeks or conventional doses every 3 weeks with prophylactic granulocyte growth factors every 3 weeks is unclear. EMP is associated with significant gastrointestinal and thromboembolic toxicities that have led to decreased usage, despite one meta-analysis demonstrating a modest improvement in survival by the addition of EMP to multiple partnering agents [14]. The rate of arterial and venous thromboembolic events in men with CRPC who are treated with EMP-based regimens was 7 % and was not related to the dose of EMP [15]. Moreover, the value of concurrent anticoagulation to prevent such events is unclear.

The toxicities of chronic daily prednisone may raise the question of its value. However, the potential value of combining with prednisone is provided by the ASCENT-2 and VITAL-2 trials that compared conventional 3-week docetaxel in combination with DN-101 (high-dose calcitriol) or GVAX (an investigational vaccine), respectively [16, 17]. Both of these trials suggested poorer outcomes in the experimental arms that did not administer daily prednisone; additionally, ASCENT-2 administered weekly docetaxel in the experimental arm only. Hence, the combination of docetaxel plus prednisone may be the preferred regimen in the absence of prohibitive contraindications for administering low-dose daily oral prednisone. Conversely, in patients that are not candidates for chemotherapy or other biologic options, a palliative role may exist for daily low-dose prednisone alone. Prednisone alone may induce ≥50 % PSA declines in up to 22 % of patients and palliative responses in ~15 % of patients [18].

Value of Intermittent Docetaxel and Continuing Beyond 10–12 Cycles

The concept of intermittent treatment was evaluated in the ASCENT-1 trial, where patients could suspend therapy if PSA declined ≥50 % and to ≤4 ng/mL [19]. Docetaxel was resumed upon clinical progression or if the PSA increased by ≥50 %

and to ≥2 ng/mL. Of the 250 patients on this trial, 18 % of patients underwent intermittent chemotherapy after a median of 22 weeks. The median duration of the first chemotherapy holiday was 18 weeks (range, 4–70 weeks), and on resuming therapy, 45.5 % of patients displayed a ≥50 % PSA decline. It is reasonable to hypothesize that intermittent chemotherapy may be a valuable strategy in vulnerable or frail elderly patients (Fig. 13.1). In a retrospective analysis of 39 patients, the interval between the last cycle of first-line docetaxel and progression was associated with PFS with second-line re-administration of docetaxel [20]. The median PFS with second-line docetaxel was 3.4 months and 6.3 months in patients with an interval <3.0 months and ≥3.0 months, respectively. A phase 3 trial, PON-PC-02, is comparing 10 cycles of DP with intermittent DP after at least 4 cycles if PSA declines >50 % and is powered for demonstrating non-inferiority of intermittent therapy.

The optimal number of cycles is empiric with TAX327 allowing up to 10 cycles and SWOG-9916 allowing up to 12 cycles. The numbers of cycles were arbitrarily chosen due to concern for cumulative cardiotoxicity of mitoxantrone and neurotoxicity of docetaxel, although a recent retrospective analysis suggests that the impact of continuing docetaxel beyond 10 cycles may be marginal [21]. In addition, this retrospective analysis suggested a trend for reduced survival with fewer than 10 cycles. Intriguingly, data indicate that the clearance of docetaxel in the castrate environment may be substantially accelerated, suggesting that the currently employed dose (which was developed in a non-castrate environment) may be less than the optimal biologic dose in CRPC patients [22].

Second-Line Docetaxel Following Prior Mitoxantrone

Treatment with second-line docetaxel following prior MP and retreatment in those displaying an excellent prior response to docetaxel appear to be reasonable strategies. In the TAX327 trial, 232 patients crossed over to docetaxel after mitoxantrone and vice versa [23]. Median survival for the entire group was ~10 months and did not depend on direction of crossover. PSA response occurred in fewer men (15 % of 71) receiving mitoxantrone after docetaxel, compared to those receiving docetaxel after mitoxantrone (28 % of 25 men). Moreover, docetaxel demonstrated activity with PSA responses in 36 % of patients following ixabepilone [24].

Docetaxel in Elderly Men with Metastatic CRPC

As already alluded to, the TAX327 trial demonstrated similar improvements in outcomes for men 65 years or older compared to younger than 65 years. Among 335 patients in TAX327 treated with DP every 3 weeks, 38 % were <65 years old, 42 % were 65–74 years, and 20 % were ≥75 years. There were nonsignificant associations of poorer tolerability and efficacy with advancing age among men receiving DP (Ian

Tannock, M.D., Ph.D., personal communication 2012). Among men ≥75 years, DP was associated with more frequent dose reductions, but tolerability was otherwise comparable to weekly docetaxel. However, given that every-3-week DP was associated with better survival but similar tolerability compared to weekly docetaxel, it should probably remain the preferred regimen. Weekly docetaxel may continue to play a role in selected patients with a significant concern for myelosuppression and indeed is still employed in the community. The caveat is that these patients were eligible for a phase III trial and were likely "healthy" elderly patients. Hence, in the community, a greater proportion of vulnerable or frail elderly patients may be expected to be treated off-protocol. The implication may be that dose and schedule modifications and aggressive supportive care may be necessary in such elderly patients in the community.

Another small study reported the efficacy of docetaxel 70 mg/m^2 every 3 weeks for 20 CRPC patients aged 75 or higher (older group) and 31 patients younger than 75 years (younger group) [25]. The median relative dose intensity of both groups was 0.84, while the median dose intensity and the number of treatment cycles of the younger and older groups were 14.6 versus 12.3 mg/m^2/week ($P=0.021$) and 9 versus 8 cycles ($P=0.15$), respectively. No significant differences were observed in outcomes or adverse events in both groups.

Impact of Comorbidities on Outcomes with Docetaxel-Based Chemotherapy

Comorbidities, especially cardiovascular and pulmonary diseases, are common in the elderly. The impact of baseline comorbidities was analyzed in a randomized phase III trial of men who received docetaxel and prednisone with or without bevacizumab [26, 27]. Fourteen comorbid conditions including cardiovascular, hypertension, diabetes, arthritis, thrombosis, AIDS, renal disease, liver disease, and peptic ulcer were prospectively collected at baseline, and the proportional hazards model was used to test if comorbidity number (CON) predicted survival after adjusting for treatment arm, age, race, and body mass index and predicted survival probability at 24 months using the CALGB nomogram [28]. There was a statistically significant association between comorbidity number and death, and the hazard ratio (HR) for death for one unit increase in CON was 1.09 ($P=0.0008$).

Docetaxel as the Platform to Develop Combination Regimens

Preliminary evidence of enhanced outcomes has been demonstrated with multiple classes of novel agents in combination with docetaxel. Unfortunately, the addition of bevacizumab, lenalidomide, or endothelin receptor antagonists (atrasentan, zibotentan) to docetaxel has not yielded benefits in phase III trials [27]. Agents targeting the stroma (aflibercept, tasquinimod) and novel molecular targets (Src, clusterin antisense oligonucleotide) are being evaluated in phase III trials that utilize a docetaxel backbone (Table 13.1). The exploration of doublet chemotherapy-based combinations with biologic agents usually does not exclude elderly men with satisfactory performance status and no serious uncontrolled comorbidities.

Cabazitaxel Chemotherapy

Efficacy of Cabazitaxel

Cabazitaxel, a novel semisynthetic taxane, stabilizes microtubules as potently as docetaxel, is preclinically active in both docetaxel-sensitive and docetaxel-resistant cell lines, demonstrated resistance to the P-gp efflux pump, and was able to penetrate the blood-brain barrier. Cabazitaxel plus prednisone was compared with MP for progressive mCRPC following prior docetaxel in the TROPIC trial, which enrolled 755 patients (Table 13.1) [1]. The Eastern Cooperative Oncology Group (ECOG) performance status was required to be 0–2 and prior radiotherapy to $\geq 40\%$ of the bone marrow, and peripheral neuropathy > grade 1 were not allowed.

Patients were randomized to a maximum of 10 cycles of cabazitaxel 25 mg/m^2 intravenously over one hour every 3 weeks ($n=378$) or mitoxantrone 12 mg/m^2 every 3 weeks, and both groups received prednisone 10 mg daily ($n=377$). Premedication was required when administering cabazitaxel including an antihistamine, corticosteroid, and H2 antagonist due to the polysorbate-80 solvent. One dose reduction (cabazitaxel 20 mg/m^2 or mitoxantrone 10 mg/m^2) was allowed, and prophylactic granulocyte colony-stimulating factor was not allowed during the first cycle, but was allowed (at physicians' discretion) after first occurrence of neutropenia lasting ≥ 7 days or for neutropenic infection. Complete blood counts were measured weekly each treatment cycle. Patients continued therapy until 10 cycles or progression defined by PSA or clinical criteria, i.e., PCWG-2 guidelines were not employed.

The median age of patients in the 2 arms was 67–68 years, and 18–19 % were ≥ 75 years old. The vast majority of patients had a performance status of 0–1 (91–93 %). The patients had received a median of 7 cycles of prior docetaxel, and the median time from prior docetaxel to progression was 0.7–0.8 months, suggesting a docetaxel-resistant population. The median survival was significantly prolonged by cabazitaxel plus prednisone as compared to MP (15.1 vs. 12.7 months; hazard ratio 0.70, $P<0.0001$). The extension of survival was observed irrespective of performance status, number of prior chemotherapy regimens, time to progression from prior docetaxel, and age. Secondary endpoints demonstrated improvements with cabazitaxel: progression-free survival 2.8 versus 1.4 months, $P<0.001$; measurable tumor response rate 14.4 versus 4.4 %, $P=0.005$; PSA response rates 39.2 versus 17.8 %, $P=0.002$; and time to PSA progression 6.4 versus 3.1 months, $P=0.0010$;

however, pain response was similar (9.2 vs. 7.7 %, $P=0.6286$). This drug has now been approved in both the USA and Europe. A randomized phase III trial is comparing frontline chemotherapy with docetaxel or cabazitaxel 25 mg/m^2 or 20 mg/m^2.

Toxicities of Cabazitaxel

The prominent grade ≥ 3 toxicities with cabazitaxel were febrile neutropenia (8 vs. 1 %), diarrhea (6 vs. <1 %), and fatigue (5 vs. 3 %). Deaths due to adverse events occurred in 5 % in the cabazitaxel arm, as compared to 2 % in the mitoxantrone arm. Grade ≥ 3 neutropenia occurred in 82 % of patients with cabazitaxel versus 58 % with mitoxantrone. Owing to the substantial myelosuppression, weekly blood cell counts are recommended during the first cycle of cabazitaxel, and prophylactic granulocyte growth factor support is advocated in accordance with ASCO (American Society of Clinical Oncology) guidelines. Grade 3 peripheral neuropathy was reported in 3 (1 %) patients in each arm, and peripheral neuropathy of all grades was reported in 52 (14 %) on cabazitaxel and 12 (3 %) on mitoxantrone. Peripheral edema occurred in 34 (9 %) patients in each arm. Statistical trends for differences ($P<0.1$) in rates of adverse events were observed by age, previous radiotherapy, and geographical region: neutropenia by age <65 versus ≥ 65 years (17.6 vs. 24.2 %); neutropenia by region, North America (25.7 %), Europe (16.1 %), and other (35.1 %); diarrhea by age <75 versus ≥ 75 years (44.5 vs. 55.7 %); and diarrhea by prior radiotherapy versus no radiotherapy (50 vs. 41.4 %).

Abiraterone acetate is also approved for the post-docetaxel setting and is felt to possess a more favorable toxicity profile and may be more tolerable in those with a borderline performance status [29]. The most optimal outcomes may be attained by sequential administration of all active agents. In this context, MDV3100, an oral androgen receptor antagonist, recently demonstrated improved survival following docetaxel and does not require concurrent prednisone. Moreover, radium-223 extended survival for symptomatic patients with bone metastases. Given the excellent tolerability for both MDV3100 and radium-2234, both of these novel agents, once approved, may be excellent options following docetaxel in the elderly.

Mitoxantrone Plus Prednisone

Efficacy of Mitoxantrone-Prednisone

Although mitoxantrone was inferior to docetaxel as first-line chemotherapy, a palliative role may still exist following prior chemotherapy. In the 1990s, combination mitoxantrone plus prednisone (MP) was established as the conventional first-line chemotherapy regimen for men with metastatic CRPC based on palliative benefits demonstrated in two randomized trials (Table 13.1) [18, 30]. The Canadian open-label trial randomized 161 symptomatic metastatic CRPC patients to prednisone 5 mg twice daily versus mitoxantrone 12 mg/m^2 every 3 weeks plus prednisone 5 mg twice daily. A cumulative mitoxantrone dose of 140 mg/m^2 was stipulated to mitigate cardiac toxicity. Palliative response defined by a $\geq$2-point decline in pain on the 6-point McGill pain questionnaire was the major endpoint. Palliative response occurred significantly more often with MP compared to prednisone alone (29 vs. 12 %, $P < 0.01$). In addition, a significantly longer duration of response of 43 weeks versus 18 weeks ($P = <0.001$) was also attained. Overall survival was not different with a median survival of approximately 1 year in both groups, potentially due to crossover or limited power.

The second trial, CALGB-9182, accrued 242 patients with or without pain and had a primary endpoint of overall survival. This trial evaluated hydrocortisone 30 mg in the morning and 10 mg in the afternoon with or without mitoxantrone 14 mg/m^2 every 3 weeks, and crossover was not permitted. Overall survival was not significantly different with a median of approximately 1 year. The duration of response with chemotherapy was significantly longer (3.7 vs. 2.3 months, $P = 0.025$), and improvement in pain control was also observed. These studies established mitoxantrone chemotherapy as a viable option for palliative treatment in patients with metastatic CRPC.

PSA response has been demonstrated in 15 % of patients receiving MP following prior docetaxel in the TAX327 trial [23]. Corroborative evidence for modest activity was provided by another randomized phase II trial [31]. Given the excellent toxicity profile, MP may be considered a reasonable salvage chemotherapy option in patients following prior docetaxel and/or cabazitaxel. However, the decision to institute MP as salvage chemotherapy needs to be made in the context of multiple approved (abiraterone acetate) and emerging agents (MDV3100, radium-223) and the option of enrolling patients in clinical trials evaluating other promising agents (e.g., ipilimumab, cabozantinib). Notably, one planned phase III trial that evaluates cabozantinib is employing MP as the standard arm following prior docetaxel and cabazitaxel.

Toxicities of Mitoxantrone

Among 130 patients in the Canadian trial who received mitoxantrone (including crossover), 5 patients receiving cumulative doses of 116–214 mg/m^2 developed cardiac dysfunction [18]. Two of these five patients displayed symptomatic congestive heart failure, but none died of cardiac causes. Notably, cardiac dysfunction from anthracyclines may develop at a delayed time point after completion of therapy. Only 9 of 130 patients experienced neutropenic fever, and alopecia and emesis were rare. In the CALGB trial, cardiac dysfunction and neutropenic infections were infrequent with mitoxantrone therapy.

Table 13.2 Selected chemotherapeutic agents with activity in phase II trials of metastatic CRPC

Chemotherapy regimen (references)	Class of agent	Mechanism of action	PSA response rate (%)
Ixabepilone [31, 34]	Epothilone	Microtubule stabilizer	First line: 33
			Second line: 17
Ixabepilone-mitoxantrone [36]	Epothilone	Microtubule stabilizer	Second line: 31
Eribulin mesylate [39]	Halichondrin B analogue	Microtubule inhibitor	First line: 22.4
			Second line: 8.5
Nab-paclitaxel [65]	Taxane	Microtubule stabilizer	First line: 25
Patupilone [37]	Epothilone	Microtubule stabilizer	Second line: 45
Sagopilone [38]	Epothilone	Microtubule stabilizer	First line: 42
Carboplatin-docetaxel [33]	Platinum	Cross-links DNA	Second line: 18

Other Chemotherapeutic Agents with Activity in CRPC

Platinum Agents

Satraplatin, a third-generation orally available investigational platinum analogue, demonstrated a 33 % reduction in the risk of progression or death following one prior chemotherapy regimen in the phase III placebo-controlled SPARC (Satraplatin and Prednisone Against Refractory Cancer) trial (Table 13.1) [32]. Satraplatin also demonstrated beneficial effects on pain and biologic activity with PSA declines and objective responses. However, satraplatin and prednisone did not extend median survival compared to placebo and prednisone (14.3 months in both groups). Data suggest a possible increment in activity by employing docetaxel in combination with platinum agents as evidenced by modest activity demonstrated by the combination of carboplatin with docetaxel in patients progressing following docetaxel alone (Table 13.2) [33]. The combination of carboplatin with docetaxel yielded PSA declines ≥50 % in 18 % of patients and measurable responses in 14 % of patients progressing within 45 days following docetaxel alone [33]. Patients more likely to respond to the combination were those that had previously responded to docetaxel.

Tubulin Targeting Agents

Epothilones stabilize tubulin assembly and have demonstrated activity in phase II trials. Ixabepilone has demonstrated antitumor activity similar to that of docetaxel as monotherapy or in combination with EMP in the first-line setting (Table 13.2) [34, 35]. While single-agent ixabepilone yields PSA responses in 15–20 % of patients following prior docetaxel, the combination of ixabepilone and mitoxantrone appears to have additive activity in the second-line setting (Table 13.2) [31, 36]. Patupilone is being compared with docetaxel in a randomized phase II trial for metastatic CRPC based on preliminary activity (Table 13.2) [37]. Sagopilone in combination with prednisone has demonstrated activity similar to docetaxel-prednisone as first-line therapy for metastatic CRPC [38]. Eribulin, a halichondrin B analogue, without concurrent daily prednisone demonstrated activity similar to docetaxel in a nonrandomized phase II trial in both taxane-naïve and taxane-pretreated patients with metastatic CRPC [39]. Given the similar long-term outcomes compared to docetaxel and the lack of requirement for steroid premedication and somewhat lower neurotoxicity (when comparing across trials), eribulin may warrant further development in elderly patients.

Metastatic CRPC with Neuroendocrine Differentiation

Small-cell neuroendocrine carcinoma occurs in 0.5–2.0 % of prostatic cancer primary tumor and may be more common in the castration-resistant state. Visceral metastasis especially in the setting of a relatively low PSA and elevated serum neuron-specific enolase or chromogranin A may raise suspicion for the small-cell variant. These tumors may secrete adrenocorticotropic hormone or antidiuretic hormone. Therapy for advanced small-cell carcinomas of the prostate is extrapolated from therapy for small-cell carcinomas of the lung. Small studies have demonstrated the activity of platinum- and etoposide-based regimens [40].

Predicting Chemotherapy-Induced Toxicities in Elderly Patients

Emerging data indicate that toxicities may precipitate geriatric syndromes and older patients discontinue chemotherapy sooner. In a recent prospective trial, the following variables independently predicted grade ≥ 3 toxicities from chemotherapy in a range of advanced malignancies in patients aged ≥65 years: age ≥72 years, cancer type (gastrointestinal or genitourinary), standard dosing of chemotherapy, polychemotherapy, hemoglobin (males: <11 g/dL; females: <10 g/dL), creatinine clearance <34 mL/min, hearing impairment, ≥1 fall in the last 6 months, limited in walking one block, need for assistance in taking medications, and decreased social activities [41]. Moreover, this model outperformed performance status in the ability to predict toxicities. Older adults at low (30 %), intermediate (52 %), and high risk (83 %) of chemotherapy-induced grade 3–5 toxicities were identified based on a scoring system. Notably, increasing comorbidities (Charlson comorbidity score > 2) correlated with early discontinuation of chemotherapy in advanced lung cancer [42].

Another prospective trial devised the Chemotherapy Risk Assessment Scale for High-Age Patients (CRASH) score to predict hematologic and non-hematologic toxicities, although a global model to predict all toxicities did not attain significance [43]. The CRASH score stratified patients into four risk categories (low, medium low, medium high, and high). Predictors of hematologic toxicity were lymphocytes, aspartate aminotransferase level, IADL score, lactate dehydrogenase level, diastolic blood pressure, and chemotherapy. Predictors of non-hematologic toxicity were hemoglobin, creatinine clearance, albumin, self-rated health, performance status, mini-mental status score, Mini-nutritional Assessment score, and chemotherapy.

Notably, the majority of initial episodes of neutropenic infections appear to occur during the first cycle [44]. In this prospective study, after adjustment for cancer type and age, risk factors for neutropenic infection included prior chemotherapy, abnormal hepatic and renal function, low white blood count, and chemotherapy and planned delivery ≥85 %. Among non-hematologic toxicities, peripheral neuropathy is difficult to predict, and lack of baseline neuropathy may not necessarily mitigate the risk of severe neuropathy. Moreover, baseline sarcopenia is emerging as a parameter that predicts chemotherapy toxicities [45].

Management and Mitigation of Toxicities in the Elderly

Most toxicities of chemotherapy, e.g., diarrhea, nausea, anorexia, and fatigue, can be managed by non-pharmacologic and/or pharmacologic intervention. However, myelosuppression and neurotoxicity may deserve more attention given their potential impact on survival and quality of life.

Myelosuppression

Given the higher risk of neutropenic infections in the elderly, which appear to be exacerbated by comorbidities, functional impairments and organ dysfunction, dose reductions, or prophylactic growth factors are an important consideration in such patients. It is noteworthy that docetaxel, cabazitaxel, and mitoxantrone are primarily metabolized through the hepatic route. A strategy of initial docetaxel dose of 60 mg/m^2 in patients with functional impairments may be considered followed by dose escalation if tolerability is demonstrated. Similarly, a starting dose of cabazitaxel of 20 mg/m^2 should be considered in selected patients and is being evaluated formally. Unfortunately, no definite criteria exist to guide this decision. Furthermore, no definitive evidence exists to support prophylactic antibiotics or growth factors that are frequently employed [46].

In this context, patients with minimally symptomatic disease also qualify for sipuleucel-T, which is characterized by excellent tolerability. Intriguingly, patients in the IMPACT trial that received the sequence of initial sipuleucel-T followed by docetaxel after clinical progression exhibited the longest median survival (28.5 months) [47]. It is also noteworthy that in the IMPACT trial, the median time to clinical progression was only 14.5 weeks, which suggests that observation alone is unlikely to be an effective strategy in the majority of patients with minimally symptomatic metastatic CRPC who are candidates for systemic therapy.

Neurotoxicity

The neurotoxicity of docetaxel, although generally manageable, warrants special attention in the elderly. If clinical evaluation for neuropathy is unclear, nerve conduction studies and an electromyogram may be considered. Neuropathy may lead to falls, difficulty driving and walking, which can lead to serious injuries [48]. Neuropathy and falls may occur after a latent period following completion of chemotherapy. In this context, bone health targeting agents (zoledronic acid, denosumab) in combination with calcium and vitamin D replacement are imperative in those with bone metastases, given the proven benefit for alleviating the risk of skeletal-related events [49]. Those without bone metastases also warrant attention to bone health owing to ongoing androgen deprivation.

Walking assist devices, an alerting system in the event of falls, and home safety evaluation should be considered. Balance and mobility exercises and physical therapy during chemotherapy are a consideration in those at risk. Other functional derangements that may contribute to falls such as vision problems and psychoactive medications need to be addressed if feasible. Scant data exist for the prevention of neuropathy with vitamin E, glutamine, glutathione, *N*-acetylcysteine, and antiseizure medications. Reversible causes of neuropathy (e.g., vitamin B12 deficiency) should be aggressively rectified.

Marginal efficacy may exist for amitriptylene, nortriptylene, gabapentin, and lamotrigine in the management of neuropathy. Prevention of sarcopenia may involve exercise (including resistance training), nutrition, and pharmacologic intervention (e.g., selective estrogen receptor modulators, anti-myostatin, creatine, anabolic hormones). Finally, polypharmacy for comorbidities or intake of over-the-counter medications is commonplace in the elderly, and attention should be paid to potential interactions with chemotherapy.

Prostate Cancer Working Group-2 Guidelines for Management

The Prostate Cancer Working Group (PCWG)-2 criteria recommend at least 4 cycles or 12 weeks of therapy before objective radiologic evaluation, which address the difficulty of assessing early bone scan flares [50]. Discontinuation of therapy for isolated PSA increases in the absence of clinical progression is not recommended, given the early PSA flares as well as suboptimal association of PSA changes with outcomes. While the less frequently observed measurable disease is assessed by conventional RECIST (Response Evaluation Criteria in Solid Tumors), objective evaluation of the typical patient with bone metastases is problematic. PCWG-2 guidelines define bone progression as ≥2 new lesions followed by further new lesions ≥6 weeks later on a bone scan [50].

Prognostic Factors and Intermediate Surrogates for Outcomes

Clinical Prognostic Factors at Baseline

Prognostic nomograms and risk groupings assist in estimating prognosis in men with metastatic CRPC undergoing chemotherapy [28, 51, 52]. The variables included in the nomogram developed from the TAX327 trial include pain, performance status, alkaline phosphatase, number of metastatic sites, liver metastasis, hemoglobin, PSA, and time since diagnosis [51]. Four clinical factors (visceral metastasis, anemia, bone scan progression at baseline, pain) predicted the probability of PSA response and survival and were employed to construct risk groups [52]. One retrospective analysis of the TAX327 trial that studied outcomes in the post-docetaxel setting demonstrated the association of survival with pretreatment factors, the number of progression factors (PSA, pain, and tumor size), the duration of first-line chemotherapy, and whether progression occurred during chemotherapy [53]. Notably, none of these prognostic groupings include age as an independently prognostic variable, although these prognostic classifications were developed from patients enrolled in a prospective phase III trial, who tend to be generally more functional than patients in the community.

Intermediate Clinical Surrogates for Outcomes

Prostate cancer is characterized by a poor ability to measure response and progression due either to immeasurable bone-only metastases or PSA-only disease. Retrospective studies demonstrated that a PSA decline 30 % or ≥ 50 % within 3 months had a moderate degree of surrogacy for OS in the setting of chemotherapy [54, 55]. Retrospective analyses of these trials have also demonstrated that PSA increase ≥ 25 % at 3 months correlates with poor OS [53, 56]. Progression-free survival (PFS) defined by a composite endpoint (progression by bone scan, PSA criteria, and measurable tumor progression) also correlated with poorer OS [57]. Another recent retrospective analysis of the TAX327 trial identified an association of objective measurable tumor responses by WHO criteria and favorable OS [58].

Circulating Tumor Cells (CTCs)

Prospective studies in the setting of chemotherapy have demonstrated that patients with unfavorable baseline CTCs (≥ 5 CTCs/7.5 mL) exhibited shorter median OS (11.5 vs. 21.7 months) [59]. Patients with unfavorable baseline CTCs who converted to favorable CTCs (<5 CTCs/7.5 mL) improved (6.8–21.3 months), while the prognosis for those with favorable baseline CTCs who converted to unfavorable worsened (>26–9.3 months). These data led to U.S. Food and Drug Administration approval of CTCs for the evaluation of CRPC. Prospective validation of CTC alterations in the setting of chemotherapy is awaited from prospective randomized trials, although validation in the setting of abiraterone acetate following docetaxel was recently presented [60]. The utility of early changes in CTCs to guide therapy will be investigated in a trial planned by SWOG.

Chemotherapy for Nonmetastatic or Hormone-Sensitive Prostate Cancer

Multiple trials are evaluating the role of chemotherapy in those with lower stages of prostate cancer in order to enhance long-term outcomes. These trials do not explicitly exclude elderly patients that otherwise qualify based on eligibility criteria. Trials that evaluated docetaxel preceding radical prostatectomy have demonstrated biologic activity without pathologic complete responses [61]. However, in combination with androgen deprivation, a marginal pCR rate has been shown [62]. Randomized trials are evaluating the benefit of adding docetaxel to ADT for metastatic and/or nonmetastatic castration-sensitive prostate cancer. Unfortunately, adjuvant mitoxantrone therapy following radical prostatectomy for high-risk localized prostate cancer induced an increase in acute myeloid leukemia, which led to premature termination of the trial [63]. Another phase III trial comparing adjuvant versus delayed ADT with or without docetaxel was terminated prematurely due to poor accrual. Randomized trials are evaluating the role of adjuvant docetaxel alone without ADT for patients with high-risk localized prostate cancer following radical prostatectomy. Trials are evaluating docetaxel and ADT versus ADT alone after radiation therapy (RT) in high-risk locally advanced patients. Combination of docetaxel and ADT prior to local therapy is also being evaluated.

Conclusions

In this era of biologic agents, immunotherapy (sipuleucel-T), antiandrogen agents (abiraterone acetate, MDV3100), osteoclast targeting agents (denosumab), and radiopharmaceuticals (radium-223) have all recently improved outcomes. Conversely, docetaxel and cabazitaxel are established as first- and second-line chemotherapy for metastatic CRPC, and mitoxantrone may continue to play a palliative role.

In general, elderly age alone does not preclude chemotherapy or other therapies in patients that qualify based on a satisfactory biologic age, i.e., with no serious uncontrolled comorbidities, ECOG performance status 0–2, adequate organ and cognitive function, and satisfactory nutritional status and social support. The International Society of Geriatric Oncology (SIOG) recommends that older men with prostate cancer be managed according to health status, which is primarily influenced by comorbidities and not chronological age [64]. Despite trends for increasing toxicities, selected elderly patients appear to generally tolerate chemotherapy and derive benefits similar to their younger counterparts. However, given the increased prevalence of comorbidities, functional impairments, and organ dysfunctions in the elderly, careful selection of patients coupled with dose modifications and prophylactic measures to avoid toxicities are necessary (Fig.13.2). Convenient and useful geriatric assessments in the clinic are undergoing evaluation, and further validation of emerging scales is warranted to enable implementation in the clinic.

Administration of several active agents may optimize survival. Therefore, optimal sequencing of agents and selection of patients hopefully in the future based on validated predictive proteomic and genomic profiles are necessary in conjunction with clinical models and patient preferences. Clinical trials should remain a priority, and age alone does not preclude eligibility for trials in patients that otherwise qualify.

Grants, Research Support and Financial Disclosures Guru Sonpavde, M.D., receives research support from Eli Lilly-Imclone, Pfizer, BMS, Novartis, Teva, Celgene, Cytogen and Astrazeneca and is on the speakers' bureau or advisory board for Pfizer, Novartis, GSK, Dendreon, Amgen, Astellas and Sanofi-Aventis.

Cora N. Sternberg, M.D. has received research support from Sanofi-Aventis, Cougar Biotech, and Astellas.

References

1. de Bono JS, Oudard S, Ozguroglu M, et al. Prednisone plus cabazitaxel or mitoxantrone for metastatic castration-resistant prostate cancer progressing after docetaxel treatment: a randomised open-label trial. Lancet. 2010;376(9747):1147–54.
2. Mohile SG, Xian Y, Dale W, et al. Association of a cancer diagnosis with vulnerability and frailty in older Medicare beneficiaries. J Natl Cancer Inst. 2009;101(17):1206–15.
3. Extermann M, Hurria A. Comprehensive geriatric assessment for older patients with cancer. J Clin Oncol. 2007;25(14):1824–31.
4. Balducci L, Extermann M. Management of the frail person with advanced cancer. Crit Rev Oncol Hematol. 2000;33(2):143–8.
5. Min LC, Elliott MN, Wenger NS, Saliba D. Higher vulnerable elders survey scores predict death and functional decline in vulnerable older people. J Am Geriatr Soc. 2006;54(3):507–11.
6. Hurria A, Cirrincione CT, Muss HB, et al. Implementing a geriatric assessment in cooperative group clinical cancer trials: CALGB 360401. J Clin Oncol. 2011;29(10):1290–6.
7. Read WL, Tierney RM, Page NC, et al. Differential prognostic impact of comorbidity. J Clin Oncol. 2004;22(15):3099–103.
8. Charlson ME, Pompei P, Ales KL, MacKenzie CR. A new method of classifying prognostic comorbidity in longitudinal studies: development and validation. J Chronic Dis. 1987;40(5):373–83.
9. Piccirillo JF, Tierney RM, Costas I, Grove L, Spitznagel Jr EL. Prognostic importance of comorbidity in a hospital-based cancer registry. JAMA. 2004;291(20):2441–7.
10. Tannock IF, de Wit R, Berry WR, et al. Docetaxel plus prednisone or mitoxantrone plus prednisone for advanced prostate cancer. N Engl J Med. 2004;351(15):1502–12.

11. Petrylak DP, Tangen CM, Hussain MH, et al. Docetaxel and estramustine compared with mitoxantrone and prednisone for advanced refractory prostate cancer. N Engl J Med. 2004;351(15):1513–20.

12. Berthold DR, Pond GR, Soban F, de Wit R, Eisenberger M, Tannock IF. Docetaxel plus prednisone or mitoxantrone plus prednisone for advanced prostate cancer: updated survival in the TAX 327 study. J Clin Oncol. 2008;26(2):242–5.

13. Berthold DR, Pond GR, Roessner M, de Wit R, Eisenberger M, Tannock AI. Treatment of hormone-refractory prostate cancer with docetaxel or mitoxantrone: relationships between prostate-specific antigen, pain, and quality of life response and survival in the TAX-327 study. Clin Cancer Res. 2008;14(9):2763–7.

14. Fizazi K, Le Maitre A, Hudes G, et al. Addition of estramustine to chemotherapy and survival of patients with castration-refractory prostate cancer: a meta-analysis of individual patient data. Lancet Oncol. 2007;8(11):994–1000.

15. Lubiniecki GM, Berlin JA, Weinstein RB, Vaughn DJ. Thromboembolic events with estramustine phosphate-based chemotherapy in patients with hormone-refractory prostate carcinoma: results of a meta-analysis. Cancer. 2004;101(12):2755–9.

16. Cell Genesys Halts VITAL-2 GVAX trial in advanced prostate cancer. 2010. http://phx.corporate-ir.net/phoenix.zhtml?c=98399&p=irol-newsArticle&ID=1191052. Accessed 3 Jan 2010.

17. Scher HI, Jia X, Chi K, et al. Randomized, open-label phase III trial of docetaxel plus high-dose calcitriol versus docetaxel plus prednisone for patients with castration-resistant prostate cancer. J Clin Oncol. 2011;29(16):2191–8.

18. Tannock IF, Osoba D, Stockler MR, et al. Chemotherapy with mitoxantrone plus prednisone or prednisone alone for symptomatic hormone-resistant prostate cancer: a Canadian randomized trial with palliative end points. J Clin Oncol. 1996;14(6):1756–64.

19. Beer TM, Ryan CW, Venner PM, et al. Intermittent chemotherapy in patients with metastatic androgen-independent prostate cancer: results from ASCENT, a double-blinded, randomized comparison of high-dose calcitriol plus docetaxel with placebo plus docetaxel. Cancer. 2008;112(2):326–30.

20. Loriot Y, Massard C, Gross-Goupil M, et al. The interval from the last cycle of docetaxel-based chemotherapy to progression is associated with the efficacy of subsequent docetaxel in patients with prostate cancer. Eur J Cancer. 2010;46(10):1770–2.

21. Pond GR, Armstrong AJ, Wood BA, et al. Evaluating the value of number of cycles of docetaxel and prednisone in men with metastatic castration-resistant prostate cancer. Eur Urol. 2012;61:363–9.

22. Franke RM, Carducci MA, Rudek MA, Baker SD, Sparreboom A. Castration-dependent pharmacokinetics of docetaxel in patients with prostate cancer. J Clin Oncol. 2010;28(30):4562–7.

23. Berthold DR, Pond GR, de Wit R, Eisenberger M, Tannock IF. Survival and PSA response of patients in the TAX 327 study who crossed over to receive docetaxel after mitoxantrone or vice versa. Ann Oncol. 2008;19(10):1749–53.

24. Rosenberg JE, Galsky MD, Rohs NC, et al. A retrospective evaluation of second-line chemotherapy response in hormone-refractory prostate carcinoma: second line taxane-based therapy after first-line epothilone-B analog ixabepilone (BMS-247550) therapy. Cancer. 2006;106(1):58–62.

25. Takaha N, Okihara K, Kamoi K, et al. Feasibility of tri-weekly docetaxel-based chemotherapy for elderly patients (age 75 and older) with castration-resistant prostate cancer. Urol Int. 2011;87(3):263–9.

26. Halabi S, Kelly WK, George DJ, et al. Comorbidities predict overall survival (OS) in men with metastatic castrate-resistant prostate cancer (CRPC). J Clin Oncol. 2011;9 (suppl 7; abstr 189).

27. Kelly W, Halabi S, Carducci MA, et al. A randomized, double-blind, placebo-controlled phase III trial comparing docetaxel, prednisone, and placebo with docetaxel, prednisone, and bevacizumab in men with metastatic castration-resistant prostate cancer (mCRPC): survival results of CALGB 90401. J Clin Oncol. 2010;28:18s (suppl; abstr LBA4511).

28. Halabi S, Small EJ, Kantoff PW, et al. Prognostic model for predicting survival in men with hormone-refractory metastatic prostate cancer. J Clin Oncol. 2003;21(7):1232–7.

29. de Bono JS, Logothetis CJ, Molina A, et al. Abiraterone and increased survival in metastatic prostate cancer. N Engl J Med. 2011;364(21):1995–2005.
30. Kantoff PW, Halabi S, Conaway M, et al. Hydrocortisone with or without mitoxantrone in men with hormone-refractory prostate cancer: results of the cancer and leukemia group B 9182 study. J Clin Oncol. 1999;17(8):2506–13.
31. Rosenberg JE, Weinberg VK, Kelly WK, et al. Activity of second-line chemotherapy in docetaxel-refractory hormone-refractory prostate cancer patients: randomized phase 2 study of ixabepilone or mitoxantrone and prednisone. Cancer. 2007;110(3):556–63.
32. Sternberg CN, Petrylak DP, Sartor O, et al. Multinational, double-blind, phase III study of prednisone and either satraplatin or placebo in patients with castrate-refractory prostate cancer progressing after prior chemotherapy: the SPARC trial. J Clin Oncol. 2009;27(32):5431–8.
33. Ross RW, Beer TM, Jacobus S, et al. A phase 2 study of carboplatin plus docetaxel in men with metastatic hormone-refractory prostate cancer who are refractory to docetaxel. Cancer. 2008;112(3):521–6.
34. Hussain M, Tangen CM, Lara Jr PN, et al. Ixabepilone (epothilone B analogue BMS-247550) is active in chemotherapy-naive patients with hormone-refractory prostate cancer: a Southwest Oncology Group trial S0111. J Clin Oncol. 2005;23(34):8724–9.
35. Galsky MD, Small EJ, Oh WK, et al. Multi-institutional randomized phase II trial of the epothilone B analog ixabepilone (BMS-247550) with or without estramustine phosphate in patients with progressive castrate metastatic prostate cancer. J Clin Oncol. 2005;23(7):1439–46.
36. Harzstark AL, Rosenberg JE, Weinberg VK, et al. Ixabepilone, mitoxantrone, and prednisone for metastatic castration-resistant prostate cancer after docetaxel-based therapy: a phase 2 study of the department of defense prostate cancer clinical trials consortium. Cancer. 2010 December 29 [Epub ahead of print].
37. Chi KN, Beardsley E, Eigl BJ, et al. A phase 2 study of patupilone in patients with metastatic castration-resistant prostate cancer previously treated with docetaxel: Canadian Urologic Oncology Group study P07a. Ann Oncol. 2012;23:53–8.
38. Beer TM, Smith D, Hussain M, et al. Phase II study of first-line sagopilone combined with prednisone in patients with metastatic castration-resistant prostate cancer. J Clin Oncol. 2009;27:15s (suppl; abstr 5059).
39. de Bono JS, Molife LR, Sonpavde G, et al. Phase II study of eribulin mesylate (E7389) in patients with metastatic castration-resistant prostate cancer stratified by prior taxane therapy. Ann Oncol. 2012;23:1241–9.
40. Papandreou CN, Daliani DD, Thall PF, et al. Results of a phase II study with doxorubicin, etoposide, and cisplatin in patients with fully characterized small-cell carcinoma of the prostate. J Clin Oncol. 2002;20(14):3072–80.
41. Hurria A, Togawa K, Mohile SG, et al. Predicting chemotherapy toxicity in older adults with cancer: a prospective multicenter study. J Clin Oncol. 2011;29(25):3457–65.
42. Frasci G, Lorusso V, Panza N, et al. Gemcitabine plus vinorelbine versus vinorelbine alone in elderly patients with advanced non-small-cell lung cancer. J Clin Oncol. 2000;18(13):2529–36.
43. Extermann M, Boler I, Reich RR, et al. Predicting the risk of chemotherapy toxicity in older patients: the chemotherapy risk assessment scale for high-age patients (CRASH) score. ;Cancer. doi:10.1002/cncr.26646.
44. Lyman GH, Kuderer NM, Crawford J, et al. Predicting individual risk of neutropenic complications in patients receiving cancer chemotherapy. Cancer. 2011;117(9):1917–27.
45. Prado CM, Baracos VE, McCargar LJ, et al. Sarcopenia as a determinant of chemotherapy toxicity and time to tumor progression in metastatic breast cancer patients receiving capecitabine treatment. Clin Cancer Res. 2009;15(8):2920–6.
46. Herbst C, Naumann F, Kruse EB, et al. Prophylactic antibiotics or G-CSF for the prevention of infections and improvement of survival in cancer patients undergoing chemotherapy. Cochrane Database Syst Rev. 2009;1:CD007107.
47. Kantoff PW, Higano CS, Shore ND, et al. Sipuleucel-T immunotherapy for castration-resistant prostate cancer. N Engl J Med. 2010;363(5):411–22.

48. Mohile SG, Fan L, Reeve E, et al. Association of cancer with geriatric syndromes in older Medicare beneficiaries. J Clin Oncol. 2011;29(11):1458–64.
49. Fizazi K, Carducci M, Smith M, et al. Denosumab versus zoledronic acid for treatment of bone metastases in men with castration-resistant prostate cancer: a randomised, double-blind study. Lancet. 2011;377(9768):813–22.
50. Scher HI, Halabi S, Tannock I, et al. Design and end points of clinical trials for patients with progressive prostate cancer and castrate levels of testosterone: recommendations of the Prostate Cancer Clinical Trials Working Group. J Clin Oncol. 2008;26(7):1148–59.
51. Armstrong AJ, Garrett-Mayer ES, Yang YC, de Wit R, Tannock IF, Eisenberger M. A contemporary prognostic nomogram for men with hormone-refractory metastatic prostate cancer: a TAX327 study analysis. Clin Cancer Res. 2007;13(21):6396–403.
52. Armstrong AJ, Tannock IF, de Wit R, George DJ, Eisenberger M, Halabi S. The development of risk groups in men with metastatic castration-resistant prostate cancer based on risk factors for PSA decline and survival. Eur J Cancer. 2010;46(3):517–25.
53. Armstrong AJ, Garrett-Mayer E, de Wit R, Tannock I, Eisenberger M. Prediction of survival following first-line chemotherapy in men with castration-resistant metastatic prostate cancer. Clin Cancer Res. 2010;16(1):203–11.
54. Petrylak DP, Ankerst DP, Jiang CS, et al. Evaluation of prostate-specific antigen declines for surrogacy in patients treated on SWOG 99–16. J Natl Cancer Inst. 2006;98(8):516–21.
55. Armstrong AJ, Garrett-Mayer E, Ou Yang YC, et al. Prostate-specific antigen and pain surrogacy analysis in metastatic hormone-refractory prostate cancer. J Clin Oncol. 2007;25(25):3965–70.
56. Hussain M, Goldman B, Tangen C, et al. Prostate-specific antigen progression predicts overall survival in patients with metastatic prostate cancer: data from Southwest Oncology Group Trials 9346 (Intergroup Study 0162) and 9916. J Clin Oncol. 2009;27(15):2450–6.
57. Halabi S, Vogelzang NJ, Ou SS, Owzar K, Archer L, Small EJ. Progression-free survival as a predictor of overall survival in men with castrate-resistant prostate cancer. J Clin Oncol. 2009;27(17):2766–71.
58. Sonpavde G, Pond GR, Berry WR, et al. The association between radiographic response and overall survival in men with metastatic castration-resistant prostate cancer receiving chemotherapy. Cancer. 2011;117:3963–71.
59. de Bono JS, Scher HI, Montgomery RB, et al. Circulating tumor cells predict survival benefit from treatment in metastatic castration-resistant prostate cancer. Clin Cancer Res. 2008;14(19):6302–9.
60. Scher H HG, Molina A, Kheoh T, Attard G, Moreira J, Sandhu S, Parker C, Logothetis C, McCormack R, Fizazi K, Anand A, Danila D, Fleisher M, Olmos D, Haqq C, De Bono J. Evaluation of circulating tumor cell (CTC) enumeration as an efficacy response biomarker of overall survival (OS) in metastatic castration-resistant prostate cancer (mCRPC): planned final analysis (FA) of COU-AA-301, a randomized double-blind, placebo-controlled phase III study of abiraterone acetate (AA) plus low-dose prednisone (P) post docetaxel. J Clin Oncol. 2011;29 (suppl; abstr LBA4517^).
61. Magi-Galluzzi C, Zhou M, Reuther AM, Dreicer R, Klein EA. Neoadjuvant docetaxel treatment for locally advanced prostate cancer: a clinicopathologic study. Cancer. 2007;110(6):1248–54.
62. Chi KN, Chin JL, Winquist E, Klotz L, Saad F, Gleave ME. Multicenter phase II study of combined neoadjuvant docetaxel and hormone therapy before radical prostatectomy for patients with high risk localized prostate cancer. J Urol. 2008;180(2):565–70; discussion 570.
63. Flaig TW, Tangen CM, Hussain MH, et al. Randomization reveals unexpected acute leukemias in Southwest Oncology Group prostate cancer trial. J Clin Oncol. 2008;26(9):1532–6.
64. Droz JP, Balducci L, Bolla M, et al. Management of prostate cancer in older men: recommendations of a working group of the International Society of Geriatric Oncology. BJU Int. 2010; 106(4):462–9.
65. Kolevska T, Rayan C, Huey V, et al. Phase II trial of nab-paclitaxel as first-line therapy of hormone refractory metastatic prostate cancer. J Clin Oncol. 2009;27:15s (suppl; abstr 5152).

Chapter 14
Clinical Management of Elderly Patients' Metastatic Prostate Cancer: Other Treatments and Supportive Care

Helen Boyle and Aude Fléchon

Abstract Prostate cancer is a frequent disease, especially in elderly men. Treatment of metastatic prostate cancer is palliative at any age. It requires a global oncological approach with the input of several teams: urologists, medical oncologists, radiotherapists, other surgeons etc. Hormone deprivation is the main treatment for hormone-sensitive metastatic disease. Chemotherapy is the standard treatment for metastatic castration-resistant disease, but new drugs, mainly new hormonal treatments, are being developed. Other treatment modalities can be used to treat patients in these situations, such as bone-targeted agents, radiopharmaceutics etc. Evolution of the disease is variable, but some problems, such as pain, fractures, compressions, etc., occur frequently and need a specific approach.

Keywords Prostate cancer • Metastases • Androgen deprivation • Chemotherapy • Radiopharmaceutics • Bone • Elderly • Radiotherapy • Palliation • Pain

Introduction

Prostate cancer is a frequent tumor. Incidence increases with age. In 2008, there were around 65,000 new cases in France [1]. Median age at diagnosis is 68 years, and 27 % of patients are 75 or more [2].

Most deaths from prostate cancer occur in men over 75.

Treatment of metastatic prostate cancer is palliative at any age. It requires a global oncological approach with the input of several teams: urologists, medical oncologists, radiotherapists, other surgeons etc.

H. Boyle, M.D. (✉) • A. Fléchon, M.D., Ph.D.
Department of Medicine, Center Léon-Bérard,
Lyon, France
e-mail: helen.boyle@lyon.unicancer.fr; aude.flechon@lyon.unicancer.fr

J.-P. Droz, R.A. Audisio (eds.), *Management of Urological Cancers in Older People*,
Management of Cancer in Older People,
DOI 10.1007/978-0-85729-999-4_14, © Springer-Verlag London 2013

Evolution of the disease is variable, but some recurrent problems occur frequently such as pain, fractures, compressions etc.

Treatment options for metastatic disease are changing. Chemotherapy still plays an important role in the management of metastatic castration-resistant disease, but new drugs, mainly new hormonal treatments, are being developed (see corresponding chapter in this book).

In this chapter, we will try and review the management of metastatic disease in elderly patients, focusing on some of the other drugs (nonchemotherapy) that are used.

Role of Geriatric Evaluation

Elderly patients are not a homogenous group of patients. Aging is a quite variable, individual process.

The impact of cancer in this population varies greatly depending on the general health of these patients. It is important to evaluate comprehensively patients' global health status to offer the most adequate treatment and to prevent possible treatment related side effects. This should be done for any patient but more importantly in elderly patients [3].

Several tools have been developed. The comprehensive geriatric assessment (CGA) is a multidisciplinary process. It assesses several domains such as comorbidities, nutrition, cognition, emotional conditions, function, geriatric syndromes, pharmacy and socioeconomic conditions. It involves diagnostic procedures, specific treatment plans, and geriatric intervention. It aims to evaluate the multiple problems of elderly patients and allow physicians to make the best decision for the treatment of the cancer taking into account the balance between underlying conditions, prostate cancer death risk, and the side effects of treatment.

In the SIOG evaluation for patients with prostate cancer, the CIRS-G grid was used to evaluate comorbidity [2]. Nutrition status was evaluated by weight loss in the last 3 months. ADL (activities of daily living) include bathing, dressing, toileting, transferring, continence, and feeding. IADL (instrumental activities of daily living) correspond to tasks that require a higher level of cognition and judgement such as preparation of meals, shopping, light housework, financial management, medication management, use of transportation, and use of the telephone. In the SIOG evaluation for prostate cancer, only the last four IADL in the list above were considered.

Patients were classified according to four groups after CGA:

- Fit patients with no serious comorbidity who are able to perform activities of daily living (ADL) and instrumental activities of daily living (IADL) and who have no malnutrition.
- Vulnerable patients, i.e., with reversible problems. They are dependant in one or more IADL (but have no dependence for any ADL) or one uncontrolled comorbidity (CISG-R grade3) or who are at risk for malnutrition.
- Frail patients, i.e., with nonreversible problems. They are dependant in one or more ADL or have more than one uncontrolled comorbidity (at least two CISG-R

grade 3 comorbidities or at least one CISG-R grade 4 comorbidity) or showing major malnutrition.

- Patients who "are too sick." These patients have a very poor health status, usually due to several impairments. Patients with severe cognition impairment are classified in this group; however, cases of patients with signs of dementia should be discussed on individual basis.

Hormone-Sensitive Metastatic Disease

Treatment of metastatic hormone-sensitive prostate cancer is based on androgen suppression [4–6]. There are several treatment options [7, 8]:

- Chemical castration with use of LHRH agonists
- Surgical castration with bilateral orchidectomy

Patients should be given antiandrogens for a month to avoid initial flare-up at the initiation of LHRH agonists [9]. However, there is no additional benefit from complete androgen blockade compared to single agent LHRH agonist [10].

Both chemical and surgical castration are effective. The most frequently used treatment is chemical castration because of the physical and psychological consequences of bilateral castration. However, the decision is based on patients' choice and ability and desire to undergo regular injections.

Hormone therapy should be offered to all patients with symptomatic metastatic disease to improve symptom control and reduce risk of severe complications (bone fracture, cord compression, urine retention etc.). Early initiation of hormone therapy in asymptomatic metastatic patients can prevent the development of symptoms and severe complications [2, 11]. Patients who progress after first-line hormone therapy can benefit from further hormonal manipulations (adjunction of antiandrogens, withdrawal of antiandrogens etc.) [2]

Early side effects of androgen deprivation (ADT) are hot flushes, decreased libido, gynecomastia, and asthenia. Long-term effects of androgen deprivation can be of concern especially in elderly patients. ADT is associated with increased cardiovascular disease, diabetes, osteoporosis, muscle wasting, and cognitive decline.

NCCN recommends that patients with surgical or medical castration should be evaluated for osteoporosis (calcemia, vitamin D levels, and determination of bone mineral density) [12]. Patients on ADT should receive calcium and vitamin D. If osteoporosis is diagnosed, patients should be treated (see Chap. 6).

Taylor et al. published a review on long-term side effects of androgen deprivation [13]. Three studies showed a decrease of bone mineral density with the use of androgen deprivation therapy. Fracture risk is also increased with a relative risk of 1.23 (IC 95 % = 1.1–1.38) for skeletal fractures and of 1.29 (IC 95 % = 1.2–1.6) for vertebral fractures.

In the same review, they found an increase of diabetes and cardiovascular morbidity, ranging from 20 to 49 % depending on the studies. Cardiovascular mortality was also increased with an RR = 1.17 (IC 95 % = 1.07–1.29). ADT increases insulin resistance and lipid levels. It also increases body fat and decreases lean mass. The American Heart Association, American Cancer Society, and American Urological Association published a Science Advisory in 2010 [14]. It was also endorsed by the American Society for Radiation Oncology. The benefit-risk balance of introducing ADT should be evaluated in patients with cardiovascular disease. Patients on ADT should be regularly monitored by their primary care physician. Patients who develop cardiovascular complications on ADT should receive secondary prevention measures too.

Cardiovascular risk increases with age, and this should be noted when starting elderly patients on ADT.

Patients on androgen deprivation therapy will progress despite this treatment. Median time to hormone resistance is between 18 and 24 months.

Castration-Resistant Metastatic Disease: First-Line Chemotherapy

The standard first-line treatment of metastatic castration-resistant disease is docetaxel chemotherapy. In the pivotal TAX 327 trial, there was an overall survival benefit with docetaxel 75 mg/m^2 administered every 3 weeks compared to mitoxantrone (19.2 months (95 % IC 17.5–21.3)) versus 16.3 months (95 % IC 14.3–17.9). There was no survival benefit with weekly administration of docetaxel compared to mitoxantrone. Median age in the trial was 68 years (36–92); 20 % of patients were ≥75 years [15].

Subgroup analysis in this trial shows that patients ≥ 69 years benefit from 3-weekly docetaxel. However, inclusion criteria required an IK ≥ 60 %, no other serious medical condition, normal cardiac function, and creatinine levels < 1.5 upper limit of normal. Therefore, most of the patients included would be considered "fit" according to the previously described categories.

Fossa et al. published a randomized phase II trial comparing weekly docetaxel + prednisolone to prednisolone alone. Median age was 70 years (range: 52–84). Patients needed to have an ECOG PS of less than 2, serum creatinine ≤ 1.5 ULN, and liver functional tests ≤ 2.5 ULN. Median overall survival was 27 months (IC 95 % (19.8–34.2)) with docetaxel plus prednisolone and 18 months (IC 95 % (15.2–20.8)) with prednisolone alone [16].

Fit elderly patients can receive standard chemotherapy. Vulnerable and frail patients should undergo geriatric evaluation before deciding on the choice of treatment. If possible, vulnerable patients should receive standard 3-weekly docetaxel after geriatric intervention [2].

Chemotherapy in frail patients should be adapted, probably with a weekly administration.

A French collaborative trial is ongoing to study docetaxel administration (weekly or 3-weekly). This phase II randomized trial is aimed to evaluate the feasibility of these 2 schedules in patients with metastatic castration-resistant prostate cancer, older than 75, that are considered vulnerable or frail according to the SIOG criteria.

Other Treatments

Supportive Care

Erythropoietin and G-CSF can be used in elderly patients to reduce the side effects of chemotherapy, especially the risk of neutropenic fever. As described in the EORTC 2010 recommendations, age over 65 is a high risk factor to be taken into account when deciding to give primary prophylaxis with G-CSF for patients receiving chemotherapy when the estimated risk of neutropenic fever is between 10 and 20 % [17]. However, neutropenic fever incidence with 3-weekly docetaxel in the TAX 327 trial was 2.7 % [15].

Patients should be informed of side effects of chemotherapy and how to manage them. Symptomatic treatments, such as antiemetics and antidiarrhea drugs, should be prescribed to treat side effects.

Bone-Targeted Treatments

Bisphosphonates

Zoledronic acid was the first agent to decrease skeletal-related events in patients with metastatic castration-resistant prostate cancer. In a phase III trial, two doses of zoledronic acid were compared to placebo. Due to more frequent increased creatinine levels in the higher dose (8 mg) of zoledronic acid, an amendment was passed to continue with the 4-mg dose, every 3 weeks, in a 15-min IV perfusion. The primary end point was the proportion of patients with at least one skeletal-related event (SRE), defined as a pathologic fracture, spinal cord compression, radiation therapy or surgery to bone, or change in the antineoplastic therapy to treat bone pain. The trial was built to detect a 16 % difference in the proportion of patients receiving zoledronic acid at 4 mg or placebo who reported any skeletal-related event during the 15 months of the trial. Median age in the zoledronic acid arms was 72 years; more than 90 % of patients were over 60. Patients with severe cardiovascular disease, uncontrolled hypertension, symptomatic coronary disease, or severe renal failure (serum creatinine >265 mmol/l) were excluded [18, 19].

During the entire 24-month study, fewer patients in the 4-mg zoledronic acid group than in the placebo group had at least one SRE (38 vs. 49 %, $p=0.028$). Median time to first SRE was 488 days with zoledronic acid versus 321 days in the placebo arm ($p=0.009$).

Main side effects with 4 mg of zoledronic acid were fatigue (32.7 %), myalgia (24.8 %), fever (32.7 %), anorexia (20.1 %), anemia (26.6 %), and hypocalcemia (2 % grade 3–4). Grade 3 serum creatinine increases occurred in 3.3 % of patients in the 4-mg arm.

Before prescribing zoledronic acid, patients should undergo teeth assessment and dental care if necessary. It is important, especially in elderly patients, to evaluate renal function and calcium levels. If renal function is impaired, zoledronic acid dosage must be reduced and perfusion time increased.

Denosumab

Denosumab is a humanized monoclonal antibody against RANK ligand. RANK ligand plays a major role in osteoclast formation, function, and survival. Denosumab has been tested in a phase III trial against zoledronic acid in patients with metastatic castration-resistant disease [20]. It was a double-blind randomized trial with double dummy placebos, as zoledronic acid is administered by intravenous infusion and denosumab by a subcutaneous injection. Intravenous treatment (zoledronic acid or placebo) doses were adapted to renal function. Calcium and vitamin D supplementation was recommended.

Primary end point was time to first on study skeletal event. It was a non-inferiority study.

Median age in the zoledronic acid arm was 71 years (66–77) and 71 years (64–77) in the denosumab arm. Seventy-seven percent of patients in the zoledronic acid were 65 or older and 73 % in the denosumab arm. Denosumab significantly delayed first SRE by 18 % compared to zoledronic acid, with a difference of 3.6 months. Denosumab also delayed subsequent events. There was no difference in overall survival with a median of 19.4 months (95 % IC 18.1–21.7) in the denosumab arm versus 19.8 months (95 % IC 18.1–20.9) in the zoledronic acid arm.

The main side effects were anemia, back pain, decreased appetite, nausea, fatigue, constipation, and bone pain. Hypocalcemia occurred in 13 % in the denosumab arm and 6 % in the zoledronic arm with grade ≥3 events in 5 and 1 % of patients, respectively. Osteonecrosis of the jaw occurred in 2 % of patients on denosumab and 1 % on zoledronic acid. Most cases occurred after dental extraction.

This trial shows that denosumab can delay occurrence of skeletal-related events. It does not cause renal function impairment, and there is no need for dose adjustments if renal function is impaired. Patients should receive calcium and vitamin D supplementation. Dental care should be performed before starting treatment. This drug has recently been approved by the FDA and the EMA.

Radiopharmaceutics

Several radiopharmaceutics have been used to treat pain related to bone metastases [21].

Strontium-89 has shown some benefit in palliating pain symptoms in patients with metastatic prostate cancer [22–27]. Main side effects were hematological toxicity. Several phase III trials have been performed. Strontium-89 has been studied as an adjuvant treatment to local radiotherapy: it improves quality of life and pain control and reduces incidence of new sites of pain and the need for further radiotherapy. In another phase III trial, Strontium-89 was compared to radiotherapy. Overall survival was better in the radiotherapy arm (borderline significance). There was no difference in progression-free survival. Subjective response rates were similar in both arms (about 1/3 of patients). Studies of combination with chemotherapy have been performed with conflicting results. These combinations are not routinely used in the clinic.

Samarium-153 is the other radiopharmaceutical used in this setting [28–31]. In a phase III trial, radioactive 153Sm-lexidronam at the dose of 1 mCi/kg was compared to nonradioactive 152Sm-lexidronam in patients with hormone-refractory prostate cancer and painful bone metastases [32]. It showed an increase in pain relief compared within 1–2 weeks and a reduction in narcotic use at weeks 3 and 4. The main toxicity was mild myelosuppression. Blood count recovered at 8 weeks.

Several trials combining samarium with chemotherapy have been conducted. Combination with docetaxel is feasible [33, 34]. In a phase II trial, consolidation therapy with 153Sm-lexidronam and docetaxel allows long-term pain control in patients with metastatic castration-resistant prostate cancer that respond to docetaxel.

A new radionucleotide has been recently developed. In a phase III trial, Radium-223 (Alpharadin®) was compared to placebo in patients with castration-resistant prostate cancer and symptomatic bone metastases and no visceral metastases who had progressed after docetaxel or could not receive docetaxel [35]. Radium-223 is a calcium mimetic and an alpha-emitting particle. Radium-223 is excreted by the digestive tract and has a low penetration into adjacent tissues. Primary end point was overall survival. Mean age in this trial was 70.2 years. Five hundred and eight patients received Radium-223, and 254 received placebo. Patients enrolled in the study were given up to six intravenous treatments with radium-223 chloride or placebo. Results of the interim analysis show that median overall survival was 14 months in the Alpharadin® arm and 11.2 months in the placebo arm (HR = 0.695; p = 0.00185). Median time to first SRE was also delayed with Alpharadin®: 13.6 months versus 8 months (HR = 0.61; p = 0.0046). Tolerance was quite good. Main side effects were bone pain (43 % with radium-223 vs. 58 % with placebo), gastrointestinal toxicity such as diarrhea (22 % with radium-223 vs. 13 % with placebo), nausea (34 % with radium-223 vs. 32 % with placebo), and vomiting (17 % with radium-223 vs. 13 % with placebo). Anemia was the main hematological side effect (27 % in both arms, with grade 3–4 events in 11 % patients on radium and 12 % on placebo).

This could be an interesting drug for elderly patients with bone metastases from hormone-resistant cancer. It has not yet been approved.

New Treatments

Several new drugs are being developed in patients with metastatic castration-resistant prostate cancer. Some of the phase III trials are finished, and some have been published. There was not an upper age limit in these trials: older patients could be enrolled.

In the Cougar 301 study comparing abiraterone acetate + prednisone to placebo + prednisone, there was a benefit in overall survival with the use of abiraterone acetate. Median overall survival was 14.8 months with abiraterone and 10.9 months with placebo (hazard ratio = 0.65; 95 % confidence interval = 0.54–0.77; $p < 0.001$) (see Chap. 15). Subgroup analyses show a benefit in patients <65 years, in patients ≥65 years, and in patients ≥75 years too. Tolerance is good and therefore the drug can be used even in elderly patients. Blood pressure and potassium levels should be monitored [36].

Cabazitaxel is a new taxane that has shown a benefit in overall survival for patients with metastatic castration-resistant prostate cancer who have progressed after docetaxel, compared to mitoxantrone, in a phase III randomized trial [37]. In the cabazitaxel arm, median age was 68 years (95 % IC: 62–73); 18 % were ≥75 years. Subgroup analysis shows a benefit also in patients ≥65 years. However, toxicity is more important than with docetaxel (neutropenic fever, diarrhea, fatigue). This leads to carefully prevent and monitor side effect in elderly patients.

Disease-Related Complications

Pain

Pain is a frequent problem in patients with metastatic prostate cancer. It can be related to bone metastases or enlarged lymph nodes.

Management is based on pain killers. Nonsteroidal anti-inflammatory drugs should be avoided because of the gastrointestinal and renal side effects.

Often, morphine is necessary. When starting patients on narcotic drugs, dose must be adapted to renal function and be started slowly to avoid side effects, such as nausea and delirium. Constipation should be systematically prevented to avoid neurological complications.

Radiotherapy is a good treatment for palliating pain in patients. Data from phase III trials suggest that one fraction (8 Gy) can control bone pain as standard schemes [38, 39]. Most of these trials included patients with prostate cancer. This can allow treating elderly patients without many visits to the hospital.

Data from a retrospective trial on patients with symptomatic bone metastases showed a similar benefit from radiotherapy for patients ≥65, ≥70, and ≥75 years, compared to younger patients [40].

Specific treatments, such as chemotherapy, can also improve pain.

Bone Fractures and Cord Compressions

These are also frequent problems that can cause pain and disability.

Orthopedic surgery is the main treatment for bone fractures, usually followed by radiotherapy, to avoid local recurrence.

Cord compression is a more complex situation. Surgical treatment can be offered to patients. However, it is not always possible if the disease is progressive, if there are several vertebral metastases and if the patients have lots of comorbidities. The MD Anderson team published a retrospective series of 44 patients with metastatic prostate cancer who had stable enough condition to undergo surgery and who had obvious spinal deformity with intractable pain or significant spinal cord compression or prior irradiation of the site of progressive spinal involvement, or medically intractable mechanical or neurological pain [41]. Median age at surgery was 68 years (range 51–85 years). All patients had castration-resistant disease.

Out of the 12 patients that were not ambulatory before surgery, 8 regained their ability to ambulate. Eighty-four percent were continent after surgery. Two patients died. Median postoperative narcotic dose was lower than before surgery. The median length of stay after surgery was 12 days (range 1–46 days). Complications occurred in 15 of the 47 procedures (32 %). There were nine major complications (19 %) and six minor (13 %). Median overall survival was 5.4 months (95 % CI 0.8–10.1). In a multivariate analysis, age ≥ 65 years was associated with an increased risk of complications.

Radiotherapy can be used to treat spinal cord compression. Patchell et al. compared radiotherapy to surgery + radiotherapy in 101 patients with cord compression caused by metastases [42]. Nineteen patients had prostate cancer. The primary end point was ability to walk. More patients in the surgery group were able to walk (42/50, 84 % vs. 29/51, 57 %: odds ratio = 6.2 (95 % CI 2.0–19.8) $p=0.001$). They walked longer (median 122 vs. 13 days, $p=0.003$) and required less corticosteroids and opioid drugs. Thirty-two patients were unable to walk at study entry. Significantly more patients in the surgery group regained the ability to walk than patients in the radiation group (10/16 [62 %] vs. 3/16 [19 %], $p=0.01$).

In a matched paired analysis, Rades et al. found no difference in results with surgery + radiotherapy compared to radiotherapy alone [43]. One hundred and twenty-two patients with cord compression were treated with surgery followed by radiotherapy. Each patient was matched to 2 patients from a cohort of 2,296 patients treated by radiotherapy alone. They were matched for 11 prognosis factors. One hundred and eight groups were found, representing 324 patients. Thirty-three patients in the series had prostate cancer. In these 33 patients, 6-month and 12-month control rates were 100 and 93 %, respectively. Six-month and 12-month survival rates were 53 and 32 %, respectively

In the whole series, there was no difference in ambulatory rates, in the number of patients who regained ability to walk and local control rates according to the treatment.

In the multivariate analysis, survival was significantly associated with ECOG performance status, tumor type, number of involved vertebrae, visceral metastases, interval between tumor diagnosis and cord compression, and time developing motor deficits.

Hematological Complications

Patients with prostate cancer can develop pancytopenia or, more frequently, anemia and thrombocytopenia because of bone medullar involvement. Treatment is based on transfusion and general treatment of prostate cancer (hormone therapy, chemotherapy).

Another hematological complication is disseminated intravascular coagulation. This is a rare complication that usually arises late in the history of patients; however, in some patients, it is the first presenting symptom. Traditionally, estrogens were considered effective, in combination with low-dose heparin, platelet transfusion, and factor transfusion.

The MSKCC have recently reported their experience on 42 patients with prostate cancer and who met the following criterion: a fibrinogen level < 150 mg/dl and two of the following criteria: platelets < $150 \times 10(9)$/l, D-dimer > 0.5 µg/ml, prothrombin time, and activated partial thromboplastin time exceeding normal values, hemorrhage, and/or thrombosis [44].

Most patients had a Gleason score ≥ 7. Thirty-nine patients developed the syndrome in a context of metastatic disease; 93 % had castration-resistant disease. There was no thrombosis, but bleeding was frequent. Prognosis is poor with a median overall survival of 4 months. However, 20 % with metastatic patients had reversal of disseminated intravascular coagulation with excessive fibrinolysis, mainly after receiving chemotherapy. In that group, median survival was 26 months.

Urinary Complications

Patients who have received treatment for their primary tumor can have urinary long-term side effects, such as incontinence, urinary retention, urgency, and hematuria (radiotherapy-induced cystitis). Incontinence is more frequent when patients are treated at an older age.

In other cases, patients can develop urinary symptoms because of local (and regional) evolution. Patients can develop urinary retention that may require transurethral resection or indwelling catheters. Ureteral obstruction is frequent; it can be caused by compression by the primary prostate tumor or metastatic lymph nodes. It usually requires ureteral stenting or in some cases nephrostomies.

Sometimes, bladder invasion by the primary tumor can be responsible for hematuria. Resection can sometimes improve symptoms. Palliative hemostatic radiotherapy can be offered.

Palliative radiotherapy can be used in patients with metastatic castration disease and symptomatic local tumor. Din et al. reported their experience on 58 patients who received palliative short course radiotherapy for troublesome pelvic symptoms, such as hematuria, urinary obstruction symptoms, rectal obstruction symptoms, and pelvic pain [45]. Most patients received 20 Gy. More than half of the patients had metastases when they received irradiation, and 97 % had received androgen deprivation therapy. Median age was 76.6 years (54–91). At 4 months, 89 % of patients had complete or partial symptom resolution. Median overall survival from radiotherapy was 13.6 months. Toxicity was manageable.

Elderly patients with metastatic castration-resistant will probably die from disease progression. Chemotherapy and hormonal therapy improve symptom control and overall survival but do not cure patients. Palliative symptom control is important, especially in patients with terminal disease.

Conclusions

Metastatic prostate cancer occurs frequently in elderly men. Treatment of hormone-sensitive disease is based in androgen deprivation.

Management of castration disease in elderly patients requires evaluation of the balance between the risk/symptoms related to the disease, the expected benefit of the treatment, and its side effects and the underlying medical and social conditions of the patient. First-line chemotherapy with docetaxel can be used in elderly patients. Administration modalities may need to be adjusted in vulnerable patients and must be adapted in frail patients. Some patients can benefit from new treatments, such as abiraterone.

Prevention of skeletal-related events is important, especially in elderly patients so that they do not become dependent.

Many complications can occur in the evolution of metastatic prostate cancer. It is important that patients' symptoms be palliated; sometimes, it will require multimodality approaches.

References

1. Ferlay J, Shin HR, Bray F, Forman D, Mathers C, Parkin DM. GLOBOCAN 2008 v1.2, cancer incidence and mortality worldwide: IARC CancerBase No. 10 [Internet]. Lyon: International Agency for Research on Cancer; 2010.
2. Droz JP, Balducci L, Bolla M, Emberton M, Fitzpatrick JM, Joniau S, Kattan MW, Monfardini S, Moul JW, Naeim A, van Poppel H, Saad F, Sternberg CN. Background for the proposal of SIOG guidelines for the management of prostate cancer in senior adults. Crit Rev Oncol Hematol. 2010;73(1):68–91.
3. Extermann M, Hurria A. Comprehensive geriatric assessment for older patients with cancer. J Clin Oncol. 2007;25(14):1824–31. Review.
4. Huggins C, Hodges CV. Studies on prostatic cancer. I. The effect of castration, of estrogen and of androgen injection on serum phosphatase in metastatic carcinoma of the prostate. J Urol. 2002;167(2P 2):948–51, discussion 952.
5. Huggins C, Stevens Jr RE, Hodges CV. Studies on prostate cancer. II. The effect of castration on advanced carcinoma of the prostate gland. Arch Surg. 1941;43:209.
6. Mottet N, Bellmunt J, Bolla M, Joniau S, Mason M, Matveev V, Schmid HP, Van der Kwast T, Wiegel T, Zattoni F, Heidenreich A. EAU guidelines on prostate cancer. Part II: treatment of advanced, relapsing, and castration-resistant prostate cancer. Eur Urol. 2011;59(4):572–83.

7. Soloway MS, Chodak G, Vogelzang NJ, Block NL, Schellhammer PF, Smith Jr JA, Scott M, Kennealey G, Gau TC. Zoladex versus orchiectomy in treatment of advanced prostate cancer: a randomized trial. Zoladex Prostate Study Group. Urology. 1991;37(1):46–51.

8. Peeling WB. Phase III studies to compare goserelin (Zoladex) with orchiectomy and with diethylstilbestrol in treatment of prostatic carcinoma. Urology. 1989;33(5 Suppl):45–52.

9. Labrie F, Dupont A, Bélanger A, Emond J, Monfette G. Simultaneous administration of pure antiandrogens, a combination necessary for the use of luteinizing hormone-releasing hormone agonists in the treatment of prostate cancer. Proc Natl Acad Sci USA. 1984;81(12):3861–3.

10. Maximum androgen blockade in advanced prostate cancer: an overview of the randomised trials. Prostate Cancer Trialists' Collaborative Group. Lancet. 2000;355(9214):1491–8.

11. Nair B, Wilt T, MacDonald R, Rutks I. Early versus deferred androgen suppression in the treatment of advanced prostatic cancer. Cochrane Database Syst Rev. 2002;(1):CD003506.

12. http://www.nccn.org/professionals/physician_gls/pdf/prostate.pdf. November 2011.

13. Taylor LG, Canfield SE, Du XL. Review of major adverse effects of androgen-deprivation therapy in men with prostate cancer. Cancer. 2009;115(11):2388–99.

14. Levine GN, D'Amico AV, Berger P, Clark PE, Eckel RH, Keating NL, Milani RV, Sagalowsky AI, Smith MR, Zakai N, American Heart Association Council on Clinical Cardiology and Council on Epidemiology and Prevention, the American Cancer Society, and the American Urological Association. Androgen-deprivation therapy in prostate cancer and cardiovascular risk: a science advisory from the American Heart Association, American Cancer Society, and American Urological Association: endorsed by the American Society for Radiation Oncology. Circulation. 2010;121(6):833–40.

15. Tannock IF, de Wit R, Berry WR, Horti J, Pluzanska A, Chi KN, Oudard S, Théodore C, James ND, Turesson I, Rosenthal MA, Eisenberger MA, TAX 327 Investigators. Docetaxel plus prednisone or mitoxantrone plus prednisone for advanced prostate cancer. N Engl J Med. 2004;351(15):1502–12.

16. Fosså SD, Jacobsen AB, Ginman C, Jacobsen IN, Overn S, Iversen JR, Urnes T, Dahl AA, Veenstra M, Sandstad B. Weekly docetaxel and prednisolone versus prednisolone alone in androgen-independent prostate cancer: a randomized phase II study. Eur Urol. 2007;52(6):1691–8.

17. Aapro MS, Bohlius J, Cameron DA, Dal Lago L, Donnelly JP, Kearney N, Lyman GH, Pettengell R, Tjan-Heijnen VC, Walewski J, Weber DC, Zielinski C, European Organisation for Research and Treatment of Cancer. 2010 Update of EORTC guidelines for the use of granulocyte-colony stimulating factor to reduce the incidence of chemotherapy-induced febrile neutropenia in adult patients with lymphoproliferative disorders and solid tumours. Eur J Cancer. 2011;47(1):8–32.

18. Saad F, Gleason DM, Murray R, Tchekmedyian S, Venner P, Lacombe L, Chin JL, Vinholes JJ, Goas JA, Chen B, Zoledronic Acid Prostate Cancer Study Group. A randomized, placebo-controlled trial of zoledronic acid in patients with hormone-refractory metastatic prostate carcinoma. J Natl Cancer Inst. 2002;94(19):1458–68.

19. Saad F, Gleason DM, Murray R, Tchekmedyian S, Venner P, Lacombe L, Chin JL, Vinholes JJ, Goas JA, Zheng M, Zoledronic Acid Prostate Cancer Study Group. Long-term efficacy of zoledronic acid for the prevention of skeletal complications in patients with metastatic hormone-refractory prostate cancer. J Natl Cancer Inst. 2004;96(11):879–82.

20. Fizazi K, Carducci M, Smith M, Damião R, Brown J, Karsh L, Milecki P, Shore N, Rader M, Wang H, Jiang Q, Tadros S, Dansey R, Goessl C. Denosumab versus zoledronic acid for treatment of bone metastases in men with castration-resistant prostate cancer: a randomised, double-blind study. Lancet. 2011;377(9768):813–22.

21. Bauman G, Charette M, Reid R, Sathya J. Radiopharmaceuticals for the palliation of painful bone metastasis-a systemic review. Radiother Oncol. 2005;75(3):258–70. Review.

22. Nilsson S, Strang P, Ginman C, Zimmermann R, Edgren M, Nordström B, Ryberg M, Kälkner KM, Westlin JE. Palliation of bone pain in prostate cancer using chemotherapy and strontium-89. A randomized phase II study. J Pain Symptom Manage. 2005;29(4):352–7.

23. Oosterhof GO, Roberts JT, de Reijke TM, Engelholm SA, Horenblas S, von der Maase H, Neymark N, Debois M, Collette L. Strontium(89) chloride versus palliative local field

radiotherapy in patients with hormonal escaped prostate cancer: a phase III study of the European Organisation for Research and Treatment of Cancer, Genitourinary Group. Eur Urol. 2003;44(5):519–26.

24. Smeland S, Erikstein B, Aas M, Skovlund E, Hess SL, Fosså SD. Role of strontium-89 as adjuvant to palliative external beam radiotherapy is questionable: results of a double-blind randomized study. Int J Radiat Oncol Biol Phys. 2003;56(5):1397–404.

25. Pagliaro LC, Delpassand ES, Williams D, Millikan RE, Tu SM, Logothetis CJ. A phase I/II study of strontium-89 combined with gemcitabine in the treatment of patients with androgen independent prostate carcinoma and bone metastases. Cancer. 2003;97(12):2988–94.

26. Akerley W, Butera J, Wehbe T, Noto R, Stein B, Safran H, Cummings F, Sambandam S, Maynard J, Di Rienzo G, Leone L. A multiinstitutional, concurrent chemoradiation trial of strontium-89, estramustine, and vinblastine for hormone refractory prostate carcinoma involving bone. Cancer. 2002;94(6):1654–60.

27. Sciuto R, Festa A, Rea S, Pasqualoni R, Bergomi S, Petrilli G, Maini CL. Effects of low-dose cisplatin on 89Sr therapy for painful bone metastases from prostate cancer: a randomized clinical trial. J Nucl Med. 2002;43(1):79–86.

28. Serafini AN. Samarium Sm-153 lexidronam for the palliation of bone pain associated with metastases. Cancer. 2000;88(12 Suppl):2934–9. Review.

29. Menda Y, Bushnell DL, Williams RD, Miller S, Thomas MO. Efficacy and safety of repeated samarium-153 lexidronam treatment in a patient with prostate cancer and metastatic bone pain. Clin Nucl Med. 2000;25(9):698–700.

30. Sartor O. Overview of samarium sm 153 lexidronam in the treatment of painful metastatic bone disease. Rev Urol. 2004;6 Suppl 10:S3–12.

31. Sartor O, Reid RH, Bushnell DL, Quick DP, Ell PJ. Safety and efficacy of repeat administration of samarium Sm-153 lexidronam to patients with metastatic bone pain. Cancer. 2007;109(3):637–43.

32. Sartor O, Reid RH, Hoskin PJ, Quick DP, Ell PJ, Coleman RE, Kotler JA, Freeman LM, Olivier P, Quadramet 424Sm10/11 Study Group. Samarium-153-lexidronam complex for treatment of painful bone metastases in hormone-refractory prostate cancer. Urology. 2004;63(5):940–5.

33. Morris MJ, Pandit-Taskar N, Carrasquillo J, Divgi CR, Slovin S, Kelly WK, Rathkopf D, Gignac GA, Solit D, Schwartz L, Stephenson RD, Hong C, Delacruz A, Curley T, Heller G, Jia X, O'Donoghue J, Larson S, Scher HI. Phase I study of samarium-153 lexidronam with docetaxel in castration-resistant metastatic prostate cancer. J Clin Oncol. 2009;27(15):2436–42.

34. Fizazi K, Beuzeboc P, Lumbroso J, Haddad V, Massard C, Gross-Goupil M, Di Palma M, Escudier B, Theodore C, Loriot Y, Tournay E, Bouzy J, Laplanche A. Phase II trial of consolidation docetaxel and samarium-153 in patients with bone metastases from castration-resistant prostate cancer. J Clin Oncol. 2009;27(15):2429–35.

35. Parker C, et al. First phase III trial of an alpha-pharmaceutical shows improved survival in patients with bone metastases and advanced prostate cancer. The 2011 European Multidisciplinary Cancer Congress is the 16th congress of the European CanCer Organisation (ECCO), the 36th congress of the European Society for Medical Oncology (ESMO) and the 30th congress of European Society for Therapeutic Radiology and Oncology (ESTRO), Stockholm.

36. de Bono JS, Logothetis CJ, Molina A, Fizazi K, North S, Chu L, Chi KN, Jones RJ, Goodman Jr OB, Saad F, Staffurth JN, Mainwaring P, Harland S, Flaig TW, Hutson TE, Cheng T, Patterson H, Hainsworth JD, Ryan CJ, Sternberg CN, Ellard SL, Fléchon A, Saleh M, Scholz M, Efstathiou E, Zivi A, Bianchini D, Loriot Y, Chieffo N, Kheoh T, Haqq CM, Scher HI, COU-AA-301 Investigators. Abiraterone and increased survival in metastatic prostate cancer. N Engl J Med. 2011;364(21):1995–2005.

37. de Bono JS, Oudard S, Ozguroglu M, Hansen S, Machiels JP, Kocak I, Gravis G, Bodrogi I, Mackenzie MJ, Shen L, Roessner M, Gupta S, Sartor AO, TROPIC Investigators. Prednisone plus cabazitaxel or mitoxantrone for metastatic castration-resistant prostate cancer progressing after docetaxel treatment: a randomised open-label trial. Lancet. 2010;376(9747):1147–54.

38. Nielsen OS, Bentzen SM, Sandberg E, Gadeberg CC, Timothy AR. Randomized trial of single dose versus fractionated palliative radiotherapy of bone metastases. Radiother Oncol. 1998;47(3):233–40.
39. Hartsell WF, Scott CB, Bruner DW, Scarantino CW, Ivker RA, Roach 3rd M, Suh JH, Demas WF, Movsas B, Petersen IA, Konski AA, Cleeland CS, Janjan NA, DeSilvio M. Randomized trial of short- versus long-course radiotherapy for palliation of painful bone metastases. J Natl Cancer Inst. 2005;97(11):798–804.
40. Campos S, Presutti R, Zhang L, Salvo N, Hird A, Tsao M, Barnes EA, Danjoux C, Sahgal A, Mitera G, Sinclair E, DeAngelis C, Nguyen J, Napolskikh J, Chow E. Elderly patients with painful bone metastases should be offered palliative radiotherapy. Int J Radiat Oncol Biol Phys. 2010;76(5):1500–6.
41. Williams BJ, Fox BD, Sciubba DM, Suki D, Tu SM, Kuban D, Gokaslan ZL, Rhines LD, Rao G. Surgical management of prostate cancer metastatic to the spine. J Neurosurg Spine. 2009;10(5):414–22.
42. Patchell RA, Tibbs PA, Regine WF, Payne R, Saris S, Kryscio RJ, Mohiuddin M, Young B. Direct decompressive surgical resection in the treatment of spinal cord compression caused by metastatic cancer: a randomised trial. Lancet. 2005;366(9486):643–8.
43. Rades D, Huttenlocher S, Dunst J, Bajrovic A, Karstens JH, Rudat V, Schild SE. Matched pair analysis comparing surgery followed by radiotherapy and radiotherapy alone for metastatic spinal cord compression. J Clin Oncol. 2010;28(22):3597–604.
44. Hyman DM, Soff GA, Kampel LJ. Disseminated intravascular coagulation with excessive fibrinolysis in prostate cancer: a case series and review of the literature. Oncology. 2011;81(2):119–25.
45. Din OS, Thanvi N, Ferguson CJ, Kirkbride P. Palliative prostate radiotherapy for symptomatic advanced prostate cancer. Radiother Oncol. 2009;93(2):192–6.

Chapter 15
New Treatment Developments Applied to Elderly Patients

Deborah Mukherji, Carmel J. Pezaro, and Johann S. De-Bono

Abstract Metastatic prostate cancer remains a considerable therapeutic challenge; however, recent advances in clinical research have resulted in five new treatments with positive phase III trial results in the last 2 years. The immunotherapy sipuleu-cel-T, the cytotoxic cabazitaxel, the androgen biosynthesis inhibitor abiraterone acetate, the radioisotope Alpharadin, and the antiandrogen MDV3100 have all been shown to improve survival in randomized, phase III studies for patients with metastatic castration-resistant prostate cancer (CRPC). This chapter will discuss clinical trials in elderly patients with prostate cancer and review the clinical data regarding new developments as applied to the elderly population.

Keywords Prostate cancer • Abiraterone • Sipuleucel-T • Cabazitaxel • MDV3100 • Alpharadin • Denosumab

Introduction

Metastatic prostate cancer remains a considerable therapeutic challenge; however, recent advances in clinical research have resulted in five new treatments with positive phase III trial results in the last 2 years. The immunotherapy sipuleucel-T, the cytotoxic cabazitaxel, the androgen biosynthesis inhibitor abiraterone acetate, the

D. Mukherji, B.Sc., M.B.B.S., Ph.D., MRCP • C.J. Pezaro, BHB, MBChB, FRACP, DMedSc
J.S. De-Bono, MBChB, M.Sc., Ph.D., FRCP (✉)
Drug Development Unit and Prostate Targeted Therapy Group,
The Royal Marsden Foundation Trust,
Sutton, Surrey, UK
e-mail: Deborah.mukherji@icr.ac.uk; Carmel.pezaro@icr.ac.uk; Johann.de-bono@icr.ac.uk

J.-P. Droz, R.A. Audisio (eds.), *Management of Urological Cancers in Older People*, 217
Management of Cancer in Older People,
DOI 10.1007/978-0-85729-999-4_15, © Springer-Verlag London 2013

radioisotope Alpharadin, and the antiandrogen MDV3100 have all been shown to improve survival in randomized, phase III studies for patients with metastatic castration-resistant prostate cancer (CRPC) [1–5]. This chapter will discuss clinical trials in elderly patients with prostate cancer and review the clinical data regarding new developments as applied to the elderly population.

Abiraterone

Abiraterone acetate (Zytiga®, Janssen) is an oral inhibitor of CYP17A1, a key enzyme in the testosterone biosynthesis pathway. Inhibition of CYP17A1 results in reduction of testosterone from adrenal steroid precursors and also interferes with intratumoral testosterone production. In a partnership with Cancer Research UK, scientists at the Institute of Cancer Research designed abiraterone acetate as a more specific CYP inhibitor than the previously utilized agent ketoconazole, a nonspecific CYP inhibitor with significant associated toxicity [6, 7]. In a pivotal phase III study published in 2011, abiraterone acetate was proven to prolong survival in men with CRPC who had progressive disease following docetaxel chemotherapy [3]. Approval from the US Food and Drug Administration (FDA) for the use of abiraterone acetate in the post-docetaxel setting for CRPC followed in April 2011. From the outset, the clinical testing of abiraterone acetate has included elderly men. Phase I testing included men in their 70s and 80s, and no age-specific issues were identified in terms of pharmacokinetic profile or adverse effects [8, 9]. In a dedicated renal impairment trial, renal dysfunction had no appreciable impact on pharmacokinetic parameters [10]. Phase II studies in both chemo-naïve and post-docetaxel patients suggested similar rates of PSA decline and radiological response in elderly men compared to their younger counterparts [11–13]. In the randomized, phase III trial COU-AA-301, 331 of the 1,195 participants were at least 75 years of age, and the median age of the overall study population was 69 years. The eligibility criteria reflected a representative "real-world" population, including 10 % of participants with a baseline Eastern Cooperative Oncology Group (ECOG) performance status of 2. The main exclusion criteria were significant liver dysfunction, uncontrolled hypertension, and clinically significant cardiac dysfunction.

In early testing, abiraterone acetate was given as a single agent, with glucocorticoids added for the management of toxicity or at initial progression. Although no dose-limiting toxicities were identified, side effects relating to the accumulation of upstream steroid precursors with potent mineralocorticoid effects led to the recommendation for combination treatment of abiraterone acetate with prednisone (or prednisolone) 5 mg twice daily. The phase III study was a double-blind, randomized study comparing abiraterone acetate with prednisone versus matched placebo with prednisone.

The primary end point of the COU-AA-301 study was overall survival, and the study was halted when prespecified criteria for efficacy were met at the planned interim analysis. The initial analysis reported a 3.9-month improvement in median survival, but at the final analysis, the benefit had extended to 4.6 months [14]. All secondary efficacy end points favored the experimental arm at the time of study unblinding, including time to PSA progression (10.2 vs. 6.6 months, $p < 0.001$), progression-free survival (5.6 vs. 3.6 months, $p < 0.001$), and PSA response rate (29 vs. 6 %, $p < 0.001$) [3].

An important exploratory end point in COU-AA-301 was quality of life assessment using the functional assessment of cancer therapy (prostate version) (FACT-P) and the brief pain inventory (short form) (BPI). Pain palliation was shown to be significantly superior in patients who received abiraterone acetate, but FACT-P results have yet to be formally reported. Participants also completed brief fatigue inventory (BFI), and again, there was significant improvement in men who received abiraterone acetate compared to placebo [15].

Despite the addition of prednisone, the most common side effects in patients receiving abiraterone acetate related to mineralocorticoid excess include hypertension, fluid retention, and hypokalemia. These toxicities were managed with increased glucocorticoid doses or by using the specific mineralocorticoid antagonist eplerenone. The incidence of hypertension was 10 % in the abiraterone acetate group compared to 8 % in the placebo group with the incidence of grade 3 hypertension 1 % and <1 % in each group, respectively. The incidence of fluid retention and edema was higher in the abiraterone acetate group (31 vs. 22 % in the placebo group, $p = 0.04$); however, most of these events were grades 1 or 2 and easily managed. Hypokalemia occurred more commonly in the group receiving abiraterone acetate (17 vs. 8 % in the placebo group, $p < 0.001$) with 27 patients experiencing grade 3 and 3 patients experiencing grade 4 hypokalemia in the abiraterone group. The frequency of cardiac adverse events was not significantly different in the abiraterone acetate group compared with the placebo group (13 vs. 11 %, respectively, $p = 0.14$). For elderly patients who may be more likely to suffer from common comorbidities such as hypertension and reduced cardiac function, evaluation and optimization of cardiac status prior to commencing abiraterone therapy is recommended. Careful monitoring of blood pressure and potassium once abiraterone treatment is started with proactive management of treatment-related hypertension, hypokalemia, and fluid overload should minimize treatment-related morbidity.

Abiraterone acetate treatment has been associated with elevated aminotransferase levels; however, in the randomized, phase III study, abnormalities in liver function blood tests occurred at a similar frequency in both groups. Despite this, it has been recommended that liver function tests are closely monitored, particularly during the first 12 weeks of abiraterone acetate treatment.

Abiraterone acetate is orally administered once daily at a recommended dose of 1,000 mg (four 250 mg tablets). It is recommended that it is taken on an empty stomach with no food consumed for at least 2 h pre-dose and 1 h post-dose, although clinical trial data indicate that abiraterone given in the fed state increases drug absorption [9]. This may have implications for patients on multiple other tablets. Abiraterone is given in combination with low-dose corticosteroids, most commonly prednisone or prednisolone 5 mg twice daily; however, dexamethasone 0.5 mg daily can also be used and has much less mineralocorticoid activity. Concomitant corticosteroids may be problematic for certain patients, particularly those with diabetes. It is not yet known whether longer-term abiraterone acetate therapy will be associated with development of clinically important late toxicities. Certainly, the further lowering of testosterone in castrate patients, so-called super castration, may be associated with further morbidity in terms of bone and cardiovascular health which will need careful monitoring. In general, abiraterone acetate is an extremely well-tolerated treatment in patients of all ages.

Abiraterone has also been tested in chemotherapy-naïve patients in the phase III COU-AA-302 study which randomized 1088 patients to receive abiraterone plus prednisone or placebo plus prednisone. The co-primary endpoints of this study were radiographic PFS (rPFS) and OS. The study was unblinded and patients receiving placebo offered abiraterone when a planned interim analysis showed a statistically significant improvement in rPFS and a strong trend for increased OS in the abiraterone arm. Median rPFS was 8.3 months in the placebo arm and had not been reached in the abiraterone arm; median OS was 27.2 months in the placebo arm and again had not been reached in the abiraterone arm [16]. Full results from this study are awaited; however, if abiraterone is approved for use before docetaxel chemotherapy, it may offer an attractive therapeutic option for elderly patients reluctant or unable to tolerate toxicities associated with cytotoxic chemotherapy.

Cabazitaxel

In 2010, the novel taxane agent cabazitaxel (Jevtana®, Sanofi-Aventis) was shown to significantly prolong survival for men with metastatic CRPC who had previously received docetaxel chemotherapy. Cabazitaxel was initially investigated in early phase studies that enrolled patients up to the age of 80 years, one of whom had advanced prostate cancer and whose partial response led to further investigation in prostate cancer patients. Thus far, there has been limited experience using cabazitaxel in elderly patients. Pharmacokinetic analysis from phase I testing showed no difference in patients 75 years or older, compared to those younger than 65. In addition, there was no significant difference in the clearance of cabazitaxel in patients with mild or moderate renal impairment (creatinine clearance >30 ml/min) [17]. Cabazitaxel is minimally excreted through the kidney, but has not been tested in patients with severe renal impairment. Cabazitaxel is extensively metabolized by the liver, so hepatic impairment would be expected to increase plasma concentration and exaggerate toxicity.

The most detailed clinical information for cabazitaxel is that from the pivotal, randomized, phase III TROPIC study, the results of which led to US Food and Drug Administration (FDA) approval in June 2010. This study enrolled 755 patients with progressive CRPC after docetaxel chemotherapy and tested cabazitaxel and prednisolone against a standard therapy comparator of mitoxantrone and prednisolone [2]. The median age of participants receiving cabazitaxel was 67 years. Seventy of the men enrolled were at least 75 years old (9 %). The trial specifically excluded patients with significant preexisting renal, hepatic, or cardiac dysfunction.

The TROPIC study demonstrated a 2.4-month improvement in median survival for subjects receiving cabazitaxel, correlating with a hazard ratio of 0.7 ($p < 0.0001$) [2]. In the planned subgroup analysis, the survival advantage was preserved for men >65 years. Additional efficacy parameters such as progression-free survival, tumor response, and PSA response also favored the cabazitaxel group overall, but subgroup information on responses in elderly patients has not been published to date.

Toxicity was observed to be greater in older patients who participated in the TROPIC trial. All-grade neutropenia was observed in 24.2 % of the 240 patients ≥65 years, compared to 17.6 % in 131 patients <65 years. Febrile neutropenia also occurred more frequently in the older population (8 % compared to 6 %, respectively). Other adverse events that were reported more commonly in patients ≥65 years included fatigue (40 % compared to 30 %), asthenia (24 % compared to 15 %), pyrexia (15 % compared to 8 %), dizziness (10 % compared to 5 %), urinary tract infection (10 % compared to 3 %), and dehydration (7 % compared to 2 %) [18].

Toxic deaths (defined as deaths within 30 days of receiving chemotherapy that were not related to disease progression) occurred in 18 patients who participated in the TROPIC study. Seven of these were ascribed to neutropenia or sepsis, five to cardiac dysfunction, and three to renal failure [2]. Only three of the deaths occurred in younger patients, making the toxic death rate in patients ≥65 years a rather concerning 6 % (15 of 240 patients) [18]. It is unclear whether the use of gold standard supportive management including growth-factor support and febrile neutropenia pathways will improve the on-treatment mortality.

It is hoped that the safety of cabazitaxel in elderly patients will be further defined in data from the completed expanded access program and from two large (approximately 1,200 patient) trials currently recruiting. The expanded access program was conducted in multiple countries worldwide and collected safety and quality of life data on participants; this is likely to be published in the near future. The PROSELICA study (clinicaltrials.gov identifier NCT01308580) is enrolling patients with metastatic CRPC fit for second-line chemotherapy and randomizing them between the cabazitaxel dose of 25 mg/m^2 used in the TROPIC trial and the lower dose of 20 mg/m^2, which was recommended as the maximum tolerated dose in one of the two conducted phase I trials [17]. The FIRSTANA trial (clinicaltrials.gov identifier NCT01308567) is a first-line chemotherapy trial, randomizing men with metastatic CRPC between one of the two cabazitaxel doses and to the current standard of docetaxel chemotherapy at 75 mg/m^2. Appropriately, neither study has an upper age criterion, meaning that fit elderly patients will be offered the choice to participate. In addition, a phase I study examining safety and pharmacokinetics of cabazitaxel in patients with liver impairment (clinicaltrials.gov identifier NCT01140607) is likely to provide useful information.

Considering the utility of cabazitaxel in elderly patients outside of clinical trials, the recommendations of the International Society of Geriatric Oncology are likely to prove most appropriate: patients will need to be managed according to individual health status rather than chronological age [19]. The data available thus far support the assertion that elderly men who are healthy seem able to tolerate cabazitaxel as well as younger men, whereas men who have significant comorbidities are likely to suffer more severe toxicity and to gain less benefit from treatment.

Sipuleucel-T

The approval of sipuleucel-T (Provenge®, Dendreon) by the US Food and Drug Administration (FDA) for the treatment of minimally symptomatic CRPC in April 2010 heralded the first immunotherapy to be approved for cancer treatment. In a randomized, phase III trial involving 512 patients with asymptomatic or minimally symptomatic CRPC, median OS was 25.8 months in the sipuleucel-T group, compared with 21.7 months in the placebo group (unadjusted HR for death in the sipuleucel-T group 0.77, 95 % CI 0.61–0.97, $p=0.02$) [1]. There was no difference in time to objective or clinical disease progression between the two study arms. The median age of patients enrolled within this study was 71 (range 40–91 years), and all were minimally symptomatic with an Eastern Cooperative Group (ECOG) performance status of 0 or 1. Previous studies had suggested an increase in cerebrovascular adverse events associated with sipuleucel-T [20], and in the pivotal phase III study, cerebrovascular events were reported for 8 of 338 patients (2.4 %) in the sipuleucel-T arm and 3 of 168 patients (1.8 %) in the placebo arm ($p=1.00$ by Fisher's exact test). The incidence rate was 1.33 cerebrovascular events per 100 person years (95 % CI 0.58–2.62) in the sipuleucel-T group and 1.11 per 100 person years (05 % CI 0.23–3.24) in the placebo group. Although adverse effects were reported in most patients on trial, treatment was generally well tolerated with few reported grade 3–4 events (31.7 % sipuleucel-T vs. 35.1 % placebo arm). Toxicities reported more commonly in sipuleucel-T patients were generally self-limiting grade 1–2 events that often occurred shortly after the infusion. The most common of these toxicities included chills (51.2 %), nausea (28.1 %), fever (22.5 %), headache (16 %), and pain (13 %). In a survival analysis of all randomized studies investigating sipuleucel-T, 78.3 % of randomized patients were ≥65 years of age. The median survival of patients in the sipuleucel-T group ≥65 years of age was 23.4 months (95 % CI 22.0–27.1), compared with 17.3 months in the control group (95 % CI 13.5–21.5). There were no apparent differences in the safety of sipuleucel-T between patients ≥65 years of age and younger patients [21]. Sipuleucel-T may be an attractive option for asymptomatic or minimally symptomatic CRPC pre-docetaxel; however, the high costs of over \$93,000 for the 1-month course of treatment are likely to impact its use [22].

Alpharadin

Radium-223 chloride (Alpharadin®, Bayer) is a novel bone-targeting alpha-emitting agent which has recently been reported to improve overall survival in patients with CRPC and symptomatic bone metastasis. Following a planned interim analysis of a phase III trial showing mean overall survival in the Alpharadin arm of 14 months compared to 11.2 months for placebo (two-sided $p=0.0033$, HR=0.699), the trial was stopped, and patients on the placebo arm were offered treatment with Alpharadin

[4]. Patients were eligible for the phase III ALSYMPCA study if they had prostate cancer with confirmed symptomatic bone metastasis and no evidence of visceral disease or significant lymphadenopathy and were either post-docetaxel or unfit for docetaxel chemotherapy. The mean age in both arms was 70 years. At baseline, 13 % of the Alpharadin group and 14 % of the placebo group had an Eastern Cooperative Oncology Group (ECOG) performance status of 2, and 42 % of patients randomized within the study had not received prior docetaxel therapy. Alpharadin appeared to be well tolerated; however, thrombocytopenia and diarrhea were seen more frequently in the Alpharadin group compared to the placebo group. Alpharadin treatment significantly prolonged time to first skeletal-related adverse event (HR = 0.610, 95 % CI 0.461–0.807, p = 0.00046), time to PSA progression and both ALP response, and time to ALP progression. Alpharadin has yet to be granted regulatory approval for use; however, this is anticipated in 2012. For elderly patients with significant comorbidities unfit for docetaxel chemotherapy, Alpharadin may be an important palliative treatment option.

MDV3100

MDV3100 is an oral novel AR antagonist that binds to the AR more avidly than currently available antiandrogens. MDV3100 prevents DNA binding, induces apoptosis, and has no agonist activity when AR is overexpressed [23]. In a phase I/II study of MDV3100 involving 140 men with progressive, metastatic CRPC, antitumor effects were noted at all doses used, and there was a decrease in serum PSA of 50 % or more in 78 patients (56 %). In this study, the mean age was 58 years, and nine patients were over 80 years old [24]. MDV3100 was generally well tolerated with fatigue, the most common adverse event reported in the phase I/II trial. A significant proportion of patients required dose reductions for fatigue at doses of 240 mg/day and above. Concern has been raised regarding MDV3100 lowering seizure threshold which may be relevant for elderly patients. There were two witnessed seizures at doses of 600 and 360 mg/day and one possible seizure at 480 mg/day. Both patients with witnessed seizures were taking concurrent medications that could have contributed to a lowered seizure threshold. Despite this, patients with a history of seizure have been excluded from phase III clinical trials evaluating MDV3100. Concurrent steroids are not required with MDV3100 treatment; however, surgical castration or maintenance of LHRH agonists has been mandated for phase III studies of MDV3100 in CRPC.

The phase III AFFIRM study of MDV3100 160 mg daily versus placebo for metastatic CRPC in patients who have progressed after docetaxel chemotherapy has shown a significant survival benefit associated with MDV3100 treatment. A planned interim analysis of the study showed a 4.8-month improvement in median overall survival associated with MDV3100 treatment compared to placebo (18.4 vs. 13.6 months, HR = 0.631, p < 0.0001) [5]. Regulatory approval for MDV3100 in the post-chemotherapy setting is anticipated; however, it is expected that MDV3100 will also benefit patients at earlier stages of disease. The phase III PREVAIL study is examining the overall survival and progression-free survival benefits in patients with progressive, metastatic prostate cancer who have failed androgen deprivation therapy but have not yet received chemotherapy (ClinicalTrials.gov identifier: NCT01212991). An advantage of MDV3100 for elderly patients over androgen bio-synthesis inhibitors such as abiraterone acetate is the fact that concurrent steroids are not required with MDV3100.

Denosumab

Bone is the most common site of prostate cancer metastasis, and these are a major cause of prostate cancer-specific morbidity and mortality [25]. Elderly patients are also at increased risk of complications secondary to reduced bone mineral density associated with normal aging and accelerated by androgen deprivation therapies [26]. Prior standard of care for the treatment of osteoporosis and palliation of bone metastasis was the bisphosphonate zoledronic acid [27]. RANK (receptor activator of nuclear factor kappa B) signaling has been identified as a potent stimulus for osteoclast proliferation and bone resorption. Denosumab (Xgeva®, Amgen) is a fully humanized monoclonal antibody targeting RANK ligand (RANKL) that has recently been shown to be superior to zoledronic acid in preventing or delaying skeletal-related events (SREs) in patients with bone metastases from CRPC in a phase III trial [28]. This large, double-blind study of non-inferiority design random-ized 1,904 patients to denosumab 120 mg subcutaneously monthly or zoledronic acid 4 mg intravenously monthly. The primary composite end point was time to SRE as defined by pathological fracture, radiotherapy to bone, surgery to bone, or spinal cord compression. The median age of participants was 71 years. The adverse event profile was similar in both arms. There were significantly more cases of hypocalcemia in the group of patients receiving denosumab. Patients with a creati-nine clearance of less than 0.5 ml/s were excluded from the trial due to the contrain-dication of zoledronic acid for patients with this level of renal impairment. Denosumab was shown to be superior to zoledronic acid for prevention of SRE in this population of patients with median time to SRE 20.7 months in the denosumab arm compared to 17.1 months in the zoledronic acid arm giving a hazard ratio of 0.82, $p=0.008$ [28]. In an earlier study, denosumab was tested against placebo at a lower dose of 60 mg subcutaneously every 6 months in men receiving androgen deprivation therapy for prostate cancer. The primary end point in this study was the percentage change in bone mineral density in the lumbar spine at 24 months. The median age of participants receiving denosumab was 75.3 years. Treatment was generally well tolerated, and denosumab therapy resulted in increased bone mineral density and reduced the incidence of new vertebral fractures [29].

Donosumab has advantages over zoledronic acid in ease of subcutaneous administration versus intravenous infusion and reduced requirement for renal monitoring; however, drug-related costs are significantly higher. The cost per quality of life adjusted year (QALY) gained with denosumab has been estimated at $1.25 million [30]. Since the impact on SRE was not followed by an improvement in overall survival, it is unclear whether denosumab will replace zoledronic acid as the standard of care for patients with symptomatic bone metastasis from prostate cancer.

Clinical Trials in Elderly Patients with Prostate Cancer

The incidence of prostate cancer increases with age, and it is appropriate that potential new therapies are tested in a representative patient population. Clinical trials no longer exclude patients on the basis of increasing age; however, many elderly patients with prostate cancer are excluded from participating due to comorbidities such as cardiac and renal dysfunction. It is encouraging that recent phase III studies have included a population of patients over 70 years of age allowing valid extrapolation of results to the community clinic setting. Overall survival rather than prostate cancer-specific survival remains the most concrete end point in prostate cancer trials, particularly in an elderly population where treatment can carry morbidity, for example, the potential to increase cardiovascular risk. An example of a study demonstrating an improvement in prostate cancer-specific survival with no improvement in overall survival was the large cohort study evaluating primary androgen deprivation therapy in elderly men with localized prostate cancer [31].

Polypharmacy is a particular concern for clinicians treating elderly patients. Medications used for the treatment of common comorbid conditions may impact on prostate cancer growth or interact with anticancer treatment. An example of this is the diuretic spironolactone which has been shown to bind and activate the wild-type androgen receptor [32]. The effects of strong inhibitors or inducers of CPY3A4 have yet to be evaluated with respect to drugs such as abiraterone acetate and MDV3100, and their concurrent use is discouraged. Drug interactions with many novel therapies have yet to be determined, and particular caution should be exercised with drugs likely to prolong the cardiac QT interval such as antiarrhythmic agents, some antihistamines, and antidepressants. The inclusion of comprehensive geriatric assessment as part of the routine multidisciplinary care of older cancer patients may help to rationalize unnecessary medication and highlight potential drug interactions.

Conclusions

Elderly patients have been well represented in recent clinical trials of novel agents for advanced prostate cancer. With optimization of comorbid conditions and an awareness of potential drug interactions, age should not be a barrier to patients benefiting from the rapid pace of drug development in this field.

References

1. Kantoff PW, Higano CS, Shore ND, Berger ER, Small EJ, Penson DF, et al. Sipuleucel-T immunotherapy for castration-resistant prostate cancer. N Engl J Med. 2010;363(5):411–22.
2. de Bono JS, Oudard S, Ozguroglu M, Hansen S, Machiels JP, Kocak I, et al. Prednisone plus cabazitaxel or mitoxantrone for metastatic castration-resistant prostate cancer progressing after docetaxel treatment: a randomised open-label trial. Lancet. 2010;376(9747):1147–54.
3. de Bono JS, Logothetis CJ, Molina A, Fizazi K, North S, Chu L, et al. Abiraterone and increased survival in metastatic prostate cancer. N Engl J Med. 2011;364(21):1995–2005.
4. Cea P. Overall survival benefit of radium-223 chloride (Alpharadin) in the treatment of patients with symptomatic bone metastases in castration-resistant prostate cancer (CRPC): a phase III randomized trial (ALSYMPCA). European Multidsiciplinary Cancer Congress, Stockholm; 2011.
5. MEDIVATION. Medivation and astellas announce positive survival data from nterim analysis of phase 3 AFFIRM trial of MDV3100 in men with advanced prostate cancer. 2011. Available from: http://investors.medivation.com/releasedetail.cfm?ReleaseID=620500. Cited 03/11/2011.
6. Potter GA, Barrie SE, Jarman M, Rowlands MG. Novel steroidal inhibitors of human cyto-chrome P45017 alpha (17 alpha-hydroxylase-C17,20-lyase): potential agents for the treatment of prostatic cancer. J Med Chem. 1995;38(13):2463–71.
7. Barrie SE, Potter GA, Goddard PM, Haynes BP, Dowsett M, Jarman M. Pharmacology of novel steroidal inhibitors of cytochrome P450(17) alpha (17 alpha-hydroxylase/C17-20 lyase). J Steroid Biochem Mol Biol. 1994;50(5–6):267–73.
8. Attard G, Reid AH, Yap TA, Raynaud F, Dowsett M, Settatree S, et al. Phase I clinical trial of a selective inhibitor of CYP17, abiraterone acetate, confirms that castration-resistant prostate cancer commonly remains hormone driven. J Clin Oncol. 2008;26(28):4563–71.
9. Ryan CJ, Smith MR, Fong L, Rosenberg JE, Kantoff P, Raynaud F, et al. Phase I clinical trial of the CYP17 inhibitor abiraterone acetate demonstrating clinical activity in patients with castration-resistant prostate cancer who received prior ketoconazole therapy. J Clin Oncol. 2010;28(9):1481–8.
10. Marbury T, Stonerock R, Tran N, Gonzalez M. A phase 1 single dose open-label reduced/staged pharmacokinetic (PK) and safety study of abiraterone acetate (AA) in men with impaired renal function. Eur J Cancer. 2011;47 Suppl 1:S502.
11. Ryan CJ, Shah S, Efstathiou E, Smith MR, Taplin ME, Bubley GJ, et al. Phase II study of abiraterone acetate in chemotherapy-naive metastatic castration-resistant prostate cancer dis-playing bone flare discordant with serologic response. Clin Cancer Res. 2011;17(14):4854–61.
12. Danila DC, Morris MJ, de Bono JS, Ryan CJ, Denmeade SR, Smith MR, et al. Phase II multi-center study of abiraterone acetate plus prednisone therapy in patients with docetaxel-treated castration-resistant prostate cancer. J Clin Oncol. 2010;28(9):1496–501.
13. Reid AH, Attard G, Danila DC, Oommen NB, Olmos D, Fong PC, et al. Significant and sus-tained antitumor activity in post-docetaxel, castration-resistant prostate cancer with the CYP17 inhibitor abiraterone acetate. J Clin Oncol. 2010;28(9):1489–95.
14. Scher HI, Heller G, Molina AS, et al. Evaluation of circulating tumor cell (CTC) enumeration as an efficacy response biomarker of overall survival (OS) in metastatic castration-resistant prostate cancer (mCRPC): planned final analysis (FA) of COU-AA-301, a randomized double-blind, placebo-controlled phase III study of abiraterone acetate (AA) plus low-dose prednisone (P) post docetaxel. J Clin Oncol. 2011;29(Suppl):LBA4517 [Abstract].
15. Sternberg CN, Scher HI, Molina A, North S, Mainwaring P, Hao Y, Gagnon D, Kheoh T, Haqq CM, de Bono J, et al. Fatigue improvement/reduction with abiraterone acetate in patients with metastatic castration-resistant prostate cancer (mCRPC) post-docetaxel – results from the COU-AA-301 phase 3 study. EJC. 2011;47(Supplement 1):S488–9.
16. Ryan CJ, Sith MR, De Bono JS, Molina A, Logothetis C, De Souza PL, Fizazi K, Mainwaring P, Piulats Rodriguez JM, Ng S, Carles J, Mulders P, San Kheoh T, Griffin J, Small EJ,

Scher HI, Rathkopf DE. Interim analysis (IA) results of COU-AA-302, a randomized, phase III study of abiraterone acetate (AA) in chemotherapy-naive patients (pts) with metastatic castration-resistant prostate cancer (mCRPC). JClin Oncol. 2012;30(Suppl):LBA4518.

17. Mita AC, Denis LJ, Rowinsky EK, Debono JS, Goetz AD, Ochoa L, et al. Phase I and pharmacokinetic study of XRP6258 (RPR 116258A), a novel taxane, administered as a 1-hour infusion every 3 weeks in patients with advanced solid tumors. Clin Cancer Res. 2009;15(2):723–30.

18. Aventis S. Jevtana prescribing information. 2011. Available from: http://www.provenge.com/pdf/prescribing-information.pdf. Accessed Dec 2011.

19. Droz JP, Balducci L, Bolla M, Emberton M, Fitzpatrick JM, Joniau S, et al. Management of prostate cancer in older men: recommendations of a working group of the International Society of Geriatric Oncology. BJU Int. 2010;106(4):462–9.

20. Higano CS, Schellhammer PF, Small EJ, Burch PA, Nemunaitis J, Yuh L, et al. Integrated data from 2 randomized, double-blind, placebo-controlled, phase 3 trials of active cellular immunotherapy with sipuleucel-T in advanced prostate cancer. Cancer. 2009;115(16):3670–9.

21. Dendreon. Provenge prescribing information. 2011. Available from: http://www.provenge.com/pdf/prescribing-information.pdf. Cited Dec 2011.

22. Longo DL. New therapies for castration-resistant prostate cancer. N Engl J Med. 2010;363(5):479–81.

23. Tran C, Ouk S, Clegg NJ, Chen Y, Watson PA, Arora V, et al. Development of a second-generation antiandrogen for treatment of advanced prostate cancer. Science. 2009;324(5928):787–90.

24. Scher HI, Beer TM, Higano CS, Anand A, Taplin ME, Efstathiou E, et al. Antitumour activity of MDV3100 in castration-resistant prostate cancer: a phase 1-2 study. Lancet. 2010;375(9724):1437–46.

25. Saad F, Lipton A, Cook R, Chen YM, Smith M, Coleman R. Pathologic fractures correlate with reduced survival in patients with malignant bone disease. Cancer. 2007;110(8):1860–7.

26. Shahinian VB, Kuo YF, Freeman JL, Goodwin JS. Risk of fracture after androgen deprivation for prostate cancer. N Engl J Med. 2005;352(2):154–64.

27. Saad F, Gleason DM, Murray R, Tchekmedyian S, Venner P, Lacombe L, et al. A randomized, placebo-controlled trial of zoledronic acid in patients with hormone-refractory metastatic prostate carcinoma. J Natl Cancer Inst. 2002;94(19):1458–68.

28. Fizazi K, Carducci M, Smith M, Damiao R, Brown J, Karsh L, et al. Denosumab versus zoledronic acid for treatment of bone metastases in men with castration-resistant prostate cancer: a randomised, double-blind study. Lancet. 2011;377(9768):813–22.

29. Smith MR, Egerdie B, Hernandez Toriz N, Feldman R, Tammela TL, Saad F, et al. Denosumab in men receiving androgen-deprivation therapy for prostate cancer. N Engl J Med. 2009;361(8):745–55.

30. Snedecor SJ, Carter JA, Kaura S, Botteman M. Cost-effectiveness of zoledronic acid (ZOL) versus denosumab (Dmab) in prevention of skeletal-related events (SREs) in castration-resistant prostate cancer metastatic to the bone (mCRPC). J Clin Oncol. 2011;29(Suppl): abstr 4581.

31. Lu-Yao GL, Albertsen PC, Moore DF, Shih W, Lin Y, DiPaola RS, et al. Survival following primary androgen deprivation therapy among men with localized prostate cancer. JAMA. 2008;300(2).173–81.

32. Luthy IA, Begin DJ, Labrie F. Androgenic activity of synthetic progestins and spironolactone in androgen-sensitive mouse mammary carcinoma (shionogi) cells in culture. J Steroid Biochem. 1988;31(5):845–52.

Part V
Bladder Cancer

Chapter 16
Management of Superficial Bladder Cancer in Elderly Patients

Marco Oderda, Paolo Gontero, and Steven Joniau

Abstract The management of non-muscle-invasive bladder cancer (NMIBC) in the elderly is complex and must be tailored to the individual needs and the physical capacity of this particular group of patients, taking into account the frailty status and life expectancy. On one hand, treatments that may be required might further stress an already vulnerable organism, carrying the risk of being more harmful to the patient than the disease itself. On the other hand, a surprisingly high cancer-specific mortality has been shown even in this old age group, which makes active treatment, and not only palliative approach, advised in fit categories. The issue of reduced efficacy of intravesical therapy, such as BCG, with advancing age further complicates the picture. More radical treatment such as early cystectomy has been shown to be feasible also in octogenarians, keeping in mind that the risk of intraoperative death or major complications becomes relevant in advanced age groups. In this respect, device-assisted administration of intravesical therapies will play an increasing role in the future. Unfortunately, up-to-date, no specific guidelines exist to guide the physician choosing the optimum management of these older patients, who too often end up receiving substandard care.

Keywords Non-muscle-invasive bladder cancer • Elderly • Frailty • BCG • Intravesical therapy

M. Oderda, M.D. • P. Gontero, M.D.
Department of Urology, A.O.U. San Giovanni Battista Molinette,
University of Turin,
Turin, Italy
e-mail: marco.oderda@libero.it; paolo.gontero@unito.it

S. Joniau, M.D. (✉)
Department of Urology, University Hospital Leuven,
Leuven, Belgium
e-mail: steven.joniau@uzleuven.be

J.-P. Droz, R.A. Audisio (eds.), *Management of Urological Cancers in Older People*,
Management of Cancer in Older People,
DOI 10.1007/978-0-85729-999-4_16, © Springer-Verlag London 2013

Introduction

Bladder cancer represents one of the most prevalent neoplasms worldwide, with an estimated 386.300 new cases and 150.200 deaths in 2008 [1]. In the USA, it is the fourth most common cancer in men and the ninth most common in women, resulting in significant morbidity and mortality [2]. Urothelial carcinoma accounts for 95 % of bladder cancers, being associated to cigarette smoking and occupational exposures. Among risk factors, however, age has been recognized as the most important one, as bladder cancer is primarily a disease of the elderly [3]. The median age at diagnosis for both men and women is 73 years [4], and incidence increases with age. Ninety percent of bladder cancer occurs in people older than 55 years, with the highest risk in those aged 75–85 years [3]. As the median life expectancy improves, a significant increase in the elderly population is expected: the 2000–2050 annual growth rate for the population aged 65 years and older is 2.4 % worldwide, and the group aged 80 years and older increases even faster, with an anticipated threefold increase by the year 2050 [5]! As a result of the aging trends and their close relationship with cancer development, a dramatic boost in the incidence of bladder cancer is expected in the years ahead, which will become a major public health challenge. This challenge is going to become even harder if we consider the difficulties in the treatment planning when we deal with elderly patients, who constitute a more vulnerable category, exposed to higher risks of side effects and complications. In the older adults, treatment has to be tailored to the individual needs and the physical capacity, taking into account the frailty status and life expectancy. Nonetheless, age alone must not preclude the possibility of a curative therapy. Treatments for non-muscle-invasive bladder cancers (NMIBC), which account for the 75–80 % of newly diagnosed bladder neoplasms, are generally well-tolerated in the elderly, although the potential complications of the intravesical therapy might not be so easy to handle in these patients [6]. Even radical cystectomy, when muscle-invasive disease is diagnosed, can be considered in selected elderly patients, having demonstrated to be safe and feasible [7]. Unfortunately, although most elderly patients with bladder cancer seem to tolerate curative therapy, they often still receive substandard care. Up-to-date, specific guidelines on the management of bladder cancer in the elderly population are lacking. Aim of this chapter is to analyze the existing literature on this subject and provide a short summary of evidence-based recommendations for the management of elderly patients with superficial bladder cancer.

Elderly and Frail Patients

Elderly, an Evolving Concept!

It is very difficult to identify a definite threshold to consider an individual to be "elderly," owing to the continuous increase in the longevity of the population. In the EU, the proportion of people aged 65 years and over is expected to increase from 16.4 % in 2004 to 22.6 % in 2025, with an annual 2.4 % growth rate for this age group worldwide. It is predicted that up to 113 millions of people will be aged 80 years or older by 2050 [5]. All these things considered, nowadays people are considered "elderly" when they fall outside the so-called working age group, past 65 years. For both healthcare and research purposes, this group is further subdivided into *young old* (65–74 years), *old old* (75–84 years), and *oldest old* (85+ years) [8]. However, broad variations still characterize even these groupings, depending on the individual performance status. Rates of frailty and disability increase with increasing age among the elders, conferring high risk for adverse health outcomes [8, 9]. Nevertheless, it seems that in the twenty-first century, people are not only living longer but are generally healthier and less frail at advanced age than were previous cohorts. As a matter of fact, today, most elders are neither frail nor incapable of independent living. Therefore, chronological age must not be synonymous of frailty in the elderly group: comorbidity, disability, and functional status might represent far better predictors of undesirable outcomes than age alone [10]. This concept is particularly relevant in the treatment planning of elderly patients with bladder cancer: there is no definite age threshold to candidate a patient in good health for a curative treatment. In the setting of bladder cancer management, a limit of 75–80 years has generally been adopted to define the elderly patients, hence excluding the so-called *young old* [7].

The Concept of "Frailty"

Even in the absence of diseases, the human body suffers a progressive decline in function of nearly all organ systems, which begins at the age of 30. This decline manifests itself in an increased vulnerability and diminished recoverability when the organism is exposed to stressors. Moreover, the elderly often suffer from one or more chronic medical pathologies that further impair their functional reserve. Functional status, comorbidity, nutrition, cognition, and disabilities have all been found to be useful predictors of survival in older adults [3]. A geriatric condition that reunites all these domains is termed "frailty." Frailty is defined as a biologic syndrome of decreased reserve and resistance to stressors, resulting from cumulative decline across multiple physiologic systems and causing vulnerability to adverse outcomes [9]. Comorbidities are etiologic risk factors for frailty, while disabilities are its outcomes. Frailty in older adults has already been demonstrated to be independently

Table 16.1 Frailty score

Shrinking	Weight loss, unintentional, of ≥10 lb in prior year or, at follow-up, of ≥5 % of body weight in prior year
Weakness	Grip strength in the lowest 20 % at baseline, adjusted for gender and body mass index
Poor endurance and energy	As indicated by self-report of exhaustion. Self-reported exhaustion is associated with stage exercise reached in graded exercise testing and is predictive of cardiovascular disease
Slowness	The slowest 20 % of the population was defined at baseline, based on time to walk 15 ft, adjusting for gender and standing height
Low physical activity level	A weighted score of kilocalories expended per week was calculated at baseline. The lowest quintile of physical activity was indentified for each gender

Adapted from Fried et al. [9]
The phenotype of frailty is identified by the presence of three or more of the following components

predictive of falls, hospitalizations, disability, and death. A frailty score, based on unintentional weight loss, self-reported exhaustion, weakness, slow walking speed, and low physical activity, has been developed and could be precious to predict the outcome of different types of treatment in elderly bladder cancer patients (Table 16.1) [9, 10]. The occurrence of bladder cancer in an elder represents another stressor that might further increase the vulnerability of its body, by both cancer development and its treatment. Therefore, the concept of frailty cannot be disregarded in the treatment planning of such patients.

Age and Bladder Cancer

Influence of Age on Bladder Cancer Incidence and Outcomes

Bladder cancer is typically a disease of the elderly [11], with a progressive increase in incidence from 28.6 % in patients under 65 years to 71.4 % in those over 65 years [1, 11]. Patients aged 70 years and older have a fourfold increased risk of developing bladder cancer compared to younger ones (Table 16.2) [2]. We refer to data on bladder cancer in general, knowing that NMIBC accounts for 75–80 % of all bladder neoplasms [11].

In 2008, a Californian Cancer Registry data analysis showed a peak in the incidence of bladder cancer in individuals 85 years or older, with a rapid increase in the rate of bladder cancer in this population [12]. This peak age is 20 years after the general retirement age and would imply a longer than usual latent period in carcinogenesis: a 10-year peak difference between lung and bladder cancers, two malignancies that share some of the same carcinogens (mainly cigarette smoking and

Table 16.2 Probability (%) of developing bladder cancer within selected age intervals by sex, United States, 2005–2007

	Birth to 39	40–59	60–69	70 and older	Birth to death
Male	0.02 (1 in 4.693)	0.38 (1 in 262)	0.93 (1 in 107)	3.67 (1 in 27)	3.80 (1 in 26)
Female	0.01 (1 in 12.116)	0.12 (1 in 836)	0.26 (1 in 390)	0.98 (1 in 102)	1.16 (1 in 87)

Adapted from Jemal et al. [1]

occupational exposure to various aromatic amines), has been demonstrated. As a possible explanation, the bladder might require longer exposure than lungs for the induction of cellular mutations by carcinogens. In addition, aging might be associated with a decreased ability to completely empty the bladder, hence prolonging the contact time of the urothelium to active carcinogens [3].

As with incidence, also bladder cancer-specific mortality is higher in the elderly [11], going from 14–18 % in the US population aged 65–69 years to 30–37 % in those aged 80–84 years [3, 11]. A correlation between aging and biological aggressiveness of bladder cancer has thus been suggested [6, 13, 14]. Advanced age would be associated with a significantly increased risk of higher stage and grade at diagnosis, even when the cancer is still superficial [4, 13, 14]. According to Shy et al., elderly patients with superficial bladder cancer are more likely to present with poorly differentiated features. At the same time, a decrease in recurrence-free survival was seen with increasing age [13]. Age was also found to be a significant predictor of both tumor recurrence and progression by Kohjimoto et al. [15]. A correlation between higher stages and grades on the hazard of death from bladder cancer has been demonstrated, both for superficial and invasive disease, justifying aggressive therapies even in the elderly, when feasible [14].

Up-to-date, the precise reason for the adverse prognosis of superficial bladder cancer in the elderly is still unclear. The high cancer-specific death even in this old group, usually afflicted by a very high risk of non-cancer-specific mortality, is certainly surprising. Several hypotheses have been advanced, including a biological, age-related aggressiveness, impaired host defenses, a delayed diagnosis in older people due to social reasons, or else the administration of less aggressive therapies.

Aging and Carcinogenesis: A Complex Relationship

Several mechanisms have been hypothesized to explain the link between cancer and aging. Advancing age might lead to an increase in the activation of some oncogenes while inhibiting the tumor-suppressor activity. Furthermore, an aged cell may have a decreased capacity for repair of mutations in its DNA, promoting the development of cancer. Molecular pathways of aging and cancer are intertwined, being both associated with the accumulation of damage, senescence, and disruption of the replicative capacity of a cell [3]. Some of the main mechanisms shared by both aging and cancer are oxidative stress, telomere shortening, apoptosis, DNA methylation, increasing genomic instability, and accumulation of errors in nuclear DNA [10]. As for bladder cancer, multiple age-related changes in mutational frequency and epigenetic have been discovered as potential triggers for carcinogenesis. Furthermore, aging would allow an increasing and cumulative exposure to carcinogens, together with the accumulation of multiple cellular events. Other factors linking age and bladder cancer might be a prolonged contact time of the urothelium to active carcinogens as a consequence of an impaired ability of emptying the bladder and a decreased ability to detoxify potential carcinogens as a result of a progressive organism deterioration with aging [3]. In considering the complex relationship between aging and bladder cancer development, we must keep in mind the concept of frailty: the progressive decline of the organism with aging leads to frailty, increasing the vulnerability to disease and death, and also to carcinogenesis. Again, age seems to be directly correlated with the development of cancer.

Age and Treatment of Superficial Bladder Cancer

General Considerations

The physician must often face difficult choices when choosing the optimum management of elderly patients with superficial bladder cancer. Treatments that may be required might further stress an already vulnerable organism, with the risk of being more harmful to the patient than the disease itself. However, not all the elderly are equal. As previously stated, the assessment of the performance status, the calculation of the frailty score (Table 16.1), and the comorbidity evaluation are warranted in order to predict the treatment feasibility and outcome. Several scales have been used in order to characterize elderly patients deemed to be in "good health," such as the American Society of Anesthesiologists (ASA) physical status classification, the age-adjusted Charlson comorbidity index (ACCI), and the Karnofsky performance status (KPS), although none of them has been specifically designed for the selection of elderly bladder cancer patients. Besides, issues related to individual independence and quality of life must be considered, as these factors may assume an importance equal as survival in the elderly [10]. The impact of treatment on such factors must be taken into account so that older patients can make informed choices regarding their treatment options [3]. Based on a simple evaluation, according to their individual health status, patients may be classified into four groups: (1) "fit" elderly, with controlled comorbidities, fully independent in daily living activities, who should receive the standard-of-care treatment, same as younger patients; (2) "vulnerable" elderly, with reversible impairment and mild dependence in their daily activities, who should receive standard treatment after medical intervention; (3) "frail" elderly, affected by nonreversible impairment, with heavy dependence in daily activities, who should receive adapted treatment; and (4) patients who are "too sick," with "terminal illness," should receive only supportive care and symptomatic palliative treatment.

Of additional importance in the treatment planning of elderly individuals with superficial bladder cancer are social factors such as the availability of a network to provide home care, transportation, and assisted living [3]. For example, it might be impossible to schedule a cycle of intravesical instillations in older patients who cannot mobilize or do not have the transportation assistance. In the setting of individual with dependence in daily activities, therefore, the decision of undergoing treatment introduces the issues of caregiving and assistance services that need to be dealt with.

Transurethral Resection (TUR) and Adjuvant Intravesical Therapy

The diagnosis of NMIBC requires consideration of all transurethral resection (TUR) specimens, assessing that the detrusor muscle is not invaded. Based on the invasion (T1) or not (Ta) of the lamina propria, on the degree of neoplasia and other tumor characteristics such as focality, size, and recurrence, NMIBC is classified into three risk groups of recurrence and progression. Single, low-grade Ta tumors fall in the low-risk group, whereas high-grade T1 or CIS lesions are considered high-risk NMIBC. Intermediate-risk group comprises all the other kinds of NMIBC [16]. Once performed, TUR can be followed or not by adjuvant intravesical chemotherapy or immunotherapy, according to the risk stratification. These treatments are generally well-tolerated in the elderly: the TUR and the anesthesia required are not particularly invasive or debilitating. Neither habitually creates scenarios that jeopardize the functions of cardiovascular, pulmonary, or renal systems.

During a TUR, elderly patients are not exposed to a higher rate of complications than the younger population, and even when they require repeated endoscopic resections, the risk of side effects is low [3]. This risk increases when large resections are needed, as severe bleeding and bladder perforation become more common [17]. Large resections, however, are not contraindicated in older patients, if they are deemed fit for the procedure. With regard to the adjuvant intravesical therapies, most of the agents are not absorbed systematically and therefore do not produce significant systemic effects to which the elderly may be more vulnerable [3].

Up-to-date, specific guidelines for the management of superficial bladder cancer in the older patients are lacking. In absence of major contraindications, the risk-adapted approach presented in the EAU guidelines can be followed also in the setting of advanced age [16], with some exceptions. In most elderly patients with low-risk tumors, for example, treatment can be safely deferred without threatening survival since these neoplasms are at low risk of progression, in respect to the advanced age. This has to be kept in mind especially in more vulnerable elderly patients, whose comorbidities may create an increased risk for anesthesia. On the contrary, the potential complications of intravesical therapy might not be as well-tolerated in older patients, especially in the case of immunotherapy [18]. As Shariat et al. assessed, even minor complications such as fever, dysuria, hematuria, clot retention, and the need for repeated catheterization can be more problematic for the elderly [6]. Therefore, intravesical therapy must be administered with caution in the elderly, and sometimes even avoided, no matter what the guidelines say.

Watchful Waiting for Small Superficial Bladder Cancers: Is It Feasible?

Low-risk NMIBC is characterized by extremely low rates of progression and cancer-specific mortality, which make room to the option of a watchful waiting protocol instead of immediate TUR [19]. This approach would be interesting especially in the elderly, who might be spared the anesthesiological and surgical risks of the TUR, being followed with flexible cystoscopy and urinary cytology. Some evidence supports the benign behavior of low-risk NMIBC: in a combined series of three EORTC studies, a marker lesion was left in place for 8–10 weeks in 185 patients with low- or intermediate-risk NMIBC, with no cases of progression [20]. The slow growth rate of low-grade Ta tumors was successively confirmed by Soloway et al. [21]. According to a recent study, the watchful waiting approach is reasonable in patients presenting with small (<10 mm), recurrent papillary bladder cancer after resection of low-grade Ta tumor [19]. Standard TUR becomes mandatory if significant changes in tumor morphology or size are noted during the follow-up.

Intravesical Chemotherapy in Elderly Patients

To our knowledge, there are no studies that specifically address the role of intravesical chemotherapy in elderly patients. In intermediate-risk non-muscle-invasive bladder cancer, the superiority of immunotherapy with BCG over chemotherapy has been established for disease recurrence but not for progression [22] and needs to be balanced against higher toxicity: a recent meta-analysis showed that approximately 30 % of patients receiving mitomycin C (MMC) developed local toxicity compared with 44 % with BCG and 12 and 19 % developed systemic side effects, respectively [23]. Therefore, according to the latest guidelines [16], the less toxic intravesical chemotherapy can be considered as an alternative to BCG as adjuvant therapy in intermediate-risk patients. Given the increased vulnerability of elderly patients to the potential side effects of the intravesical instillations, intravesical chemotherapy could be recommended as first-line therapy in this group of patients diagnosed with intermediate-risk tumors, with failures being switched to BCG.

Early Single Instillation of Chemotherapy in Elderly Patients

A single immediate instillation of chemotherapy after TUR has been suggested as the best initial option for patients of all risk categories, having shown to reduce significantly the recurrence rate at cost of mild side effects such as chemical cystitis and contact dermatitis [16]. Again, no studies have been carried out to evaluate the risk-benefit ratio of this procedure in the elderly population. On one hand, it could delay the occurrence of recurrences and hence the need of further TURs; on the other hand, it could increase the complication risk of the TUR, which is generally well-tolerated. Therefore, it is essential to individually tailor the treatment on the basis of the patient's general health conditions.

Intravesical BCG in Elderly Patients

Intravesical bacillus Calmette-Guerin (BCG) is currently the most effective agent for superficial bladder cancer, representing the first-line therapy for high-risk tumors [16]. BCG has been shown to reduce the risk of recurrence and also progression to muscle-invasive disease, both in patients with papillary tumors and in patients with CIS [24]. The antitumor activity of BCG resides in its ability to switch on a robust cellular immune response, particularly cell-mediated immunity, which is needed to maintain a therapeutic effect through continued "maintenance" instillations. Therefore, an intact and efficient immune system is required. It has been demonstrated that aging is associated with a decline in immune functions: the elderly suffer increased morbidity and mortality associated with infection, have a reduced capacity to generate high-affinity antibodies in response to vaccination, and are more likely to develop select cancers and autoimmune disorders [25]. All these things considered, the efficacy and safety of BCG have been questioned in elderly patients.

Is BCG Less Effective in Elderly Patients?

Aging progressively weakens the immune response, especially the adaptive immunity [25], on which the therapeutic efficacy of BCG depends. Therefore, older patients could be less responsive to intravesical immunotherapy. A retrospective analysis performed on 1,008 patients showed that patients older than 80 years had a poor response to BCG plus interferon compared to younger patients, with a 74 % higher likelihood of not responding to the therapy. Age was an independent risk factor for response in multivariate analysis [26]. Another study on 805 patients showed that age did not affect the initial response to BCG, but pointed out a 10 % difference in freedom from disease at 5 years after treatment with BCG for patients older than 70 years (27 %) compared with those younger than 70 years (37 %) [27]. These findings were confirmed by a recent study that reported the lowest recurrence-free and progression-free survival among age groups for patients aged 80 years and older treated with BGC [15]. On the contrary, in a retrospective analysis by Yuge et al. age was not found to be independent predictor of recurrence in a series of BCG-treated patients; unfortunately, progression was not analyzed [28]. More recently, Margel et al. demonstrated that advanced age is associated with higher progression rates despite BCG. The 2-year progression-free survival was 87 % among patients <75 years versus 65 % in patients >75 years [29]. Taken together, these data suggest that BCG efficacy is actually impaired in elderly patients, pointing in the direction of alternative treatments. Further studies should be needed to shed light on the complex relationship between aging, immunity, and BCG activity.

Is BCG Toxicity a Hazard in Elderly Patients?

Intravesical BCG is more toxic than chemotherapy and therefore might not be so well-tolerated, especially in older patients. More importantly, due to its nature of live, attenuated strain of Mycobacterium bovis, it is not recommended in immuno-compromised patients because of the theoretical risk of severe morbidity and sepsis [30]. Due to the progressive weakening of the immune system, advanced age is considered also a condition at risk for complications in patients receiving BCG therapy. Nonetheless, it has been shown that BCG remains a viable option even in several conditions of immunosuppression, such as concomitant lymphoma, chronic lymphocytic leukemia, or steroid treatment as well as in renal transplant patients [31]: an intact urothelium might provide an effective barrier against hematogenous spread of the drug. This finding would support the use of BCG even when the immune response is deteriorated, such as in the elderly.

On the other hand, there are numerous reports of serious complications in the elderly individuals. In a retrospective study on 58 patients, Heiner et al. found higher complication rates for patients older than 70 years (48.6 vs. 17.6 %) treated with maintenance BCG [18]. It was suggested caution in administering maintenance BCG in elderly patients, and even avoidance of this therapy in the octogenarians. A threefold dose reduction of BCG had been proposed in order to reduce the risk of complications, especially in this delicate setting of patients. However, the one-third dose was recently shown to be less effective than standard dose against progression [32] and is therefore less appealing. All these things considered, the optimal management of high-risk superficial bladder cancer in the elderly remains debatable. BCG represents the gold-standard therapy in this risk group but must be handled with extra care with increasing age. In alternative, early cystectomy can be considered.

Early Cystectomy in Elderly Patients: Feasibility and Indications

Some cases of high-grade superficial bladder tumors (T1G3) harbor a particularly high risk of progression to muscle-invasive disease, especially if these neoplasms are multifocal, greater than 3 cm or associated with carcinoma in situ. For such high-risk cancers and for BCG failures, early cystectomy is advocated to maximize the chance of a cure. This indication can be very controversial in the setting of elderly individuals, who are less likely to be treated with extirpative surgery even when muscle-invasive disease is diagnosed [4]. However, a growing body of evidence indicates the cystectomy, once avoided in the elderly for fear of higher morbidity and mortality, is safe and even feasible in those at high risk [7]. Recently, a statistical model was developed to estimate life expectancy in patients with T1G3 bladder cancer treated either by immediate cystectomy or by intravesical BCG: according to this model, immediate cystectomy increased the mean life expectancy only for 70-year-old men with no to mild comorbiditiy and for 75-year-old men without comorbidity, while in patients aged 80 years, neither strategy differed meaningfully in terms of life expectancy [33]. Therefore, increasing age and worsening comorbidities diminished the benefits of early cystectomy. However, this statistical approach has many limitations, linked to the uncertainty around the estimates of the model. In the setting of radical cystectomy for muscle-invasive disease, a life expectancy of 2 years, independently of chronological age, has been suggested as a cutoff [7].

Again, a careful patient selection and a treatment tailored to the needs and the physical capacity of the individual elderly patients are essential in order to obtain the best therapeutic results. If an elderly patient is deemed fit for major surgery, age alone must not preclude radical cystectomy.

Conservative Management of High-Risk NMIBC in the Elderly: Is It Safe?

Although early cystectomy is advocated in some cases of high-risk NMIBC, its feasibility and benefits are questioned in advanced age groups with significant comorbidities. Therefore, the debate between cystectomy and secondary conservative therapies becomes even more pronounced in this vulnerable setting of patients. In case of failures of previous intravesical treatments, device-assisted chemotherapy instillations can yield responses in selected cases. Although still experimental, the combination of bladder wall hyperthermia and intravesical chemotherapy with mitomycin C, delivered by means of a dedicate system (Synergo), proved to be safe and effective as adjuvant therapy in intermediate- and high-risk NMIBC patients, even when they had already failed previous intravesical treatments [34]. To our knowledge, however, no study assessed its efficacy and tolerability in the specific setting of elderly, where it could play an interesting role in the future, especially in those deemed unfit for cystectomy.

Another enigmatic condition is represented by elderly patients with carcinoma in situ (CIS), a noninvasive but highly dysplastic flat neoplasia with low risk of bleeding but a high risk of progression to muscle-invasive disease, which accounts for 54 % without any treatment [17]. Intravesical BCG can be an effective therapy for CIS; in case of BCG failure, however, the risk of progression rises up to 66 % and cystectomy is warranted [17]. Again, in advanced age groups, the risk of leaving a lesion at high risk of progression has to be balanced with the implications of aggressive surgery.

Conclusions

The management of NMIBC in the elderly is complex. Most of them (the low- and the intermediate-risk categories) will hardly ever kill the patient since their biological aggressiveness is low. Rather they carry a risk of complications, chiefly hematuria, that can threaten life or at least significantly affect the quality of life of a frail age group. For this reason, resection of the tumor (TURBT) is often mandatory, more as a palliative rather than an oncological procedure even in very high-risk patients.

The high-risk group of NMIBC is also problematic in the elderly: its prevalence is higher, and the cancer-specific mortality is not unremarkable. Palliative TURBT can be inadequate due to high recurrence risk. The issue of reduced efficacy of intravesical therapy, such as BCG, further complicates the picture. The debate between cystectomy and secondary conservative therapies becomes even more pronounced in elderly patients harboring a high-risk NMIBC. While cystectomy has been shown to be feasible also in octogenarians, intraoperative death or major complications become relevant in advanced age groups. In this respect, device-assisted administration of intravesical therapies will play an increasing role in the future. On the other side, since high-risk NMIBC is at lifelong risk of recurrence and progression, the spectrum of aging as a cut point where the therapeutic window of opportunity may be lost represents a plea for early cystectomy in younger and fitter categories.

References

1. Jemal A, Bray F, Center MM, Ferlay J, Ward E, Forman D. Global cancer statistics. CA Cancer J Clin. 2011;61:69–90.
2. Siegel R, Ward E, Brawley O, Jemal A. The impact of eliminating socioeconomic and racial disparities on premature cancer deaths. CA Cancer J Clin. 2011;61:212–36.
3. Shariat SF, Milowsky M, Droller MJ. Bladder cancer in the elderly. Urol Oncol. 2009;27:653–67.
4. Prout Jr GR, Wesley MN, Yancik R, Ries LA, Havlik RJ, Edwards BK. Age and comorbidity impact surgical therapy in older bladder carcinoma patients: a population-based study. Cancer. 2005;104(8):1638–47.
5. United Nations Department of Economic and Social Affairs/Population Division. World Population to 2300. www.unpopulation.org.
6. Shariat SF, Sfakianos JP, Droller MJ, Karakiewicz PI, Meryn S, Bochner BH. The effect of age and gender on bladder cancer: a critical review of the literature. BJU Int. 2009;105:300–8.
7. Froehner M, Brausi MA, Herr HW, Muto G, Studer UE. Complications following radical cystectomy for bladder cancer in the elderly. Eur Urol. 2009;56:443–54.
8. Crews DE, Zavotka S. Aging, disability, and frailty: implications for universal design. J Physiol Anthropol. 2006;25:113–8.
9. Fried LP, Tanged CM, Walston J, Newman AB, Hirsch C, Gottdiener J, Seeman T, Tracy R, Kop WJ, Burke G, McBurnie MA. Frailty in older adults: evidence for a phenotype. J Gerontol. 2001;56A(3):M146–56.

10. Taylor III JA, Kuchel GA. Bladder cancer in the elderly: clinical outcomes, basic mechanisms, and future research direction. Nat Clin Pract Urol. 2009;6(3):135–44.
11. Messing EM. Urothelial tumors of the bladder (chapter 75). In: Campbell-Walsh urology. 9th ed. Philadelphia: Saunders Elsevier; 2008. p. 2407–746.
12. Schultzel M, Saltzstein SL, Downs TM, Shimasaki S, Sanders C, Sadler GR. Late age (85 years or older) peak incidence of bladder cancer. J Urol. 2008;179:1302–6.
13. Shi B, Zhang K, Zhang J, Chen J, Zhang N, Xu Z. Relationship between patient age and superficial transitional cell carcinoma characteristics. Urology. 2008;71:1186–90.
14. Scosyrev E, Wu G, Golijanin D, Messing E. Non-bladder cancer mortality in patients with urothelial cancer of the bladder. Urol Oncol. 2011 May 6. [Epub ahead of print].
15. Kohjimoto Y, Iba A, Shintani Y, Inagaki T, Uekado Y, Hara I. Impact of patient age on outcome following bladder-preserving treatment for non-muscle-invasive bladder cancer. World J Urol. 2010;28:425–30.
16. Babjuk M, Oosterlinck W, Sylvester R, Kaasinen E, Böhle A, Palou-Redorta J, Rouprêt M. EAU guidelines on non-muscle-invasive urothelial carcinoma of the bladder, the 2011 update. Eur Urol. 2011;59(6):997–1008.
17. Blandy JP, Notley RG, Reynard JM. Complications occurring during transurethral resection (chapter 10). In: Transurethral resection. 5th ed. London: Taylor & Francis; 2005. p. 182–6.
18. Heiner JG, Terris MK. Effect of advanced age on the development of complications from intravesical bacillus Calmette-Guérin therapy. Urol Oncol. 2008;26:137–40.
19. Gofrit ON, Pode D, Lazar A, Katz R, Shapiro A. Watchful waiting policy in recurrent TaG1 bladder tumours. Eur Urol. 2006;49:303–7.
20. Oosterlinck W, Bono AV, Mack D, et al. Frequency of positive biopsies after visual disappearance of superficial bladder cancer marker lesions. Eur Urol. 2001;40:515–7.
21. Soloway MS, Bruck DS, Kim SS. Expectant management of small, recurrent, noninvasive papillary bladder tumours. J Urol. 2003;170:438–41.
22. Gontero P, Bohle A, Malmstrom PU, O'Donnel MA, Oderda M, Sylvester R, Witjes F. The role of bacillus Calmette-Guérin in the treatment of non-muscle-invasive bladder cancer. Eur Urol. 2010;57:410–29.
23. Huncharek M, Kupelnick B. Impact of intravesical chemotherapy versus BCG immunotherapy on recurrence of superficial transitional cell carcinoma of the bladder: metaanalytic reevaluation. Am J Clin Oncol. 2003;26(4):402–7.
24. Sylvester R, Van der Meijden A, Lamm D. Intravesical bacillus Calmette-Guerin reduces the risk of progression in patients with superficial bladder cancer: a meta-analysis of the published results of randomized clinical trials. J Urol. 2002;168:1964–70.
25. DeVeale B, Brummel T, Seroude L. Immunity and aging: the enemy within? Aging Cell. 2004;3:195–208.
26. Joudi FN, Smith BJ, O'Donnell MA. Final results from a national multicenter phase II trial of combination bacillus Calmette-Guérin plus interferon α-2B for reducing recurrence of superficial bladder cancer. Urol Oncol. 2006;24:344–8.
27. Herr HW. Age and outcome of superficial bladder cancer treated with bacilli Calmette-Guérin therapy. Urology. 2007;70:65–8.
28. Yuge K, Kikuchi E, Matsumoto K, Takeda T, Miyajima A, Oya M. Could patient age influence tumor recurrence rate in non-muscle-invasive bladder cancer patients treated with BCG immunotherapy? Jpn J Clin Oncol. 2011;41(4):565–70.
29. Margel D, Alkhateeb SS, Finelli A, Fleshner N. Diminished efficacy of bacilli Calmette-Guérin among elderly patients with nonmuscle invasive bladder cancer. Urology. 2011;78:848–54.
30. Palou J, Angerri O, Segarra J, Caparrós J, Guirado L, Diaz JM, Salvador-Bayarri J, Villavicencio-Mavrich H. Intravesical bacillus Calmette-Guèrin for the treatment of superficial bladder cancer in renal transplant patients. Transplantation. 2003;76(10):1514–6.

31. Yossepowitch O, Eggener S, Bochner B, Donat M, Herr H, Dalbagni G. Safety and efficacy of intravesical bacillus Calmette-Guérin instillations in steroid treated and immunocompromised patients. J Urol. 2006;176:482–5.

32. Palou J, Solsona E, Angulo J, Fernàndez JM, Unda M, Martinez Pineiro L. Retrospective study of different options in the management of non-muscle invasive bladder cancer T1G3: maintenance BCG is here to stay. Eur Urol Suppl. 2011;10(2):149.

33. Kulkarni GS, Alibhai SMH, Finelli A, Fleshner NE, Jewett MAS, Lopushinsky AM. Cost-effectiveness analysis of immediate radical cystectomy versus intravesical bacillus Calmette-Guerin therapy for high-risk, high-grade (T1G3) bladder cancer. Cancer. 2009;115:5450–9.

34. Colombo R, Salonia A, Leib Z, Pavone-Macaluso M, Engelstein D. Long-term outcomes of a randomized controlled trial comparing thermochemotherapy with mitomycin-C alone as adjuvant treatment for non-muscle-invasive bladder cancer (NMIBC). BJU. 2010;107:912–8.

Chapter 17
Radical Cystectomy in Muscle-Infiltrative Bladder Cancer and Conservative Treatment in Localized Disease

Massimo Maffezzini

Abstract Bladder cancer (BCa) is the second most frequent cancer of the genito-urinary tract after prostate cancer. Transitional cell carcinoma (TCC), or urothelial cancer used as a synonym, is the most frequent histology accounting for 97 % of all bladder cancers. Macroscopic, asymptomatic hematuria is the most frequent and only sign of BC. Transurethral resection of bladder, or TURB, represents the only modality that allows for accurate diagnosis, grading, and staging of the disease. Radical cystectomy, or RC, is standard treatment for muscle-invasive disease, with bilateral pelvic lymphadenectomy and intestinal urinary reconstruction. The increasing age of the population has led to refinements in patient selection and perioperative management; as a result, RC is considered also in the elderly. The principles of fast-track surgery have greatly contributed to reduce the burden of surgical treatment and complications in the elderly. In such patient population, the aim of maximal long-term survival should be conveniently replaced by minimal morbidity and risk of complications. Patients aged 75 years, or older, or pre-frail, or with a reduction in life expectancy aside from BC, a completely extraperitoneal approach to the ablative part of the procedure, the cystoprostatovesiculectomy, can represent a resourceful option. Radical radiotherapy is considered as a treatment option for patients with major contraindications for surgery. The 5-year survival after RC for MIBC is generally unsatisfactory. It varies from 40 to 60 % for stage pT2 N0 M0 to around 15 % for stage pT4. Survival for patients with nodal disease found at surgery, pN, is reported to vary from 6 to 24 months.

Keywords Muscle-invasive TCC • Surgery • Elderly • Fast-track • Extraperitoneal approach

M. Maffezzini, M.D.
Department of Specialized Surgery, Galliera Hospital,
Genova, Italy
e-mail: massimo.maffezzini@galliera.it

J.-P. Droz, R.A. Audisio (eds.), *Management of Urological Cancers in Older People*,
Management of Cancer in Older People,
DOI 10.1007/978-0-85729-999-4_17, © Springer-Verlag London 2013

Incidence and Mortality

Bladder cancer (BCa) is the second most frequent cancer of the genitourinary tract in the adult after prostate cancer. More than 80,000 new diagnoses were expected for 2010, with an overall mortality >30,000 patients per year in Europe and the United States [1]. The probability of developing BCa from birth to death is 1 in 16 adult males and 1 in 84 females. The mortality rate in men is 7.5 per 100,000 in Europe, ranging from 3.3 out of 100,000 in Finland to 8.3 out of 100,000 in Spain [2]. An incidence peak is observed after 65 years of age, and 70 % of patients diagnosed with BCa are >60 years of age. BCa constitutes the ninth most frequent solid tumor, accounting for 7 % of all solid tumors and 2.5 % of all cancer deaths, whereas in the elderly population (defined as patients ≥75 years of age), it ranks fifth among cancer diagnoses and accounts for approximately 40 % of new BCa cases.

Histopathology

Transitional cell carcinoma (TCC), also called urothelial cancer, is the most frequent histology, accounting for 97 % of all bladder cancers; squamous cell and adenocarcinoma account for the majority of the remaining BCa types. Sarcomas and secondary tumors of different origins (e.g., lymphomas, breast cancers), as well as tumors invading from adjacent organs (e.g., prostate, colon, ovary), are infrequently seen. Less than 10 % of TCC cases are observed in the renal pelvis or calices, and <4 % are observed in the ureters.

Natural History and Biology

At presentation, almost two-thirds of TCC of the bladder are limited to the mucosal layer, or *lamina propria*, of the organ and are referred to as *non-muscle-invasive BCa* (NMIBC), whereas the remaining third shows a variable degree of infiltration into the muscular layer, or *detrusor muscle*, and the perivesical fat and is, therefore, defined as *muscle-invasive BCa* (MIBC). In locally advanced tumors, infiltration may involve adjacent organs (e.g., prostate, uterus, pelvic wall musculature) and structures (e.g., the peritoneum fixed to the posterior bladder wall and dome). Although the majority of NMIBC instances do not possess the ability to invade and kill the host, they can express a tendency to recur over time in different areas of the bladder mucosa (pleiochronotropism). A minority of NMIBC cases show the tendency to progress to muscle-invasive disease and finally metastasize. Altogether, the disease can display a continuum of risk—from low-grade Ta lesions with a 5 % risk of progression at one end of the spectrum to high-grade T1 lesions and carcinoma in situ (CIS) at the other end—associated with a ten times greater risk of progression.

CIS (also known as *Tis*) shows peculiar features. It consists of a poorly differentiated flat, intraepithelial lesion. Macroscopically, its recognition is inconstant. When visible, it is represented by velvety spots, reddish in color. CIS can be found in association with established high-grade invasive cancer and also with non-muscle-infiltrative disease. Although its natural history is incompletely understood, the presence of CIS bears a substantially negative influence on prognosis. Severe dysplasia found on histology or cytology is regarded with suspicion because it may show morphologic overlapping with CIS. Because of the disease's strong tendency to recur and eventually progress, BCa patients need to undergo repetitive transurethral surgery, adjuvant intravesical treatments, and follow-up tests, including invasive procedures like cystoscopy (vide infra). As a consequence, BCa is one of the most demanding solid tumors in terms of social cost [3].

Signs and Symptoms

Macroscopic, asymptomatic hematuria is the most frequent and often the only sign of BCa. Vesical irritation alone, lower urinary tract symptoms, or prostatism in the male can be the only presenting symptom associated with CIS. Similarly, signs of unstable or overactive bladder may be the only suspicious signs in the female.

Imaging, Cystoscopy, and Urinary Cytopathology

In the presence of gross or microscopic hematuria, ultrasonography is frequently employed in the initial evaluation; nevertheless, further imaging is mandatory, especially in patients with negative ultrasonography. Intravenous pyelogram (IVP) was long considered routine for its ability to show both direct and indirect signs of the presence of BCa, such as filling defects in the urinary bladder, ureter, and renal pelvis, and hydronephrosis. Currently, in most centers, IVP is being replaced by computed tomography (CT) urography, which provides greater accuracy. In selected cases and centers, MDCT can also be used for staging purposes. With regard to positron emission tomography-CT, there is currently no evidence for its role in the staging of BCa [3].

Tumors of the urothelium exfoliate cells in the urine; therefore, urinary cytopathology is helpful, especially in the diagnosis of lesions not detectable at cystoscopy (e.g., CIS).

Staging

The most widely accepted staging classification is the TNM system (2002):
- T: primary tumor
- Tx: primary not assessed
- T0: no evidence of primary
- Ta: tumor limited to the mucosa
- Tis (CIS): flat tumor, high grade, limited to the mucosa
- T1: noninvasive involvement of the basal membrane or subepithelial connective tissue
- T2: invasion of the detrusor muscle

  - T2a: inner half
  - T2b: outer half

- T3: invasion of the perivesical fat

  - T3a: microscopic
  - T3b: gross

- T4: invasion of the neighboring structures

  - T4a: prostate, uterus, vagina
  - T4b: pubic bone, muscles of the pelvic wall

- N: regional nodes
- Nx: no information on nodal status
- N0: no evidence of tumor within the examined nodes
- N1: tumor present in one node, ≤2 cm in diameter
- N2: tumor present in one node, >2 to <5 cm in diameter, or multiples nodes <5 cm in diameter
- N3: lymph node >5 cm
- M: distant metastases
- Mx: no information on M
- M0: absence of metastases
- M1: metastasis present

Staging Procedures

Accurate pathologic diagnosis, grading, and staging of BCa represent the cornerstone for treatment strategy. Transurethral resection of the bladder (TURB) represents the only modality that allows for accurate diagnosis, grading, and staging of the disease. The superficial portion of the lesions and the underlying muscular wall are sampled and sent separately to the pathologist labeled as the *endoluminal portion*, plus a full-thickness sample of the detrusor muscle underlying the tumor labeled as the *muscular layer.* The absence of orientation may negatively affect the accuracy of stage definition. In the case of small-volume papillary lesions, a partial-thickness resection of the bladder wall underlying the tumor can replace full-thickness intentional perforation.

A complete TURB—that is, when complete eradication of all visible lesions is obtained—also constitutes standard treatment for NMIBC. Morbidity and mortality after TURB are low, and 5-year survival is high. However, local control of disease is achieved in less than one-third of patients. Although TURB alone is considered sufficient treatment in patients in the low-risk category, some form of additional treatment, such as intravesical instillation with topical antitumor agents, is recommended for intermediate-risk patients, with intravesical instillation of bacillus Calmette-Guérin used in patients at high risk [3]. Laser treatment and fulguration are considered palliative treatments.

Surgical Treatment

Radical cystectomy (RC) is the standard treatment for muscle-invasive disease as well as for recurrent NMIBC stages CIS, or pTis, and pT1 G3 not controllable with conservative treatments [4]. RC includes the ablation of the bladder en bloc with the prostate and seminal vesicles in the male patient and the uterus, ovaries, and a portion of the anterior vaginal wall in the female patient. Bilateral pelvic lymphadenectomy (PLND) is considered part of the procedure. Although the boundaries of lymph-node removal may vary among different centers, there is a general consensus that considers PLND adequate when at least 14 nodes are described in the pathology report. An adequate PLND is supported by the concept of lymph-node density developed in recent years [5]. *Lymph-node density* is defined as the number of lymph nodes involved by tumor divided by the total number of lymph nodes removed. It has been reported that a lymph-node density of 20 % is of prognostic value, influencing the survival of node-positive patients. Specifically, recurrence-free 10-year survival drops from 43 % for patients with a lymph-node density ≤20 to 17 % for patients with a lymph-node density >20 %.

RC is considered the standard treatment for MIBC; however, some disparities have been observed with regard to its diffusion. The reported incidence of cystectomy in population-based studies in both the United States and Europe is <50 %, marking quite a sharp difference with teaching institutions and tertiary referral centers. In one recent study based on patients with histologically confirmed bladder carcinoma selected by stratified random sampling within the US National Cancer Institute's Surveillance, Epidemiology, and End Results Program (SEER) cancer registry, only 38 % of the lowest surgical risk patients underwent RC. One of 2 men between 54 and 74 years of age with MIBC underwent RC; the proportion dropped substantially to 1 in 6 men in the range of 75–70 years of age and dropped even further to 1 in 10 among octogenarians. Apparently, the procedure is not frequently utilized by many community urologists [6]. One potential explanation is that older patients are likely to have comorbid conditions influencing the choice of cancer therapy; however, in such studies, the influence of age was evident even when comorbidities were accounted for. In comparison with younger patients, RC was performed much less frequently in older patients.

Peculiar Features of Older Patients

Traditionally, older patients have received less aggressive surgery and little descriptive research when compared to younger patients with cancer. Older patients were also excluded or underrepresented in clinical trials; therefore, they constitute an underserved population [7, 8]. There is no agreed-upon definition for *older* or *elderly patients*. Instead of an age-based, rigid definition attached to a certain age limit—for example, 70, 75, 80 years of age, or older—considering the bigger picture of life expectancy appears to be a more reasonable alternative. Life expectancy has increased in recent decades. At 65 years of age, some 20 additional years constitute the average life expectancy, and at 75 years of age, it is more than 10 additional years. At 85 years of age, there is a 75 % chance of living 3 more years and a 25 % chance of living more than 6 years. Variations are primarily the result of functional status and the concurrent presence of different medical conditions [9]. It is noteworthy, however, that overall life expectancy does not coincide with the expectancy of *healthy* life. Data from our country, Italy, for example, showed an increase over the past decades in overall life expectancy to 84 and 78 years of age for females and males, respectively. The expectancy of healthy life, however, is slightly above 62 years of age for both sexes and has shown a consistent decline in recent years because of the increasing number of morbidities diagnosed after 60 years of age [10]. As patients live longer, they are increasingly exposed to the risk of developing a number of chronic conditions and to the consequent need for several medications. Among patients above 65 years of age, 40 % take 4–9 medications, and 18 % take 10 or more medications [11]. Consequently, drug-related adverse events occur with increased frequency with increasing age. An estimated 99 628 emergency hospitalizations for adverse drug events occur each year among older adults, and nearly half involve patients ≥80 years of age. More than 66,000 emergency hospitalizations result from the adverse effects of a few commonly prescribed antithrombotic (warfarin, oral antiplatelet agents) or antidiabetic agents (insulin, oral agents). Figure 17.1 outlines the age distribution of consecutive patients treated at our hospital for urologic diagnoses and gives an example of our population.

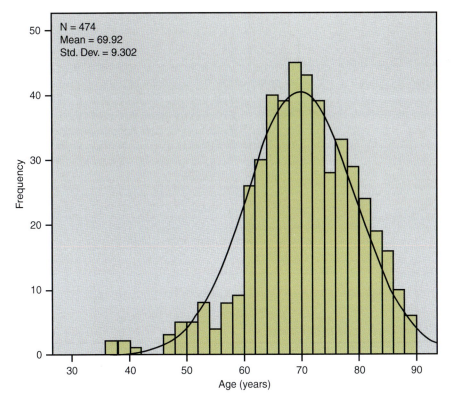

Fig. 17.1 Age distribution in a consecutive series of patients treated surgically at our hospital for urologic malignancies in 2011. *SD* standard deviation

Radical Cystectomy in Older Patients

Patient Selection

Approximately 25 % of new cancer diagnoses are for patients 65–74 years of age, 22 % are for patients in the range of 75–85 years of age, and about 7.5 % occur in those >85 years of age. The size of the population ≥65 years of age is expected to double between 2000 and 2030 [8].

The increasing age of the population has led to an increased rate of diagnosis of MIBC in the elderly. Therefore, RC is currently considered in the elderly, as well, with the contemporary refinements in patient selection in perioperative management.

The surgical treatment of MIBC is demanding—in fact, RC is included among the surgical operations at high risk for complications and death. Studies reviewing contemporary operative mortality of different cancer and cardiovascular operations in the past decade show a marked increase in the proportion of patients with comorbidities among candidates for major surgery. For RC, from 1999 through 2008, the proportion of patients with three or more comorbidities rose from 20 to 35 % [12]. In general, age may confer a degree of frailty. Although a definitive, thorough definition of *frailty* is still under study, it can be viewed as the extreme phenotype of aging [13]. The clinical criteria for frailty as proposed by the National Institutes of Ageing and American Geriatric Society include "vulnerabilities, weaknesses, instabilities, and limitations" [14]. Even in the absence of disease, *aging* implies a progressive reduction in organ reserve. The capacity to maintain physiologic homeostasis under acute stress (e.g., surgery, postoperative complications) is reduced. In other words, normal aging involves a dimming in the response to stress agents such as RC. Therefore, identifying preoperatively frail and pre-frail patients is of paramount importance.

In the multidisciplinary approach mandatory for these patients, geriatricians play a central role. Cognitive function also constitutes an essential part of preoperative assessment. Clinical studies in elderly patient candidates of different types of cancer surgery have demonstrated that reduced scoring at tests measuring cognitive function conveys a significantly higher risk of generic complications postoperatively (hazard ratio: 2.2) [15].

Perioperative Management

An increased understanding of perioperative physiology has put several tenets of traditional management of elective surgery under scrutiny, challenging their value through a critical pathway approach. Such a process inspired contemporary perioperative management plans under the principles of fast-track surgery with the aim of improving care by decreasing treatment-associated morbidity and mortality. This approach has substantially modified the postoperative course of patients submitted to colorectal surgery and, furthermore, has led to a marked reduction in overall hospital stay from 8–12 days to 2–5 days [16]. The principles of fast-track surgery have inspired and also contaminated urologic surgery and prompted the use of perioperative multimodal plans designed to minimize the adverse consequences of surgery. Detailed descriptions of such protocols can be found elsewhere [17]. A list of the most relevant interventions is summarized in Table 17.1.

Surgical Technique

The principle of *extensive resection* (i.e., eradication of all tissues neighboring the disease) may not constitute a suitable model for all patients ≥75 years of age (Fig. 17.2a). Efforts at obtaining maximal long-term survival should be replaced by efforts at inducing minimal morbidity and risk of complications. Limiting treatment interference with patients' quality of life (QoL) to the reasonable minimum also represents a critical goal. In line with these principles, in male patients ≥75 years of

Table 17.1 Perioperative treatment plan

Preoperative
Epidural thoracic cannula T9–T11
Central venous catheter
Dinner allowed before surgery
Minimal mechanical bowel preparation
Intraoperative
Combined epidural analgesia with no opioids, general anesthesia
Controlled hypotension at 80 mmHg
Timely correction of hypovolemia (500 mL EBL)
Prevention of hypoxia
Prevention of hypothermia
Jejunal cannula[a]
Postoperative
NGT early removal 6–8 h after surgery
Epidural analgesics 5 mL/h for the first 48 h
Early removal of drains
Avoidance of large amounts of saline
Artificial provision of nutrients (EN, PEN)
Soft food orally from postoperative day 1
Active/passive mobility from postoperative day 1
Defined daily care maps
Defined criteria for discharge (no tubes, restored normal diet, self-sufficient)

EBL estimated blood loss, *NGT* nasogastric tube, *EN* enteral nutrition, *PEN* parenteral nutrition
[a]Maffezzini et al. [18]

age, or who have a reduction in life expectancy aside from BCa, or in patients identified as pre-frail, a completely extraperitoneal approach to the ablative part of the procedure—the *cystoprostatovesiculectomy*—can represent a resourceful option. The advantage of leaving the peritoneum intact for the duration of the organ ablation phase consists in protecting against fluid dispersion resulting from extensive and prolonged bowel exposure. Accordingly, PLND can also be limited to the external iliac and obturator lymph nodes as well as those located medially to the obturator nerve and lateral to the bladder wall. Such limited PLND is also feasible when leaving intact the peritoneum. At the end of the ablative phase and in cases of relatively simple urinary diversions like the ureteroileal conduits (Bricker's type, vide infra), a portion of the terminal ileus can be retrieved through a limited peritoneal breach, the needed portion of about 15 cm harvested, and the ureter anastomosed to the conduit. Finally, the peritoneum can be in part reconstructed and secured with a few stitches to the mesenterium feeding the conduit, avoiding entrapment (Fig. 17.2b). Troublesome complications, such as leakage from the ureteroileal anastomoses, can be less worrisome if extraperitoneal.

Ureteral catheters (single J type) can be removed on the seventh postoperative day after obtaining a normal ureteral opacification and checking serum albumin levels. Serum albumin levels of at least 2.5 g/dL are expected before removal of the ureteral tutors but may take longer than 7 postoperative days to restore. Because of

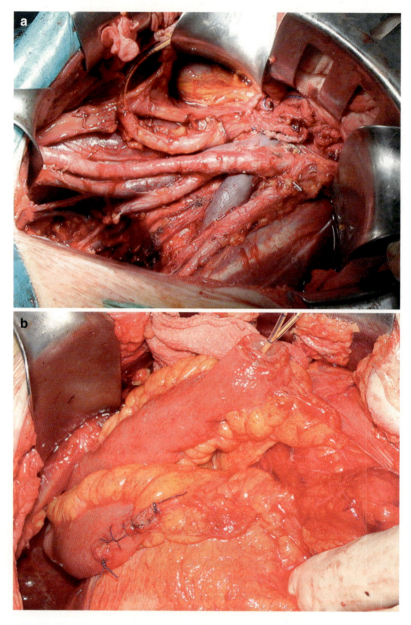

Fig. 17.2 (**a**) Unusual case of locally advanced tumor invading the anterior rectal wall and causing concomitant complete functional exclusion of the left kidney in a 62-year-old man submitted for radical cystectomy (RC) with en bloc rectal amputation, left nephrectomy, and extended pelvic lymphadenectomy. (**b**) Partial reconstruction of the peritoneum around an ileal segment (Bricker's type) after RC with an extraperitoneal approach in a 79-year-old patient. Both ureteral catheters are visible in the upper part of the figure, exiting from the distal opening of the ileal conduit. In the lower left of the image, the suture closing the proximal end of the conduit is seen lying over a portion of the reconstructed peritoneum

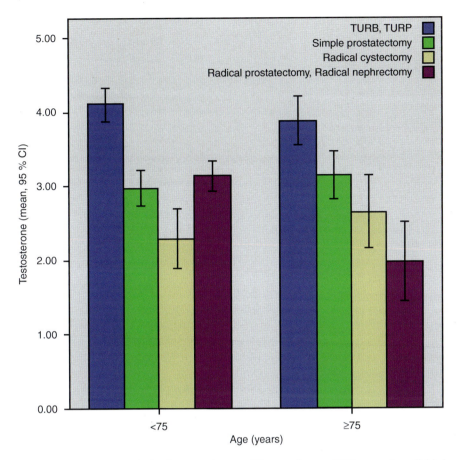

Fig. 17.3 Serum testosterone levels at entry in men <75 years of age and ≥75 years of age divided into subgroups based on the surgical treatment scheduled. Patient candidates for radical cystectomy show values at the lower range of normal. *TURB* transurethral resection of the bladder, *TURP* transurethral resection of the prostate, *CI* confidence interval

the physiologic response to surgical trauma, the protein synthesis function is temporarily abolished after RC, resulting in marked protein depletion. The supplementation of nutrients via parenteral nutrition can reduce protein catabolism; however, endogenous synthesis of proteins cannot be obtained in the first postoperative days, even by increasing the delivery of nutrients. In a previous experience, we added enteral nutrition in the postoperative period through a jejunal catheter but with no significant impact on protein depletion [18]. In an ongoing study, we found reduced testosterone levels in patients experiencing complications, and more generally, testosterone was frequently at the lower range of normal values in patents ≥75 years of age with MIBC (Fig. 17.3). The follow-up after RC should monitor the potential sites of recurrence—namely, the urethra and the pelvis as well as the upper urinary urothelium, liver, lungs, and skeletal apparatus.

Partial cystectomy (PC) consists in the surgical removal of a portion of the bladder harboring BCa. The procedure should be restricted to poor-anesthesiology-risk candidates for palliative purposes. PC's use is increasingly rare and in recent years has been almost abandoned.

Urinary Diversion

Urinary diversion encompasses several possibilities ranging from the simple ureterostomy to the creation of conduits such as the ureteroileostomy to more sophisticated forms of urinary diversion consisting of continent reservoirs obtained from intestinal segments. Such reservoirs can be implanted at the anatomic site of the native bladder, referred to as *orthotopic neobladder.* Alternatively, continent catheterizable reservoirs that can be implanted at a different site—most frequently, the lower right abdomen—are referred to as *heterotopic reservoirs.* Indications for each type of urinary diversion are based on the features of both the tumor and the host, generally leaving the simplest forms for locally advanced, poor-prognosis tumors in surgically unfit patients and the more complex continent reconstructions for organ-confined, good-prognosis tumors in surgically fit patients.

Bilateral ureterostomy constitutes the simplest and quickest form of urinary diversion. It also offers the advantage of being performed completely through an extraperitoneal approach.

Conduits are more frequently constructed using a portion of terminal ileus (Bricker-type operation) and less frequently using a portion of colon. Colon conduits were used in the past, especially in irradiated patients, to avoid using the bowel in the proximity of the boundaries of the irradiation field. The Bricker's operation, described in the second half of the last century, undeniably constitutes the form of urinary diversion with the uttermost diffusion worldwide. It consists in a tract of ileum connecting both ureters and draining the urine continuously to a cutaneous stoma, where the urine is collected into a bag. The history of the subsequent development of urinary diversion marked a substantial step forward in the 1980s, when several techniques were developed focusing on the construction of intestinal bladder substitutes to avoid stomal appliances and to improve the QoL of patients after cystectomy. Intestinal bladder substitutes can be anastomosed to the urethra, on which the external sphincter is deliberately spared at cystectomy to obtain continence, and that permits intentional voiding through the urethra. Alternatively, the reservoir is connected to a small opening in the cutaneous surface and can be voided through a catheter. Continence of heterotopic bladder substitutes is obtained using anatomic structures (i.e., ileocecal valve) with slight adaptation.

Good cognitive function is required in patient candidates for orthotopic intestinal reservoirs. Patients need to be trained to become familiar with the filling sensation of a new bladder. In addition, in the first period after discharge from hospital, patients are encouraged to void at relatively short time intervals (e.g., 2 h), in the day and at night, to avoid ureteral reflux and inadvertent voiding resulting from overdistension of the reservoir. The intervals can be increased progressively over time (e.g., 1 h every 2 weeks), allowing time for the reservoir to adapt and increase its capacity. A full 300–400 mL of capacity may take months to reach.

Intestinal segments used for the construction of urinary reservoirs retain the ability to produce intestinal mucus for the first months postoperatively. Low-pressure voiding because of the thin wall of the small bowel coupled with some degree of dehydration may cause incomplete mucous expulsion leading to "mucous plug" formation. This plug can cause obstruction and overdistension of the reservoir. Clinically, it can take the form of reflux pyelonephritis, with fever, back pain, and leukosis. To prevent mucous plug formation, patients must present once per week for bladder drainage and irrigation through a rubber catheter at least for the first 4 weeks postoperatively.

Good cognitive function and adequate manual dexterity are also required for patient candidates for heterotopic bladder substitution. Self-catheterization is needed at relatively short intervals (e.g., every 2 h) for the first 2 weeks after discharge. Intervals are gradually increased thereafter to the final number of 4—that is, every 6 h—in the majority of patients. A capacity of 300–500 mL is the most frequent capacity obtained a few months after surgery. Heterotopic reservoirs are less prone to infectious complications because mucous drainage is part of every catheterization. Furthermore, day- and nighttime continence is achieved promptly in virtually all patients.

Despite the advantages associated with continent bladder substitutes, data from the Nationwide Inpatient Sample in the United States identified 27 494 BCa patients who underwent RC with urinary diversion from 2001 to 2005. Only 16.5 % of those patients received a continent reservoir, whereas the remaining 83.5 % underwent an ileal conduit. Notably, the study also showed that continent diversion did not increase the risk of postoperative complications after RC. Again, older patients have less chance of receiving a continent urinary diversion than younger patients; in fact, in the range of 55–64 years of age, the proportion of ileal conduits to continent diversions was 4–1; in the range of 65–74 years of age, it was 5–1; and in patients >75 years of age, it was 7–1 [19]. Similar results emerged from a study based on data from SEER from 1992 to 2000, where continent neobladders were constructed in 19.9 % of patients. Age and the presence of three or more comorbidities were, among other factors, inversely related to the chance of receiving a continent diversion [20].

Complications and Mortality

BCa surgery consists of both extirpation and reconstruction of the bladder and the intestine harvested. With the exception of the rectum, all organs lying within the male and female pelvis are removed at RC. Such extensive ablation can be followed by relatively simple forms of urinary diversion or by reconstruction with intestine. Such a burdensome treatment modality may confer substantial morbidity and not negligible mortality. In general, complications of RC and urinary diversion are reported in the range of 9–62 % of cases. Short-term outcomes in elderly patients undergoing RC have been evaluated by several groups. Ninety-day mortality rates are reported to increase with age—namely, 1.2 % at ≤60 years of age, 2.1 % among patients 61–68 years of age, 5.8 % in patients 69–83 years of age, 7–9 % among patients 84–88 years of age, and 14.3 % in patients >88 years of age [21]. In patients ≥75 years of age, the 30 and 90-day mortalities are 3–4 % and 7–11 %, respectively. The 90-day complication rates in the elderly population may be up to 64 %. Such a wide range of incidence of complications is mainly because of the relatively wide range of patient general health status at presentation, tumor stages, perioperative management protocols, and the technique used in urinary reconstruction. It also reflects the lack of uniform classification systems for complications and methods of reporting. Surgical and medical complications, for example, are frequently addressed together. Similarly, early and late postoperative complications should be uniformly defined, and reasons for readmission examined in detail. Currently, the Clavien grading system for complications is gaining acceptance [22]. This system is based on the therapeutic consequences of complications, and its use may contribute substantially to facilitating comparisons among studies.

Recently, a nomogram has been built for the purpose of predicting 90-day mortality in patients ≥75 years of age based on age, Charslon comorbidity index, clinical stage, and preoperative serum albumin levels [23]. The latter was the parameter most strongly associated with the outcome, accounting for a 2.5-fold increase in the risk of 90-day mortality per 0–7 g/dL decrease in serum albumin. Although albumin may be a marker of nutritional status, it can also be influenced by factors such as inflammation and stress. The accuracy of prediction for this nomogram as reported by the authors was 71–75 %. Accurate patient selection together with the use of multimodal perioperative plans (e.g., fast-track surgery protocols) is likely to have contributed to a reduction in complication rates in recent series. Finally, cancer-specific mortality rates in patients 70–79 years of age at 5 years are 29–43 %, whereas all-cause mortality is only 15–18 %.

Organ-Sparing Treatments

With the goal of avoiding organ ablation in MIBC, organ-sparing treatments have been explored. The perspective of retaining the native bladder instead of patients having to adapt their life to a surgically reconstructed bladder substitute looks appealing indeed. Quite surprisingly, however, this approach has been studied by a limited number of centers over a relatively long period of time, giving us a sense of the difficulties inherent to the issue. Several features are involved in bladder-sparing treatment modalities, combining to make such a treatment option quite a complex choice.

Organ-sparing strategies consist primarily of trimodality treatments—namely, TURB, chemotherapy, and irradiation. Initial TURB of all respectable lesions is followed by radiation therapy (RT) with chemotherapy. Chemotherapy is used in association with external-beam RT (EBRT), with reduced doses as radiosensitizers. In patients showing complete response to initial treatment, a further session of chemoradiation is delivered for purposes of consolidation. Patients with incomplete response or relapsing after trimodality treatment should undergo salvage RC. Five-year disease-specific survival, retaining the native bladder, is reported in a range similar to RC. In the relatively limited number of studies available, the bladder is retained in about 40 % of patients treated. Reasons for salvage surgery include incomplete response to treatment, local recurrence, and in some patients, local toxicity of the combined treatments [24]. Organ sparing is considered an investigational treatment, so some critical points are worth addressing. Despite having been investigated for a relatively long time, the studies include only a few hundred patients altogether. TURB constitutes the basis for inclusion into a protocol of organ-sparing treatment. TURB can obtain an adequate sample of the lesions with the underlying muscular bladder wall—that is, a mere staging procedure—or it can completely remove the lesions, depending mainly on the volume and location of BCa and the surgeon's skill. Both variables can make generalization difficult. Some heterogeneity is observed among the studies with regard to the initial transurethral resection of bladder tumor as well as to restaging procedure, particularly after the first induction with chemotherapy and irradiation. In some studies, cystoscopy (with no tissue sampling) is considered for restaging. Although organ sparing should be reserved for select patients with clinically organ-confined disease, pT1–pT4-stage disease was included in several studies. A wide range of patient-selection criteria also contribute to making generalization of results difficult. Chemotherapy is used as a sensitizer to irradiation, with different drugs, dosages, and schedules of administration among the studies. Cisplatin is the most suitable drug for chemosensitization, and it can be used either alone or in association with other drugs (e.g., 5-fluorouracil) and on different schedules. In addition, carboplatin is used in some patients with renal function impairment, shifting the focus from intended cure to palliation. Radiation doses show also some degree of variability among protocols, and heterogeneity of dose, technique, and schedule are evident. In addition, both the technology and the techniques used in the first studies are not comparable with current standards. Modern bladder-sparing strategies in properly selected patients can obtain bladder preservation in 65 % patients, with long-term survival comparable to RC [24]. No randomized trial comparing bladder-sparing approaches to standard RC are available; however, organ sparing could represent an opportunity in properly selected patients (e.g., single lesion, organ-confined, radical TURB, complete response to the induction cycle).

Systemic Chemotherapy

Cisplatin-based chemotherapy (cisplatin, methotrexate, and vinblastine; methotrexate, vinblastine, doxorubicin, and cisplatin) administered in the neoadjuvant setting improves survival for patients with MIBC compared to RC alone (or radical RT). Specifically, data supported by the meta-analysis of more than 3,000 patients show that the use of preoperative chemotherapy resulted in a 26–33 % relative reduction in the risk of death compared to cystectomy alone (European Organization for Research and Treatment of Cancer and Southwest Oncology Group). Despite demonstration of a survival advantage, neoadjuvant chemotherapy is currently underused [25]. Elderly patients should also receive routine evaluation for chemotherapy.

References

1. Jemal A, Siegel R, Xu J, Ward E. Cancer statistics, 2010. CA Cancer J Clin. 2010;60(5):277–300.
2. Pelucchi C, Bosetti C, Negri E, Malvezzi M, La Vecchia C. Mechanisms of disease: the epidemiology of bladder cancer. Nat Clin Pract Urol. 2006;3(6):327–40.
3. Stenzl A, Cowan NC, De Santis M, European Association of Urology (EAU), et al. Treatment of muscle-invasive and metastatic bladder cancer: update of EAU guidelines. Eur Urol. 2011;59(6):1009–18.
4. Stein JP, Lieskovsky G, Cote R, et al. Radical cystectomy in the treatment of invasive bladder cancer: long-term results in 1,054 patients. J Clin Oncol. 2001;19(3):666–75.
5. Stein JP, Cai J, Groshen S, Skinner DG. Risk factors for patients with lymph node metastases following radical cystectomy with en bloc pelvic lymphadenectomy: the concept of lymph node density. J Urol. 2003;170(1):35–41.
6. Prout Jr GR, Wesley MN, Yancik R, Ries LA, Havlik RJ, Edwards BK. Age and comorbidity impact surgical therapy in older bladder carcinoma patients: a population-based study. Cancer. 2005;104(8):1638–47.
7. Raghavan D, Suh T. Cancer in the elderly population. The protection racket. J Clin Oncol. 2006;24(12):1795–6.
8. Hanson LC, Muss HB. Cancer in the oldest old: making better decisions. J Clin Oncol. 2010;28(12):1975–6.
9. Smith AK, Williams BA, Lo B. Discussing overall prognosis with the very elderly. N Eng J Med. 2011;365(23):2149–51.
10. Aspettaiva di vita sana. Effetto Cassandra web site. 2011. http://www.ugobardi.blogspot.com. Accessed 11 Oct 2011.
11. Budritz D, Lovergrove MC, Shehab N, Richards CL. Emergency hospitalizations for adverse drug events in older Americans. N Eng J Med. 2011;365(21):2002–12.
12. Finks JF, Osborne NH, Birkmeyer JB. Trends in hospital volume and operative mortality for high-risk surgery. N Eng J Med. 2011;364(22):2128–37.
13. Rodin MB, Mohile SG. A practical approach to geriatric assessment in oncology. J Clin Oncol. 2007;25(14):1936–44.
14. Walston J, Hadley EC, Ferrucci L, et al. Research agenda for frailty in older adults: towards a better understanding of physiology and etiology: summary from American Geriatric Society/ National Institute of Ageing Research conference on frailty in older adults. J Am Geriatr Soc. 2006;54(6):991–1001.

15. Audisio RA, Pope D, Ramesh HS, PACE participants, et al. Shall we operate? Preoperative assessment in elderly cancer patients (PACE) can help: a SIOG surgical task force prospective study. Crit Rev Oncol Hematol. 2008;65(2):156–63.
16. Kehlet H. Fast-track colorectal surgery. Lancet. 2008;371(9615):791–3.
17. Maffezzini M, Campodonico F, Canepa G, Gerbi G, Parodi D. Current perioperative management of radical cystectomy with intestinal urinary reconstruction for muscle-invasive bladder cancer and reduction of postoperative ileus. Surg Oncol. 2008;17(1):41–8.
18. Maffezzini M, Gerbi G, Campodonico F, Parodi D. A multimodal perioperative plan for radical cystectomy and intestinal urinary reconstruction: effects, limits and complications of early artificial nutrition. J Urol. 2006;176(3):945–9.
19. Gore JL, Yu HY, Setodji C, Hanley JM, Litwin MS, Saigal CS, Urologic Diseases in America Project. Urinary diversion and morbidity after radical cystectomy for bladder cancer. Cancer. 2010;116(2):331–9.
20. Gore JL, Saigal CS, Hanley JM, Schonlau M, Litwin MS, Urologic Diseases in America Project. Variations in reconstruction after radical cystectomy. Cancer. 2006;107(4):729–37.
21. Isbarn H, Jelders C, Zini L, et al. A population based assessment of perioperative mortality after cystectomy for bladder cancer. J Urol. 2009;182(1):70–7.
22. Dindo D, Demartines N, Clavien PA. Classification of surgical complications: a new proposal with evaluation in a cohort 6336 patients and results of a survey. Ann Surg. 2004;240(2):205–13.
23. Morgan T, Keegan KA, Barocas D, et al. Predicting the probability of 90-day survival of elderly patients with bladder cancer treated with radical cystectomy. J Urol. 2011;186(3):829–34.
24. Khosravi-Shahi P, Cabezon-Gutierrez L. Selective organ preservation in muscle-invasive bladder cancer: review of the literature. Surg Oncol. 2012;21:e17–22.
25. Bajorin DF, Herr HW. Kuhn's paradigms: are those closest to treating bladder cancer the last to appreciate the paradigm shift? J Clin Oncol. 2011;29(16):2135–7.

Chapter 18
Chemotherapy for Elderly Patients with Advanced Transitional Cell Carcinoma

Damien Pouessel and Stéphane Culine

Abstract Results from randomized trials allow concluding that cisplatin-based chemotherapy is the standard first-line treatment for patients with advanced transitional cell carcinoma of the urothelium. However, there is no standard chemotherapy regimen emerging from the literature for elderly patients as prospective studies dedicated to this population are quite rare. In daily practice, because of a better safety profile, the combination of gemcitabine and cisplatin (with G-CSF support) probably is the best choice to recommend in patients who are considered as fit for cisplatin. In patients with impaired renal function and good performance status, the combination of gemcitabine and carboplatin would be the most acceptable option. When performance status is poor, gemcitabine alone is an option along with best supportive care.

Keywords Elderly • Chemotherapy • Cisplatin • Unfit • Transitional cell carcinoma

Introduction

In 2012, cisplatin-based chemotherapy is the standard first-line treatment for patients with advanced transitional cell carcinoma (TCC) of the urothelium on the basis of randomized clinical trials. The combination of high-dose methotrexate, vinblastine, doxorubicin, and cisplatin (HD-MVAC) or gemcitabine and cisplatin (GC) is currently considered as the most effective treatments [1, 2]. Nevertheless, in spite of overall response rates of around 50 %, survival beyond 5 years is rare, with median

D. Pouessel, M.D. (✉) • S. Culine, M.D., Ph.D.
Department of Medical Oncology, Hôpital Saint-Louis,
Paris, France
e-mail: damien.pouessel@sls.aphp.fr; stephane.culine@sls.aphp.fr

J.-P. Droz, R.A. Audisio (eds.), *Management of Urological Cancers in Older People*,
Management of Cancer in Older People,
DOI 10.1007/978-0-85729-999-4_18, © Springer-Verlag London 2013

survivals of about 14 months. Moreover, TCC is largely of disease of elderly, and due to age-associated and/or disease-associated impairment in renal function and/or performance status, approximately 30–50 % of patients are ineligible for cisplatin [3]. As a result, a disconnect has emerged between the benefit of chemotherapy reported in randomized trials with selected patients (median age 61–63 years) and the efficacy observed in the whole population of patients with TCC.

Elderly Patients Fit for Cisplatin

A recently published uniform definition of unfit patients for cisplatin has been proposed from the results of a survey of genitourinary medical oncologists [3]. According to this definition, fit patients would meet all the following criteria: Eastern Cooperative Oncology Group performance status < 2, creatinine clearance > 60 mL/min, grade < 2 hearing loss, grade < 2 neuropathy, and New York Association Class I or II heart failure. No parameter related to the comprehensive geriatric assessment (CGA) has been included.

There is no standard chemotherapy regimen emerging from the literature as prospective studies dedicated to this population are quite rare. In a database analysis including 313 patients who were treated in four successive phase II studies, Bamias et al. compared the tolerability and efficacy of cisplatin-based regimens in 116 patients ≥70 years with those in younger patients. Median survival did not differ significantly (9.3 months for elderly patients vs. 10.5 months), but grade 3/4 neutropenia, neutropenic infections, and renal toxicity were more frequently observed [4]. No firm conclusion can be drawn from this study because of its design and the lack of CGA. A prospective study with gemcitabine alone (1,200 mg/m^2 on day 1 and day 8) was conducted in 25 patients of median age 76 years. Eleven (48 %) patients were considered as fully independent according to the CGA. The overall response rate was 45.5 %, including 13.5 % of complete responses. The median time to progression was 5 months, and the overall survival was 8 months. The parameters of CGA improved in 17 % of patients, remained unchanged in the great majority (74 %), and worsened in two patients (9 %). Treatment was reported as generally well tolerated [5]. The true impact of the GC combination as compared to gemcitabine alone is unknown. Finally, it should be stressed that carboplatin should not be substituted for cisplatin in patients with normal renal function since cisplatin-based chemotherapy significantly increases the likelihood of complete and objective response rates [6].

In daily practice, because of a better safety profile as compared to standard MVAC [7], the GC combination with G-CSF support probably is the best choice to recommend in elderly patients who are considered as fit for cisplatin.

Elderly Patients Unfit for Cisplatin

The results of selected prospective studies with unfit patients of median age $\geq$ 70 years are shown in Table 18.1. Most patients were considered as unfit for cisplatin because of a poor performance status and/or an impaired renal function. Three phase II studies used gemcitabine or paclitaxel in combination with carboplatin or epirubicin. A trend toward better response rates was observed with gemcitabine-based combination regimens, but median overall survivals were roughly similar [8–10]. In a French, randomized, phase II study, 44 patients (median age 76 years) were treated with gemcitabine alone or gemcitabine plus oxaliplatin. The addition of oxaliplatin to gemcitabine did not appear to improve the activity as compared with gemcitabine alone, at least in terms of response rate [11]. The unique phase III trial reported so far assessed the efficacy and toxicity of two carboplatin-based chemotherapy regimens. There were no significant differences in efficacy, but incidence of severe acute toxicities was lower in patients who received gemcitabine and carboplatin [12].

In daily practice, the median survival of patients unfit for cisplatin is clearly shorter than the one observed in fit patients. In patients with impaired renal function and good performance status, the combination of gemcitabine and carboplatin would be the most acceptable option. When performance status is poor, gemcitabine alone is an option along with best supportive care.

Future Directions

Several important issues relevant to the population of elderly patients with metastatic TCC of the urothelium need to be explored. Regarding the use of cisplatin, which estimate of renal function is the most appropriate? Which cutoff most safely defines cisplatin eligibility? Are there alternative regimens devoid of cisplatin that are beneficial? Prospective trials including CGA are required to answer these questions.

Table 18.1 Selected studies with unfit patients of median age ≥70 years

Chemotherapy	Design	Number of patients	Median age (years)	Median creatinine clearance (mL/min)	Objective response rate (%)	Progression-free survival (months)	Overall survival (months)	Reference
Gemcitabine 1,000 mg/m² d1, d8 *Epirubicin* 70 mg/m² d1 *Every 3 weeks*	Phase II	38	71.5	54	39.5	5	8	Ricci et al. [8]
Paclitaxel 225 mg/m² d1 *Carboplatin* AUC=6 *Every 3 weeks*	Phase II	37	70	35	24	3	7	Vaughn et al. [9]
Gemcitabine 1,000 mg/m² d1, d8 *Carboplatin* AUC=4 *Every 3 weeks*	Phase II	56	75	50	36	5	7	Linardou et al. [10]
Gemcitabine 1,200 mg/m² d1, d8, d15 *Every 4 weeks* *Gemcitabine* 1,000 mg/m² d1	Randomized phase II	22	77	43	43	4	5	Culine et al. [11]

Oxaliplatin 100 mg/m² d2 Every 2 weeks		22	74	48	27.5	3	8
Gemcitabine 1,000 mg/m² d1, d8 Carboplatin AUC=4.5 Every 3 weeks	Phase III	119	70	50	36	6	9	De Santis et al. [12]
Methotrexate 30 mg/m² d1, d15, d22 Vinblastine 3 mg/m² d1, d15, d22 Carboplatin AUC=4.5 Every 4 weeks		119	72	48	21	4	8

References

1. Sternberg CN, de Mulder P, Schornagel JH, et al. Seven year update of an EORTC phase III trial of high-dose intensity M-VAC chemotherapy and G-CSF versus classic M-VAC in advanced urothelial tract tumours. Eur J Cancer. 2006;42:50–4.
2. von der Maase H, Hansen SW, Roberts JT, et al. Long-term survival results of a randomized trial comparing gemcitabine plus cisplatin, with methotrexate, vinblastine, doxorubicin, plus cisplatin in patients with bladder cancer. J Clin Oncol. 2005;23:4602–8.
3. Galsky MD, Hahn NM, Rosenberg J, et al. Treatment of patients with metastatic urothelial cancer "unfit" for cisplatin-based chemotherapy. J Clin Oncol. 2011;29:2432–8.
4. Bamias A, Efstathiou E, Moulopoulos LA, et al. The outcome of elderly patients with advanced urothelial carcinoma after platinum-based combination chemotherapy. Ann Oncol. 2005; 16:307–13.
5. Castagneto B, Zai S, Marenco D, et al. Single-agent gemcitabine in previously untreated elderly patients with advanced bladder carcinoma: response to treatment and correlation with the comprehensive geriatric assessment. Oncology. 2004;67:27–32.
6. Galsky MD, Chen GJ, Oh WK, et al. Comparative effectiveness of cisplatin-based and carbo-platin-based chemotherapy for treatment of advanced urothelial carcinoma. Ann Oncol. 2012;23:406–10.
7. von der Maase H, Hansen SW, Roberts JT, et al. Gemcitabine and cisplatin versus methotrexate, vinblastine, doxorubicin, and cisplatin in advanced or metastatic bladder cancer: results of a large, randomized, multinational, multicenter, phase III study. J Clin Oncol. 2000;17:3068–77.
8. Ricci S, Galli L, Chioni A, Iannopollo M, Antonuzzo A, Francesca F, et al. Gemcitabine plus epirubicin in patients with advanced urothelial carcinoma who are not eligible for platinum-based regimens. Cancer. 2002;95:444–50.
9. Vaughn DJ, Manola J, Dreicer R, See W, Levitt R, Wilding G. Phase II study of paclitaxel plus carboplatin in patients with advanced carcinoma of the urothelium and renal dysfunction (E2896). A trial of Eastern Cooperative Oncology Group. Cancer. 2002;95:1022–7.
10. Linardou H, Aravantinos G, Efstathiou E, Kalofonos C, Anagnostopoulos A, Deliveliotis C, et al. Gemcitabine and carboplatin as first line treatment in elderly patients and those unfit for cisplatin based chemotherapy with advanced bladder carcinoma: phase II study of Hellenic Cooperative Oncology Group. Urology. 2004;64:479–84.
11. Culine S, Fléchon A, Guillot A, et al. Gemcitabine or gemcitabine plus oxaliplatin in the first-line treatment of patients with advanced transitional cell carcinoma of the urothelium unfit for cisplatin-based chemotherapy: a randomized phase 2 study of the French Genitourinary Tumor Group (GETUG V01). Eur Urol. 2011;60:1251–7.
12. De Santis M, Bellmunt J, Mead G, et al. Randomized phase II/III trial assessing gemcitabine/carboplatin and methotrexate/carboplatin/vinblastine in patients with advanced urothelial cancer who are unfit for cisplatin-based chemotherapy: EORTC study 330986. J Clin Oncol. 2012;30:191–9.

Chapter 19
Tailored Treatment for Bladder Cancer in Older Patients

Riccardo A. Audisio, Catherine Terret, Helen Boyle,
Aude Fléchon, and Jean-Pierre Droz

Abstract Bladder cancer is increasingly prevalent among older patients and requires a specific two-step approach: screening first, then the identification of geriatric problems. A good renal function is absolutely crucial for metastatic bladder cancer patients who are candidates to receiving chemotherapy. Most elderly patients with localized disease are likely to receive the same treatment options as younger patients (i.e., radical cystectomy), although specific interventions might be needed to minimize the occurrence of postoperative complications. Internationally accepted guidelines are generally valid in the population of patients with localized disease, even if more attention should be paid to health status than to life expectancy. Conversely, little knowledge is available on how best to manage metastatic disease: it is therefore mandatory to recruit patients into well-designed quality studies, after the appropriate assessment of their health status.

R.A. Audisio, M.D., FRCS (✉)
Department of Surgical Oncology, University of Liverpool,
St Helens Teaching Hospital, St Helens, UK
e-mail: raudisio@doctors.org.uk

C. Terret, M.D., Ph.D.
Geriatric Oncology Program, Department of Medical Oncology,
Center Léon-Bérard, Lyon, France
e-mail: catherine.terret@lyon.unicancer.tr

H. Boyle, M.D. • A. Fléchon, M.D., Ph.D.
Department of Medicine, Center Léon-Bérard,
Lyon, France
e-mail: helen.boyle@lyon.unicancer.fr; aude.flechon@lyon.unicancer.fr

J.-P. Droz, M.D., Ph.D.
Department of Medical Oncology, Lyon-RTH Laënnec School of Medicine,
Centre Léon-Bérard, Lyon, France
e-mail: jpdroz@orange.fr

J.-P. Droz, R.A. Audisio (eds.), *Management of Urological Cancers in Older People*,   271
Management of Cancer in Older People,
DOI 10.1007/978-0-85729-999-4_19, © Springer-Verlag London 2013

Keywords Bladder cancer • Elderly • Cystectomy • Neoadjuvant • Comorbidities • Nomogram • Decision making

Introduction

One of the most significant recent observations in public health is the population aging. A similar pattern is expected for the next decades. As life expectancy increases, the number of patients with cancer also expands. Bladder cancer ranks fourth in incidence in men older than 70 years (after prostate, lung, and colorectal cancers), and its incidence steadily increases with age [1]. Bladder cancer accounts for approximately 100,000 new cases each year in Europe (80 % are men). The median age at diagnosis is 68 years. The majority of patients (70 %) have non-muscle-invasive tumors amenable to specific surgery and intravesical instillations, and the mortality rate is low. On the contrary, bladder tumors infiltrating the muscle have a poor prognosis, and only half of the patients can be cured. Finally, metastatic bladder cancer is presently not curable, with a median overall survival of 14 months from diagnosis. About 36,000 patients died of bladder cancer in Europe in 2006, though a continuous decline of mortality rates has been reported [1].

Recently, several reviews have been published on the relationship between age and bladder cancer [2], complications of cystectomy [3], and the decision-making process of the management of bladder cancers in elderly patients [4]. The target of this chapter is to comment on the available literature and to introduce the concept of a specific geriatric oncology approach, as it has been developed for prostate cancer [5].

Standard Treatment of Bladder Cancer

Different guidelines have been published by national or international societies. We will consider here only the guidelines elaborated by the European Association of Urology [6].

Muscle-Invasive Bladder Cancer

Patients usually present with painless hematuria. Other symptoms are urgency, dysuria, increased frequency, and pelvic pain.

Diagnosis of bladder cancer is made by cystoscopy and histological analysis of transurethral bladder resection specimens. Bladder biopsies can sometimes be performed. Staging is based on physical examination and imaging. CT scan of the of the chest, abdomen, and pelvis and CT urography allow to evaluate the local extent of the tumor, the involvement of lymph nodes, the presence of metastases, and the existence of a synchronous tumor of the upper urinary tract. In some cases, MRI can be performed.

The standard curative treatment is radical cystectomy with lymph node dissection, but the extent of this dissection remains to be standardized. The urethra is generally conserved in patients with negative margins unless the primary tumor is located at the bladder neck or in the urethra (in women) or if tumor extensively infiltrates the prostate.

Orthotopic bladder substitution is proposed in the absence of contraindications such as poor general clinical condition or positive urethral margins. Otherwise, urinary diversion with ileal conduit or urine pouch is to be considered. Before surgery, neoadjuvant chemotherapy is recommended [7] since a meta-analysis has demonstrated a significant impact on overall survival. Cisplatin-based chemotherapy is generally administered [8]. Preoperative radiotherapy and adjuvant chemotherapy have not been proven to be advantageous and hence are not recommended [9]. Bladder preservation is an acceptable alternative to radical cystectomy in some patients. Multimodality treatment consists of aggressive transurethral resection (TUR) followed by chemoradiotherapy (cisplatin-based) and careful follow-up. In case of relapse, salvage radical cystectomy should be proposed. Bladder preservation is only advisable for well-informed patients with muscle-invasive bladder cancer, generally with isolated tumor, limited to the muscle and, if possible, after a complete TUR. Tumor size, presence of hydronephrosis, and CIS are prognostic factors for outcome.

Advanced and Metastatic Bladder Cancer

Palliative radical cystectomy with ileal conduit diversion is an option in case of locally advanced disease with massive bladder bleeding, fistula, and pain. The risks associated with the intervention should be weighed against the expected benefits. In some cases, upfront chemotherapy followed by either radical cystectomy or chemoradiotherapy can be proposed. These treatments have only limited indication [6].

Metastatic disease is treated with chemotherapy. The standard chemotherapy regimen is a combination of drugs including cisplatin [6]. The first regimen described was a combination of methotrexate, vinblastine, doxorubicin, and cisplatin (M-VAC). It was proven to be superior to cisplatin alone for overall survival [10], but with substantial toxicity (mainly hematological and mucositis). It also requires good cardiac and renal functions (at least a creatinine clearance >60 mL/min). A dose-dense MVAC regimen has been developed, with the drugs administered every other week with the support of hematopoietic growth factors. This modified regimen has shown good clinical activity and reduced toxicity [11, 12] and has been accepted as the standard M-VAC regimen. A randomized phase III trial comparing the original M-VAC to a combination of gemcitabine and cisplatin (GC) [13] has shown no survival benefit for GC over M-VAC, but GC has been associated with less toxicity (mainly hematological toxicity and mucositis). GC is thus generally the standard of care in the palliative treatment of metastatic bladder cancer. However, in younger patients with limited metastatic disease candidate to post-chemotherapy surgery, the modified M-VAC is widely used. None of the combinations with carboplatin or paclitaxel without platinum compounds are standard [14]. The triplet of GC plus paclitaxel has the same activity as GC and is more toxic.

Treating Bladder Cancer in Older Patients

The literature has explored different aspects of the management of elderly patients with bladder cancer. Recent published papers help understand the problems of management encountered in real life situations, outside the setting of clinical trials or without selection of patients treated in institutions. Different aspects are considered here, from a qualitative perspective rather than based on an exhaustive literature review. However, health status evaluation tools are mentioned in this section, and a complete health status assessment is performed (Chap. 2: Health status evaluation of elderly patients with GU tumors checked when the galleys are in hand).

Infiltrating Bladder Cancer

The minimum requirement of information regarding health status is often not met when reporting on urological cancers affecting older patients. As an example, one of the largest series of radical cystectomy for bladder cancer presented by the Department of Urology at Wake Forest University analyzed outcomes in a subpopulation of patients aged 70 years or more, with, respectively, 314 and 50 patients aged 70–79 years and ≥80 years [15]. Their conclusion was that "carefully selected" elderly patients have mortality and early diversion-related complication rates similar to those observed in younger patients. The question that arises is what is meant by "carefully selected elderly patients." In such studies, insufficient information is available to characterize elderly patients according to their fitness status. Treatment outcomes are not different between elderly and younger patients, since young and "fit" elderly patients are equally likely to benefit from radical cystectomy. Surveys of patient populations are interesting in this respect because they help to determine what type of information is collected.

An original approach of variations of post-cystectomy outcomes is the nomogram that provides an indirect evaluation of the impact of age and sometimes of comorbidities on the outcome itself. In the International Bladder Cancer Nomogram Consortium study [16], only age was included in the model, but other patient characteristics were not given. The age of 80 years accounted for 25 points, similar to pT1 stages, high-grade or squamous cell histology. For comparison, pelvic lymph node involvement was worth 50 points, and a 5-year progression-free survival rate of 20 % accounted for 190 points. However, the weight given to age may vary from one study to the other. A Canadian study presented a nomogram derived from a population of 958 patients aged 33–89 years (median age: 64.5) but with no information on comorbidities [17]. In the multivariate reduced model, the rate ratio for age was 1.010, while it was 1.498 for T2 stage versus T1 or lower or pT0. Interestingly, a second study from the same group [18] focusing on overall survival (OS) and cancer-specific survival (CSS) yielded very demonstrative results in a multivariate analysis on overall survival: age 70–79 versus ≤50 years had a hazard ratio of 1.78. Conversely, when the CSS was taken in account, age was not included in the model (hazard ratio 1.09 for age 70–79 versus ≤50 years). Such models, which are certainly suitable for middle-aged adult patients, do not reflect the heterogeneity of the older patients' subgroup.

Recently, Morgan et al. developed another nomogram to predict 90-day mortality after radical cystectomy [19]. They analyzed the charts of 220 consecutive patients 75 years old or older treated with radical cystectomy for bladder cancer. The median age in this series was 78.8 years. The 90-day mortality was 12.7 %. In the multivariate analysis, older age and lower preoperative albumin levels were associated with increased 90-day mortality. Muscle involvement and Charlson comorbidity index were not independent prognostic factors. However, they were also included in the nomogram that yielded with 71–75 % accuracy.

Prout et al. studied patients included in the National Cancer Institute's (NCI) Surveillance, Epidemiology, and End Results (SEER) Program [20]. Data were recorded from 820 randomly chosen bladder cancer patients (all stages), classified in three age groups (55–64, 65–74, and >74 years); comorbidity data were collected by means of the American Society of Anesthesiologists (ASA) score [21]. Their incidence was shown to increase with age. Older patients also tended to have more severe comorbidities (ASA classes 3 and 4); the most frequent comorbidities in the higher classes were cardiovascular disease (angina, arrhythmia, myocardial infarction, and other heart disease), chronic respiratory disease, deep venous thrombosis, and stroke. The study detected no difference in the management of non-muscle-invasive disease with regard to age. However, radical cystectomy was far less frequently performed as patients age increased, even when comorbidities were taken into account. Suboptimal treatments are offered to older patients, regardless of their objective health status.

The impact of the ASA classification, which is independent of age in predicting complications, has also been demonstrated in a retrospective study by Boström et al. [22]. In a population of 258 patients tested during two periods of time, ASA classes ≥3 were shown to be associated with around 40 % complications (2/3 minor complications). In this study, comorbidities were not weighted by severity, but only counted arithmetically. In a univariate analysis, the ASA class and the number of comorbidities were found to be predictive of in-hospital major complications and mortality. However in the multivariate analysis, these two factors were not independent.

In a sample of patients aged 75 years and over with ASA class 3 (34 patients) and class 4 (4 patients), no postoperative deaths were observed after radical cystectomy [23], and the rate of complications was similar to other series (29 % minor complications and 5 % major ones) [3]. All patients had a positive palliative effect of the cystectomy; 29 % of patients are alive at a mean follow-up of 22 months (3–90 months). These results contrast with the very short life expectancy of patients receiving only palliative treatment.

A more sophisticated instrument to record comorbidities is obviously needed. One of the most widely used scoring system is the Charlson index [24]. Investigators at the MD Anderson (Houston) studied 1,302 patients undergoing radical cystectomy over a 3-year period [25]. Their objective was to determine the impact of the volume of operative procedures on post-cystectomy mortality and morbidity rates. This study was the first to introduce the evaluation of comorbidities in urological series by means of the Charlson score. Multivariate analysis showed that age was the most significant predictive factor for mortality, while complications were associated with age and the Charlson index. However, the use of the Charlson index is debatable for at least two reasons: it only takes into account a limited number of comorbidities, and it has only little relevance to weigh the impact of specific comorbidities such as diabetes or stroke/hemiplegia. An alternative approach is the use of the Cumulative Illness Rating Scale Geriatrics (CIRS-G) which delineates different domains of comorbidities and weighs each domain according to its impact on functioning or to the importance of treatment [26]. This screening scale has rarely been used in urological older cancer patients.

A large survey based on 13,796 invasive bladder cancers from the University of Michigan showed that 60 % were aged >70 years (24 % >80 years). No information was provided regarding patients' health status. A wide range of treatments were delivered from aggressive surgery to conservative management (TUR, radiotherapy, watchful waiting). The interesting conclusion is that, among patients older than 80 years, after adjustment for prognostic variables and multivariate analysis, surgery is associated with the greatest reduction in the risk of death from bladder cancer or from any other cause [27]. Therefore, the questions are clearly how to carefully evaluate the risk of radical cystectomy and how to optimize patients' fitness to receive aggressive surgical treatment. This is the purpose of a geriatric approach. Interestingly, established tools for predictive screening of post-surgical morbidity and mortality, used in PACE (preoperative assessment cancer in the elderly), have not been widely used in urology [28].

The Process of Decision Making

A panel of experts took part in drafting SIOG guidelines for the management of elderly patients with prostate cancer and chose to limit the patient assessment to three domains: dependence, nutrition, and comorbidities [5]. Each domain has its own screening tools, where screening for malnourishment and comorbidities may allow prehabilitation. Patient assessment as a function of heath status should also be recommended for elderly patients with bladder cancer despite the difference between bladder and prostate cancer: untreated localized bladder cancer is a life-threatening disease, and surgery is the standard curative treatment; therefore, the main concern is to evaluate the risk for developing postoperative complications. Moreover, renal function is the most important factor limiting the administration of active chemotherapy regimens for all patients with metastatic bladder cancer. Since chemotherapy has limited activity, the treatment of these patients should be at best palliative with specifically adapted regimens and best supportive care. In the whole population of bladder cancer patients, age should be considered independently from other criteria of "unfitness": renal function, for instance, is the most important factor affecting the use of cisplatin-based chemotherapy. If renal function does not preclude cisplatin administration, a poor PS or impaired health status (particularly comorbidities) might contraindicate treatment. A two-step approach is crucially important: first, screening for unfitness by the urologist/medical oncologist and then, when needed, the administration of a proper GA by the geriatric team (geriatrician, social worker, dietician, and physiotherapist).

Prospective controlled trials are urgently needed based on accurate geriatric assessment in order to define which chemotherapy schedule achieves the best survival rate with minimal alteration of patient's QoL and less toxicity.

Conclusions

Bladder cancer is increasingly prevalent among older patients and requires a specific two-step approach: screening first, then the identification of geriatric problems. A good renal function is absolutely crucial for metastatic bladder cancer patients who are candidates to receiving chemotherapy. Most elderly patients with localized disease are likely to receive the same treatment options as younger patients (i.e., radical cystectomy), although specific interventions might be needed to minimize the occurrence of postoperative complications. Internationally accepted guidelines are generally valid in the population of patients with localized disease, even if more attention should be paid to health status than to life expectancy. Conversely, little knowledge is available on how best to manage metastatic disease: it is therefore mandatory to recruit patients into well-designed quality studies, after the appropriate assessment of their health status.

References

1. Ferlay J, Randi G, Bosetti C, Levi F, Negri E, Boyle P, La VC. Declining mortality from bladder cancer in Europe. BJU Int. 2008;101:11–9.
2. Shariat SF, Lee R, Lowrance WT, Bochner BH. The effect of age on bladder cancer incidence, prognosis and therapy. Aging Health. 2010;6:649–59.
3. Froehner M, Brausi MA, Herr HW, Muto G, Studer UE. Complications following radical cystectomy for bladder cancer in the elderly. Eur Urol. 2009;56:443–54.

4. Shalhoub PJ, Quek ML. Management of bladder cancer in the elderly: clinical decision making and guideline recommendations. Aging Health. 2010;6:607–10.
5. Droz JP, Balducci L, Bolla M, Emberton M, Fitzpatrick JM, Joniau S, Kattan MW, Monfardini S, Moul J, Naeim A, van Poppel H, Saad F, Sternberg CN. Management of prostate cancer in senior adults: recommendations of a working group of the international society of geriatric oncology (SIOG). Br J Urol Int. 2010;106:462–9.
6. Stenzl A, Cowan NC, De SM, Jakse G, Kuczyk MA, Merseburger AS, Ribal MJ, Sherif A, Witjes JA. The updated EAU guidelines on muscle-invasive and metastatic bladder cancer. Eur Urol. 2009;55:815–25.
7. Advanced Bladder Cancer (ABC) Meta-analysis Collaboration. Neoadjuvant chemotherapy in invasive bladder cancer: update of a systematic review and meta-analysis of individual patient data advanced bladder cancer (ABC) meta-analysis collaboration. Eur Urol. 2005;48:202–5.
8. Grossman HB, Natale RB, Tangen CM, Speights VO, Vogelzang NJ, Trump DL, deVere White RW, Sarosdy MF, Wood Jr DP, Raghavan D, Crawford ED. Neoadjuvant chemotherapy plus cystectomy compared with cystectomy alone for locally advanced bladder cancer. N Engl J Med. 2003;349:859–66.
9. Advanced Bladder Cancer (ABC) Meta-analysis Collaboration. Adjuvant chemotherapy in invasive bladder cancer: a systematic review and meta-analysis of individual patient data Advanced Bladder Cancer (ABC) Meta-analysis Collaboration. Eur Urol. 2005;48:189–99.
10. Saxman SB, Propert KJ, Einhorn LH, Crawford ED, Tannock I, Raghavan D, Loehrer Sr PJ, Trump D. Long-term follow-up of a phase III intergroup study of cisplatin alone or in combination with methotrexate, vinblastine, and doxorubicin in patients with metastatic urothelial carcinoma: a cooperative group study. J Clin Oncol. 1997;15:2564–9.
11. Sternberg CN, de Mulder PH, Schornagel JH, Theodore C, Fossa SD, van Oosterom AT, Witjes F, Spina M, van Groeningen CJ, Collette L, de Balincourt C. Randomized phase III trial of high-dose-intensity methotrexate, vinblastine, doxorubicin, and cisplatin (MVAC) chemotherapy and recombinant human granulocyte colony-stimulating factor versus classic MVAC in advanced urothelial tract tumors: European Organization for Tesearch and Treatment of Cancer Protocol no. 30924. J Clin Oncol. 2001;19:2638–46.
12. Sternberg CN, de Mulder PH, Schornagel JH, Theodore C, Fossa SD, van Oosterom AT, Witjes JA, Spina M, van Groeningen CJ, Duclos B, Roberts JT, de Balincourt C, Collette L. Seven year update of an EORTC phase III trial of high-dose intensity M-VAC chemotherapy and G-CSF versus classic M-VAC in advanced urothelial tract tumours. Eur J Cancer. 2006;42:50–4.
13. von der Maase H, Sengelov L, Roberts JT, Ricci S, Dogliotti L, Oliver T, Moore MJ, Zimmermann A, Arning M. Long-term survival results of a randomized trial comparing gemcitabine plus cisplatin, with methotrexate, vinblastine, doxorubicin, plus cisplatin in patients with bladder cancer. J Clin Oncol. 2005;23:4602–8.
14. Kaufman DS, Carducci MA, Kuzel TM, Todd MB, Oh WK, Smith MR, Ye Z, Nicol SJ, Stadler WM. A multi-institutional phase II trial of gemcitabine plus paclitaxel in patients with locally advanced or metastatic urothelial cancer. Urol Oncol. 2004;22:393–7.
15. Clark PE, Stein JP, Groshen SG, Cai J, Miranda G, Lieskovsky G, Skinner DG. Radical cystectomy in the elderly: comparison of clinical outcomes between younger and older patients. Cancer. 2005;104:36–43.
16. Bochner BH, Kattan MW, Vora KC. Postoperative nomogram predicting risk of recurrence after radical cystectomy for bladder cancer. J Clin Oncol. 2006;24:3967–72.
17. Karakiewicz PI, Shariat SF, Palapattu GS, Gilad AE, Lotan Y, Rogers CG, Vazina A, Gupta A, Bastian PJ, Perrotte P, Sagalowsky AI, Schoenberg M, Lerner SP. Nomogram for predicting disease recurrence after radical cystectomy for transitional cell carcinoma of the bladder. J Urol. 2006;176:1354–61.
18. Shariat SF, Karakiewicz PI, Palapattu GS, Amiel GE, Lotan Y, Rogers CG, Vazina A, Bastian PJ, Gupta A, Sagalowsky AI, Schoenberg M, Lerner SP. Nomograms provide improved accuracy for predicting survival after radical cystectomy. Clin Cancer Res. 2006;12:6663–76.

19. Morgan TM, Keegan KA, Barocas DA, Ruhotina N, Phillips SE, Chang SS, Penson DF, Clark PE, Smith Jr JA, Cookson MS. Predicting the probability of 90-day survival of elderly patients with bladder cancer treated with radical cystectomy. J Urol. 2011;186(3):829–34.
20. Prout Jr GR, Wesley MN, Yancik R, Ries LA, Havlik RJ, Edwards BK. Age and comorbidity impact surgical therapy in older bladder carcinoma patients: a population-based study. Cancer. 2005;104:1638–47.
21. Keats AS, The ASA. Classification of physical status – a recapitulation. Anesthesiology. 1978;49:233–6.
22. Boström PJ, Kossi J, Laato M, Nurmi M. Risk factors for mortality and morbidity related to radical cystectomy. BJU Int. 2009;103:191–6.
23. Farnham SB, Cookson MS, Alberts G, Smith Jr JA, Chang SS. Benefit of radical cystectomy in the elderly patient with significant co-morbidities. Urol Oncol. 2004;22:178–81.
24. Charlson ME, Pompei P, Ales KL, Mackenzie CR. A new method of classifying prognostic comorbidity in longitudinal studies: development and validation. J Chronic Dis. 1987;40:373–83.
25. Elting LS, Pettaway C, Bekele BN, Grossman HB, Cooksley C, Avritscher EB, Saldin K, Dinney CP. Correlation between annual volume of cystectomy, professional staffing, and outcomes: a statewide, population-based study. Cancer. 2005;104:975–84.
26. Linn BS, Linn MW, Gurel L. Cumulative illness rating scale. J Am Geriatr Soc. 1968;16:622–6.
27. Hollenbeck BK, Miller DC, Taub D, Dunn RL, Underwood 3rd W, Montie JE, Wei JT. Aggressive treatment for bladder cancer is associated with improved overall survival among patients 80 years old or older. Urology. 2004;64(2):292–7.
28. Audisio RA, Pope D, Ramesh HS, Gennari R, van Leeuwen BL, West C, Corsini G, Maffezzini M, Hoekstra HJ, Mobarak D, Bozzetti F, Colledan M, Wildiers H, Stotter A, Capewell A, Marshall E. Shall we operate? Preoperative assessment in elderly cancer patients (PACE) can help. A SIOG surgical task force prospective study. Crit Rev Oncol Hematol. 2008;65:156–63.

Part VI
Renal Cancer

Chapter 20
Surgery or Observation for Small Renal Masses in Older Patients?

Jean-Pierre Droz and Riccardo A. Audisio

Abstract Surgery is the standard treatment for renal cell carcinoma; however, radical nephrectomy for lesions >4 cm may be considered overtreatment as well as nephron-sparing surgery for smaller tumors. Elderly people with small renal tumors are 3.5 times more likely to have a benign lesion than younger patients; hence, careful monitoring may be considered, together with repeated bioptic sampling. Percutaneous radio-frequency ablation or cryoablation could be alternative options although no long-term follow-up data is presently available. New molecular genetic profiling techniques will hopefully be able to identify those patients which need to be managed surgically from all others.

Keywords Elderly • Kidney cancer • Small renal masses • SRM • Percutaneous radio-frequency ablation • Cryoablation • Watchful wait

Surgery is the standard of treatment for most solid tumors, including renal cell carcinoma. Active surveillance is otherwise gaining popularity for patients with kidney cancers, regardless their age [1–3]. Not only radical nephrectomy for lesions >4 cm seems overtreatment but also nephron-sparing surgery for most tumors smaller than this. New ablative techniques such as radio-frequency ablation, cryotherapy, and high-intensity focused ultrasound are gaining acceptance; however, their long-term oncologic safety remains to be proven, and a longer follow-up is needed [4, 5].

J.-P. Droz, M.D., Ph.D. (✉)
Claude-Bernard-Lyon 1 University, Department of Medical Oncology,
Centre Léon-Bérard, Lyon, France
e-mail: jpdroz@orange.fr

R.A. Audisio, M.D., FRCS
Department of Surgical Oncology, University of Liverpool,
St Helens Teaching Hospital, St Helens, UK
e-mail: raudisio@doctors.org.uk

J.-P. Droz, R.A. Audisio (eds.), *Management of Urological Cancers in Older People*,
Management of Cancer in Older People,
DOI 10.1007/978-0-85729-999-4_20, © Springer-Verlag London 2013

With an expanding number of small renal masses being detected [6], a larger proportion of patients are receiving surgery; this has surprisingly not resulted into a significant drop in mortality rates for renal cancer.

With an average age at diagnosis of 65 years, one out of two renal cancer patients is old, often presenting frailty, associated medical conditions (comorbidities), and limited physiological reserve; 25 % belong to the 65–74 age group and 25 % to the older one (≥75 years) [7].

Over the last decades, large evidence has been gained to prove underdiagnosis, under-staging, and undertreatment of senior cancer patients. This should not force us to impose inappropriate treatment modalities with no clear advantages in survival and/ or quality of life. As the barrier of overtreatment should not be crossed at any time, we advocate individualized and tailored treatment for elder patients with renal cancer.

This chapter attempts putting together the available evidence in order to facilitate the decision-making process in our clinical practice.

Chawla et al. [3] presented cumulative data in a meta-analysis published in 2006 on small renal masses (SRM) (median 2.5 cm): 286 patients were identified and followed for a median of 32 months (D3). Progression to metastatic disease was reported in only three patients (1.0 %); it was then suggested that the majority of small enhancing renal masses will grow at a very slow rate, when observed.

Serial radiologic data alone are insufficient to predict the natural course of SRMs, but an observational strategy may be appealing, particularly in the elderly group. On the other hand, an unpredictable non-negligible risk of disease progression and metastasis while on surveillance is to be kept in mind [8]. The development of meta-static deposits during the observational period is to be considered the most important negative prognostic factor in the absence of any adequate treatment for metastatic renal cancer. Fortunately, this event is rarely encountered; Youssif et al. [9] report it in 5.7 % of their observed series.

Elderly people with SRMs are up to 3.5 times more likely to have a benign lesion [10]. This group of patients can then be offered several treatment options. Surgical management is not to be neglected, whenever appropriate or feasible in all fit elderly patients; however, frail individuals could be handled more conservatively. Since 50 % of patients older than 70 have a creatinine clearance <50 ml/min, nephron sparing is to be preferred when surgical ablation is the treatment plan [11].

Careful monitoring is an option. In the meanwhile, repeated bioptic sampling is advisable, as the complication rate and the risk of seeding are negligible.

Noticeably, this gap of time is helpful in pre-abilitating unfit patients (i.e., correction of anemia, dehydration, depression, and malnourishment) in order to improve the patients' performance if surgical removal becomes advisable. Laparoscopic nephron-sparing techniques achieve similar recurrence-free and long-term survival rates in the elderly as in the younger age groups [12].

Percutaneous radio-frequency ablation or cryoablation could be alternative options. These treatments are presently considered investigational, and it is not clear whether they might interfere with the biology and the natural history of these lesions. No long-term follow-up data is available as yet, while they seem to associate to an acceptable toxicity [13–15].

Hopefully, new molecular genetic profiling techniques will soon be reliable enough to identify those patients which need to be managed surgically from all others.

References

1. Van Poppel H, Joniau S. Is surveillance an option for the treatment of small renal masses? Eur Urol. 2007;52:1323–30.
2. Kunkle DA, Egleston BL, Uzzo RG. Excise, ablate or observe: the small renal mass dilemma – a meta-analysis and review. J Urol. 2008;179:1227–33.
3. Chawla SN, Crispen PL, Hanlon AL, Greenberg RE, Chen DY, Uzzo RG. The natural history of observed enhancing renal masses: meta-analysis and review of the world literature. J Urol. 2006;175:425–31.
4. Wen CC, Nakada SY. Energy ablative techniques for treatment of small renal tumors. Curr Opin Urol. 2006;16:321–6.
5. Cambio AJ, Evans CP. Management approaches to small renal tumours. BJU Int. 2006;97:456–60.
6. Hollingsworth JM, Miller DC, Daignault S, Hollenbeck BK. Rising incidence of small renal masses: a need to reassess treatment effect. J Natl Cancer Inst. 2006;98:1331–4.
7. Edwards BK, Brown ML, Wingo PA, et al. Annual report to the nation on the status of cancer, 1972–2002, featuring population based trends in cancer treatment. J Natl Cancer Inst. 2005;97: 1407–27.
8. Phé V, Yates DR, Renard-Penna R, Cussenot O, Rouprêt M. Is there a contemporary role for percutaneous needle biopsy in the era of small renal masses? BJU Int. 2012;109:867–72. doi:10.1111/j.1464-410X.2011.10544.x. Epub 2011 Sep 2.
9. Abou Youssif T, Kassouf W, Steinberg J, Aprikian AG, Laplante MP, Tanguay S. Active surveillance for selected patients with renal masses: updated results with long-term follow-up. Cancer. 2007;110(5):1010–4.
10. Rendon RA, Stanietzky N, Panzarella T, et al. The natural history of small renal masses. J Urol. 2000;164:1143–7.
11. Duncan L, Heathcote J, Djurdjev O, Levin A. Screening for renal disease using serum creatinine: who are we missing? Nephrol Dial Transplant. 2001;16:1042–6.
12. Uzzo RG, Novick AC. Nephron-sparing surgery for renal tumors: indications, techniques and outcomes. J Urol. 2001;166:6–18.
13. Gkialas I, Kontraros M, Vassilakis P, Spanopoulos S, Theodoropoulos E, Stathouros G, Moshonas D, Doumas K. Radiofrequency ablation of renal tumors in patients unfit for surgery. Our experience. J BUON. 2011;16(2):304–8.
14. Popovic P, Surlan-Popovic K, Lukic S, Mijailovic M, Jankovic S, Kuhelj D. Percutaneous imaging-guided radiofrequency ablation of small renal cell carcinoma: techniques and outcomes of 24 treatment sessions in 18 consecutive patients. J BUON. 2011;16(1):127–32.
15. Clements T, Lin YK, Raman JD. Current status of ablative techniques for small renal masses. Expert Rev Anticancer Ther. 2011;11(6):879–91.

Chapter 21
Treatment of Metastatic Kidney Cancer in the Elderly

Helen Boyle and Sylvie Négrier

Abstract Kidney cancers are frequent tumors. Surgery is the main treatment for localized tumors. Treatment for metastatic disease is based on targeted therapies. Sunitinib, pazopanib, sorafenib, bevacizumab + interferon, temsirolimus, and everolimus are approved for the treatment of metastatic renal carcinoma. However, these drugs have quite a few side effects that can be troublesome in patients with comorbidities. There are no specific guidelines for treatment of elderly patients. This chapter will review the current data on treatment of metastatic disease focusing on elderly patients.

Keywords Kidney cancer • Elderly • Comorbidities • Antiangiogenic • Targeted therapy • Toxicity

Introduction

Kidney cancers are frequent tumors. The incidence in Europe is 13.9 per 100,000, with mortality rates of 6.2 per 100,000 [1]. Median age at diagnosis is 62 years [2]. Surgery is the main treatment for localized tumors. Until 2005, interferona was the main treatment for metastatic disease [3]. Since then, several targeted therapies have been approved in this setting.

H. Boyle, M.D. (✉)
Department of Medicine, Center Léon-Bérard,
Lyon, France
e-mail: helen.boyle@lyon.unicancer.fr

S. Négrier, M.D., Ph.D.
Department of Medical Oncology, Centre Léon-Bérard,
Lyon, France
e-mail: sylvie.negrier@lyon.unicancer.fr

J.-P. Droz, R.A. Audisio (eds.), *Management of Urological Cancers in Older People*,
Management of Cancer in Older People,
DOI 10.1007/978-0-85729-999-4_21, © Springer-Verlag London 2013

Several angiogenic mechanisms underlie the pathology of renal cancer. The three most important pathways involved in kidney cancer are the VEGF, the PDGF, and the mTOR signaling pathways [4].

Up to 75 % of tumors have VHL alterations [5]. When VHL function is lost, HIF-α accumulates and facilitates transcription of several genes such as VEGF, EGFR type 1, PDGF, TGF-α, glucose transporters, erythropoietin...This results in increased angiogenesis, cell growth, survival in difficult environments (low oxygen, low pH, low nutrient levels), and metastasis. These mitogenic growth factors bind to tyrosine kinase receptors and activate the Raf/MEK/ERK pathway. They also activate the PI3K/AKT/mTOR. mTOR regulates several biosynthetic pathways. It promotes cell growth, proliferation, and angiogenesis. It also regulates HIF-1/2 synthesis in renal cell cancer.

Current guidelines (2011) are based on phase III trials in which older patients could be enrolled if they met the other eligibility criteria. However, the drugs approved for metastatic kidney cancer have quite a few side effects that can be troublesome in patients with comorbidities. The SIOG (International Society of Geriatric Oncology) has published a position paper on the medical treatment of metastatic renal cell cancer in the elderly [6]. However, there are no specific guidelines for treatment of elderly patients.

This chapter will review the current data on treatment of metastatic disease, focusing on elderly patients.

Current Treatment Options

Several drugs have been developed to target these pathways for patients with metastatic renal cancer. Table 21.1 summarizes the current guidelines for management of metastatic renal cell carcinoma [7]. Treatment recommendations are based on the MSKCC prognostic groups [8]. There are five poor prognostic factors in this score: IK ≤ 70 %, lactate dehydrogenase level >1.5 times upper limit of normal, hemoglobin level < lower limit of normal, corrected serum calcium level >10 mg/dl (2.5 mmol/l), and time from initial diagnosis to metastases <1 year.

Patients with no risk factor are in the good-risk group, patients with 1 or 2 factors in the intermediate-risk group, and patients with ≥3 factors are in the poor-risk group.

There are four options for patients with clear cell renal carcinoma that are in the good- or intermediate-risk groups: sunitinib, bevacizumab + interferon alpha, or pazopanib. In some selected cases, high-dose interleukin-2 can still be offered.

For patients in the poor-risk group, temsirolimus or sunitinib can be used in the first-line setting.

For patients with nonclear cell, temsirolimus and sunitinib are options.

For patients who relapse after first-line cytokine, sunitinib, pazopanib, and sorafenib are options. For patients who relapse after first-line tyrosine kinase inhibitors, the only approved drug, in 2011, is everolimus [7].

Table 21.1 Current recommendations for treatment of metastatic renal cancer

	First line	Second line
Clear cell	Sunitinib	Everolimus (after TKI)
Favorable group	Bevacizumab + IFN	Sorafenib (after cytokines)
Intermediate group	Pazopanib	Sunitinib (after cytokines)
	High-dose IL2[a]	Pazopanib (after cytokines)
Clear cell	Temsirolimus	
Poor risk	Sunitinib (option)	
Non-CCC	(Sunitinib)	

[a]In selected cases

VEGF Pathway Inhibitors

Tyrosine Kinase Inhibitors

Several VEGFR (vascular endothelial growth factor receptor) inhibitors have been developed to treat patients with metastatic renal cancer. Three are approved.

Sunitinib

Introduction

Sunitinib is a small tyrosine kinase inhibitor that is administered orally. It inhibits receptor tyrosine kinase autophosphorylation. It targets VEGFR 1, 2, and 3 (vascular endothelial growth factor receptor), PDGFR α and β (platelet-derived growth factor receptor), FLT-3(FMS-like tyrosine kinase-3 receptor), CSF-1R (colony-stimulating factor-1), C-kit, and RET kinases.

Phase III Data

A phase III trial including 750 patients with treatment-naive metastatic kidney cancer compared sunitinib to interferon-α (IFNα). [9, 10].

Median age in the sunitinib arm was 62 (range 27–87 years) and 59 (range 34–85 years) in the IFNα arm.

Objective response rates were significantly higher in patients receiving sunitinib (31 vs. 6 %, $p<0.001$). Progression-free survival (PFS) was longer in the sunitinib arm compared to the IFNα arm (median PFS 11 vs. 5 months, $p<0.001$). This benefit was also seen in the group of patients that were 65 or older. Overall survival (OS) difference nearly meets statistical significance (median OS 26.4 vs. 21.8 months, $p=0.051$).

The most frequent toxicities were diarrhea (all grade: 61 %, grade 3: 9 %), fatigue (all grade: 54 %, grade 3: 11 %), nausea (52 %, grade 3: 5 %), hypertension (all grade: 31 % , grade 3: 11 %), anorexia (all grade: 34 %, grade 3: 2 %), hand–foot syndrome (all grade: 29 % with 9 % grade 3), mucosal inflammation (all grade: 26 %, grade 3: 2 %), hematological toxicity (thrombocytopenia: all grade 68 %, grade 3: 8 %; neutropenia: all grade: 78 %, grade 3: 8 %), and hypothyroidism (all grade: 14 %, grade 3: 3 %). Thirteen percent of patients experienced decrease in left ventricular function; it was grade 3 in 3 % of patients.

Expanded Access Program

Data from an international expanded access program is available [11]. The aim of this program was to provide sunitinib on a compassionate basis for patients who could not enter clinical trials and before the drug was granted approval. Out of the 4,371 patients enrolled in this program, 1,418 were 65 or older. In that population, 77 % had a clinical benefit and 60 % had stable disease for more than 3 months. Median progression-free survival and median overall survival were 11.3 months (10.7–12.3 months) and 18.2 months (16.6–19.8 months), respectively. These values are the same as to those of the whole population. Less than 1 % of patients in the expanded access program experienced cardiac failure.

There was no marked difference in the incidence of grade 3–4 toxicity between all patients and elderly patients in the expanded access program.

Other Toxicity Data

Van der Velt et al. developed a model to predict severe sunitinib toxicity. In the uni-variate analysis, female gender, high age, low BSA (body surface area), and high LDH were significantly related with severe toxicity. In the multivariate analysis, only age and gender remained significantly associated with severe toxicity. The combination of both factors was highly predictive of severe toxicity [12]. In that model, women that are 80 have a 90 % risk of developing severe toxicity on standard sunitinib dosage.

A multicentric retrospective analysis suggests that cardiac toxicity related to sunitinib is increased with history of coronary heart disease (adjusted odds ratio (OR): 18, 95 % IC 4–160, $p=0.005$) and history of hypertension (adjusted OR: 3, 95 % CI 1.5–80, $p=0.03$). Median age in patients experiencing congestive heart failure and those not were not statistically different (64 vs. 60 years, $p=0.1$) [13].

Pazopanib

Introduction

Pazopanib is another small tyrosine kinase inhibitor that targets VEGFR 1, 2, and 3 (vascular endothelial growth factor receptor), PDGFR α and β (platelet-derived growth factor receptor), and C-kit.

Efficacy

An international phase III trial compared pazopanib to placebo for patients with metastatic or locally advanced kidney cancer [14]. Four hundred and thirty-five patients were enrolled in this trial. Forty-seven percent of patients had previously received cytokine treatment. Median ages in the pazopanib arm and the placebo arm were 59 years (range 28–85) and 60 years (range 25–81), respectively. Objective response rates were significantly higher in the group treated with pazopanib compared to placebo (30 vs. 3 %, $p < 0.001$). Median progression-free survival was longer in the pazopanib arm compared to the placebo arm (9.2 vs. 4.2 months, $p < 0.001$). The benefit existed both for patients younger and older than 65.

Toxicity

The most frequent toxicities were nausea (all grade: 26 %, grade 3–4 < 1 %) and vomiting (all grade: 21 %, grade 3–4: 3 %), diarrhea (all grade: 52 %, grade 3–4: 4 %), hypertension (all grade: 40 %, grade 3–4: 4 %), anorexia (all grade: 22 %, grade 3–4: 2 %), fatigue (all grade: 19 %, grade 3–4: 2 %), hematological toxicity (neutropenia (all grade: 37 %, grade 3–4: 0 %), thrombocytopenia (all grade: 32 %, grade 3–4 < 2 %)), and hepatic toxicity (ALT increase (all grade: 53 %, grade 3–4: 12 %) and AST increase (all grade: 53 %, grade 3–4: 8 %)).

Sorafenib

Introduction

Sorafenib is also a tyrosine kinase inhibitor. It targets VEGFR 2–3, PDGFR β, FLT-3, c-Kit, RET, and RAF.

Phase III Clinical Trial Data

a-Efficacy: Sorafenib was studied in a phase III trial (TARGET) and compared to placebo in 903 patients with metastatic kidney cancer who had previously been treated with cytokines [15, 16]. Median age in the sorafenib arm was 58 years (range 19–86) and 59 in the placebo arm (range 29–84). Median progression-free survival was 5.5 months in the sorafenib arm versus 2.8 months in the placebo arm ($p < 0.001$). The median overall survival was 19.3 months for patients in the sorafenib group and 15.9 months for patients in the placebo group (hazard ratio = 0.77; 95 % CI, 0.63–0.95; $p = 0.02$). However, the analyses did not reach the prespecified O'Brien–Fleming boundaries for statistical significance. There was one complete response on sorafenib. Ten percent of patients on sorafenib reached a partial response versus 2 % in the placebo arm. Stable disease was observed in 78 % of patients on sorafenib and 53 % on placebo.

A retrospective analysis of the patients enrolled in this TARGET trial according to their age was performed (<70 or ≥70 years) [17]. In the trial, 115 patients were 70 or older, 70 received sorafenib. Sixty-six percent of the older patients had hypertension, 20 % had diabetes mellitus, and 7 % had coronary heart disease. In the older patient group, the median progression-free survival was 26.3 weeks in the sorafenib arm and 13.9 weeks in the placebo arm (HR = 0.55, 95 % CI: 0.47–0.66).

The difference was similar to that in the whole trial population and in the younger group.

Median time on sorafenib was 25.6 weeks in the younger group and 24.1 weeks in the older group.

b-Toxicity: The most frequent toxicities in the sorafenib arm were diarrhea (all grade: 48 %, grade 3–4: 3 %), nausea (all grade: 19 %, grade 3–4 < 1 %), fatigue (all grade: 29 %, grade 3–4: 3 %), hypertension (all grade: 17 %, grade 3–4: 4 %), cutaneous reactions: hand–foot syndrome (all grade: 33 %, grade 3–4: 6 %), rash and desquamation (all grade: 41 %, grade 3–4: 1 %), anorexia (all grade: 14 %, grade 3–4 < 1 %), and weight loss (all grade: 8 %, grade 3–4: 1 %).

In the subgroup analysis of the TARGET trial, adverse event rates were similar in both older and younger groups (94.2 and 98.6 %). However, grade 3–4 events were slightly more frequent in the older group (45.7 vs. 36.7 %). Older patients experienced more gastrointestinal toxicity and fatigue. There was more hypertension in younger patients. Four patients in the older group had a cardiac event: 1 had grade 4 cardiac ischemia, 2 had grade 5 cardiac ischemia, and 1 had grade 3 left ventricular systolic dysfunction.

Thirty-one patients (8.1 %) in the younger group and 15 (21.4 %) in the older group discontinued treatment because of toxicity. More patients in the older group had dose reductions (21.4 vs. 11.1 %).

Time to health deterioration was longer for younger patients in the sorafenib arm compared to the placebo arm. In the older group, the difference was not statistically different.

Expanded Access Program Data

In the European expanded access program, 1,165 patients were enrolled. Twenty-three percent of the patients were 70 or older [18]. The overall response rate was 4 % with only one patient having a complete response. The median PFS was 6.6 months (95 % IC 6.1–7.4 months). Disease control rates at 8 and 12 weeks were 85 and 78 %, respectively. A subgroup analysis by age and ECOG performance status (PS) was performed. Older patients tended to have a worse PS compared to younger patients. Tolerance was similar in older patients compared to the whole population with adverse event rates of 93.6 %. Grade 3 events occurred in 45.3 % of patients in the whole group and 49.1 % of the older patients. Older patients had more fatigue than younger patients. The other frequent side effects were hand–foot skin reaction, rash/desquamation, and diarrhea. SAE (severe adverse event) rates were similar in older and younger patients (14–16 %). Disease control rates were similar across age groups and similar to the whole group.

Results from the American access program are comparable [19, 20]. Among the 2,504 patients enrolled in this program, 736 were 70 or older. Median age in that subgroup was 75 years (range 70–93). Sixty-three percent were male. Eighty-one percent had undergone prior nephrectomy.

Main toxicities were cutaneous toxicity: hand–foot syndrome (7 % grade 2, 8 % grade ≥ 3), rash/desquamation (10 % grade 2, 5 % grade ≥ 3), fatigue (9 % grade 2,

7 % grade ≥ 3), diarrhea(6 % grade 2, 2 % grade ≥ 3), nausea (4 % grade 2, 1 % grade ≥ 3), anorexia (5 % grade 2, 1 % grade ≥ 3), hypertension (7 % grade 2, 5 % grade ≥ 3), and weight loss (3 % grade 2, <1 % grade ≥ 3). The incidence and severity of side effects were similar to those of the whole population.

No patient in the older subgroup obtained complete response, 4 % of patients reached partial response, and 80 % had stable disease for at least 8 weeks.

Median progression-free survival for the whole group was 24 weeks (95 % IC 22–25), and median overall survival was 50 weeks (95 % IC 46–52).

Anti-VEGF Antibodies

Introduction

Bevacizumab is a recombinant humanized monoclonal antibody that binds to VEGF. It therefore prevents the activation of the downstream pathway. It is administered intravenously.

Efficacy

Bevacizumab + interferon alpha (IFNα) was compared to placebo + IFNα for patients with metastatic renal clear cell carcinoma in two phase III trials [21–24].

In the AVOREN study, median age in the bevacizumab–IFNα group was 61 years (range 30–82) and 60 in the placebo–IFNα group (range: 18–81). The objective response rate was 31 % with bevacizumab versus 13 % with IFNα alone. Median progression-free survival was longer with bevacizumab (10. 2 vs. 5.4 months; $p = 0.0001$). However, there was no significant benefit in overall survival (median OS 23.3 vs. 21.3 months; $p = 0.336$). In a subgroup analysis, the HR for progression-free survival was 0.77 (95 % IC 0.58–1.03) for patients older than 65, and HR for overall survival was 1.07 (95 % IC 0.80–1.45).

The results were similar in the CALGB trial with a 25.5 % response rate for bevacizumab + IFNα and 13.1 % with IFNα ($p < 0.001$). Median PFS was significantly longer in the combination arm (8.5 vs. 5.2 months; $p < 0.001$). There again, median overall survival was not statistically different (18.3 vs. 17.4 months; $p = 0.069$). Median age in the bevacizumab–IFNα group was 61 years (interquartile range 56–70) and 62 in the IFNα group (interquartile range 55–70).

Toxicity

Main side effects were hypertension (all grade: 26–28 %, grade 3–4: 3–11 %), fatigue (all grade: 33–97 %, grade ≥ 3: 12–37 %), anorexia (all grade 36–71 %, grade ≥ 3: 3–17 %), and proteinuria (all grade: 18–71 %, grade ≥ 3: 7–15 %). Other side effects were reported, more rarely, such as ischemia, thromboembolic events, congestive heart failure, bleeding, and gastrointestinal perforation.

mTOR Inhibitors

mTOR is a multiprotein complex that is involved in cell proliferation, cell growth, cell survival, and angiogenesis. The currently available inhibitors target the serine/threonine kinase activity of mTOR complex 1 (TORC1). There are two drugs that are used in metastatic renal cancer: temsirolimus that is administered intravenously and everolimus that is an oral drug.

Temsirolimus

Introduction

Temsirolimus is an mTOR inhibitor that binds to the intracellular protein FKBP-12. It forms a complex that inhibits mTOR and causes cell cycle arrest and tumor suppression. It also contributes to angiogenesis inhibition.

Efficacy

Temsirolimus was studied in patients with treatment-naive, poor-risk metastatic renal cancer in a phase III trial [25]. Six hundred and twenty-six patients were randomly assigned to one of the three treatment arms: temsirolimus alone, temsirolimus + IFNα, or IFNα alone (standard arm). The objective response rates were 4.8 % in the IFN arm and 8.1 % in the temsirolimus arm. Thirty percent of patients in the trial were 65 or older (age interval 23–86). There was an overall survival benefit for patients in the temsirolimus-only arm compared to the IFNα arm (median OS 10.9 vs. 7.3 months, $p=0.008$) and a progression-free survival benefit too (5.5 vs. 3 months; $p<0.00$). However, in a subgroup analysis, there was no benefit in overall survival for patients 65 or older.

There was no difference between the temsirolimus + IFNα and the IFNα arms.

Toxicity

Main toxicities were hematological toxicity such as anemia (all grade: 33 %, grade 3–4: 13 %), metabolic adverse events (hyperglycemia (all grade: 18 %, grade 3–4: 9 %), hypertriglyceridemia (all grade: 25 %, grade 3–4: 3 %), hypercholesterolemia (all grade: 21 %, grade 3–4: 1 %)), pneumonitis (all grade: 2 %, grade 3–4: 1 %), creatinine increase (all grade: 11 %, grade 3–4: 2 %), cutaneous side effects such as drug-related rash and acne (all grade: 43 %, grade 3–4: 3 %), and stomatitis (all grade: 20 %, grade 3–4: 1 %) [25, 26].

Everolimus

Introduction

Everolimus is an orally administered mTOR inhibitor. As temsirolimus, it binds to the intracellular protein FKBP-12 and inhibits the mTOR and the downstream signaling pathway.

Efficacy

Everolimus was compared to placebo in a phase III trial on patients with metastatic renal cancer that had progressed on VEGF-targeted therapy [27]. Median age in the everolimus arm was 61 years (range 27–85) and 60 years in the placebo arm (range 20–79). Only one percent of patients had a partial response on everolimus, 63 % had stable disease compared to 32 % on placebo. Median progression-free survival was 4.6 months in the everolimus arm and 1.8 months in the placebo arm ($p < 0.0001$). This benefit was found in both age groups (<65 years and ≥65 years)

There was no significant difference between groups in terms of overall survival: the median was not reached in the everolimus arm and was 8.8 months in the placebo arm ($p = 0.23$).

Toxicity

Main toxicities were stomatitis (all grade: 40 %, grade 3–4: 3 %), rash (all grade: 25 %, grade 3–4 <1 %), fatigue (all grade: 20 %, grade 3–4: 3 %), pneumonitis (all grade: 8 %, grade 3–4: 3 %), hematological toxicity (anemia (all grade: 91 %, grade 3–4: 10 %), lymphopenia (all grade: 42 %, grade 3–4: 15 %)), and metabolic changes (hyperglycemia (all grade: 50 %, grade 3–4: 3 %), hypertriglyceridemia (all grade: 71 %, grade 3–4: <1 %), and hypercholesterolemia (all grade: 76 %, grade 3–4: 3 %)).

Table 21.2 summarizes the data on currently used drugs and their main side effects.

Specific Problems in the Elderly Patients: Why Could Antiangiogenic Therapies Be a Problem in Elderly Patients?

Current available data for treatment comes from phase III data. Inclusion criteria on these trials select elderly patients with few comorbidities.

Table 21.2 Summary of main side effects from the phase III trials and potential consequences

	Median age	Main side effects	Potential consequences
Sunitinib	62 years (27–87)	Hypertension	Increased cardiovascular risk
		HFS	
		Hypothyroidism	Dependence
		Fatigue	
		Nausea, diarrhea	Malnutrition
Pazopanib	59 years (28–85)	Hypertension	Increased cardiovascular risk
		Fatigue	Dependence
		Nausea, vomiting	Malnutrition
		Anorexia	
		Diarrhea	
Sorafenib	58 years (19–86)	HFS	Dependence
		Fatigue	
		Nausea, vomiting	Malnutrition
		Anorexia, weight loss	
		Diarrhea	
Bevacizumab + IFN (AVOREN)	61 years (30–82)	Hypertension	Increased cardiovascular risk
		Fatigue	Dependence
Bevacizumab + IFN (CALGB)	61 years (56–70)	Anorexia	Malnutrition
Temsirolimus	58 years (32–81)	Metabolic changes	Increased cardiovascular risk
		Stomatitis	Malnutrition
Everolimus	61 years (27–85)	Metabolic changes	Increased cardiovascular risk
		Stomatitis	Malnutrition

HFS hand–foot syndrome

Elderly patients have more comorbidities than younger patients. In a series of patients aged 75 or older with localized kidney tumors, 60 % had hypertension and 42 % had a Charlson score ≥ 2 [28].

Cardiovascular disease is more frequent in elderly patients [29]. In a prospective analysis of acute vascular events in Oxfordshire, incidence increased with age. Eighty percent of cerebrovascular attacks, 73 % of coronary events, and 78 % of peripheral events occurred in patients aged 65 or older and 54, 47, and 56 % in patients aged 75 or older. The overall yearly event rate was 0.37 per 100 people at age 45–54, 0.94 at 55–64 years, 2.4 at 65–74 years, 5.1 at 75–84 years, and 8.6 at 85 years and older.

Denys et al. analyzed the literature on metabolic syndrome in the elderly [30].

In the elderly population, the prevalence of metabolic syndrome according to the WHO criteria varied from 11 to 43 % (median 21 %) and from 23 to 55 % (median 31 %) according to NCEP (National Cholesterol Education Program). Obesity and hypertension are the most prevalent individual components. Metabolic syndrome in an elderly population is a proven risk factor for cardiovascular morbidity, especially stroke and coronary heart disease and mortality.

Osteoarticular disease is also frequent in elderly patients. The incidence increases with age. Prevalence of hip arthritis reaches up to 8 % in some series and incidence of knee arthritis up to 40 % [31]. Hand and foot syndrome that can occur as a side effect of oral antiangiogenic drugs can worsen walking difficulties in patients.

Patients with comorbidities have polymedications. The tyrosine kinase inhibitors used to treat kidney cancer are metabolized by the cytochrome 3A4. Several frequently prescribed drugs interact with that cytochrome, such as amiodarone, fluconazole … Drug interactions must be analyzed before starting patients on oral targeted therapies [32].

All of the treatments used for treating metastatic renal cancer have an impact on cardiovascular risk: they increase hypertension, they increase arterial thromboembolic events, and they have some degree of direct cardiac toxicity. Some can also increase blood glucose and lipid levels. As described above, elderly patients are at higher risk of developing cardiac disease, and giving an antiangiogenic drug may increase that risk.

The other side effects of these therapies (hand–foot syndrome, diarrhea, and fatigue) can have an impact on patients' ability to perform their daily activities.

When deciding to treat an elderly patient with metastatic kidney cancer, physicians must be aware of the possible impact of the targeted agents on the patients' global health and try and minimize it.

Conclusions

There is little specific date on the use of angiogenic treatment in elderly patients with metastatic kidney cancer. The available data comes from subgroup analysis of phase III trials. Treatment seems to be efficient also in the elderly population. It seems also that these drugs can be used safely in this population; however, patients enrolled in clinical trials are highly selected and do not always reflect "real life," with no patients over 85 in these clinical trials. Data from expanded access programs is more interesting from that point of view. There again, sorafenib and sunitinib have a manageable toxicity profile in elderly patients. Before starting treatment, patients should be evaluated for comorbidities, ability to perform ADL and IADL, and possible drug interactions. Disease aggressivity and extent must also be taken into account when deciding to treat a patient.

Elderly patients should be monitored carefully for side effects, and symptomatic treatment should be offered and treatment doses adapted if necessary.

There is still need for specific clinical trials to establish the optimal treatment for these patients.

References

1. Ferlay J, Shin HR, Bray F, Forman D, Mathers C and Parkin DM. GLOBOCAN 2008 v1.2, Cancer Incidence and Mortality Worldwide: IARC Cancer Base No. 10 [Internet].Lyon, France: International Agency for Research on Cancer; 2010. Available from: http://globocan.iarc.fr, accessed on 1 Dec 2011.
2. Aron M, Nguyen MM, Stein RJ, Gill IS. Impact of gender in renal cell carcinoma: an analysis of the SEER database. Eur Urol. 2008;54(1):133–40.

3. Motzer RJ, Bacik J, Murphy BA, Russo P, Mazumdar M. Interferon-α as a comparative treatment for clinical trials of new therapies against advanced renal cell carcinoma. J Clin Oncol. 2002;20(1):289–96.
4. Négrier S, Raymond E. Antiangiogenic treatments and mechanisms of action inrenal cell carcinoma. Invest New Drugs. 2012 Aug;30(4):1791–801.
5. Patel PH, Chadalavada RS, Chaganti RS, Motzer RJ. Targeting von Hippel-Lindau pathway in renal cell carcinoma. Clin Cancer Res. 2006;12(24):7215–20.
6. Bellmunt J, Négrier S, Escudier B, Awada A, Aapro M, SIOG Taskforce. The medical treatment of metastatic renal cell cancer in the elderly: position paper of a SIOG Taskforce. Crit Rev Oncol Hematol. 2009;69(1):64–72.
7. Ljungberg B, Cowan NC, Hanbury DC, Hora M, Kuczyk MA, Merseburger AS, Patard JJ, Mulders PF, Sinescu IC, European Association of Urology Guideline Group. EAU guidelines on renal cell carcinoma: the 2010 update. Eur Urol. 2010;58(3):398–406.
8. Motzer RJ, Bacik J, Mariani T, Russo P, Mazumdar M, Reuter V. Treatment outcome and survival associated with metastatic renal cell carcinoma of non-clear-cell histology. J Clin Oncol. 2002;20(9):2376–81.
9. Motzer RJ, Hutson TE, Tomczak P, Michaelson MD, Bukowski RM, Rixe O, Oudard S, Negrier S, Szczylik C, Kim ST, Chen I, Bycott PW, Baum CM, Figlin RA. Sunitinib versus interferon alfa in metastatic renal-cell carcinoma. N Engl J Med. 2007;356(2):115–24.
10. Motzer RJ, Hutson TE, Tomczak P, Michaelson MD, Bukowski RM, Oudard S, Negrier S, Szczylik C, Pili R, Bjarnason GA, Garcia-del-Muro X, Sosman JA, Solska E, Wilding G, Thompson JA, Kim ST, Chen I, Huang X, Figlin RA. Overall survival and updated results for sunitinib compared with interferon alfa in patients with metastatic renal cell carcinoma. J Clin Oncol. 2009;27(22):3584–90.
11. Gore ME, Szczylik C, Porta C, Bracarda S, Bjarnason GA, Oudard S, Hariharan S, Lee SH, Haanen J, Castellano D, Vrdoljak E, Schöffski P, Mainwaring P, Nieto A, Yuan J, Bukowski R. Safety and efficacy of sunitinib for metastatic renal-cell carcinoma: an expanded-access trial. Lancet Oncol. 2009;10(8):757–63.
12. van der Veldt AA, Boven E, Helgason HH, van Wouwe M, Berkhof J, de Gast G, Mallo H, Tillier CN, van den Eertwegh AJ, Haanen JB. Predictive factors for severe toxicity of sunitinib in unselected patients with advanced renal cell cancer. Br J Cancer. 2008;99(2):259–65.
13. Di Lorenzo G, Autorino R, Bruni G, Cartenì G, Ricevuto E, Tudini M, Ficorella C, Romano C, Aieta M, Giordano A, Giuliano M, Gonnella A, De Nunzio C, Rizzo M, Montesarchio V, Ewer M, De Placido S. Cardiovascular toxicity following sunitinib therapy in metastatic renal cell carcinoma: a multicenter analysis. Ann Oncol. 2009;20(9):1535–42.
14. Sternberg CN, Davis ID, Mardiak J, Szczylik C, Lee E, Wagstaff J, Barrios CH, Salman P, Gladkov OA, Kavina A, Zarbá JJ, Chen M, McCann L, Pandite L, Roychowdhury DF, Hawkins RE. Pazopanib in locally advanced or metastatic renal cell carcinoma: results of a randomized phase III trial. J Clin Oncol. 2010;28(6):1061–8.
15. Escudier B, Eisen T, Stadler WM, Szczylik C, Oudard S, Siebels M, TARGET Study Group, et al. Sorafenib in advanced clear-cell renal-cell carcinoma. N Engl J Med. 2007;356(2):125–34.
16. Escudier B, Eisen T, Stadler WM, Szczylik C, Oudard S, Staehler M, Negrier S, Chevreau C, Desai AA, Rolland F, Demkow T, Hutson TE, Gore M, Anderson S, Hofilena G, Shan M, Pena C, Lathia C, Bukowski RM. Sorafenib for treatment of renal cell carcinoma: final efficacy and safety results of the phase III treatment approaches in renal cancer global evaluation trial. J Clin Oncol. 2009;27(20):3312–8.
17. Eisen T, Oudard S, Szczylik C, Gravis G, Heinzer H, Middleton R, Cihon F, Anderson S, Shah S, Bukowski R, Escudier B, TARGET Study Group. Sorafenib for older patients with renal cell carcinoma: subset analysis from a randomized trial. J Natl Cancer Inst. 2008;100(20): 1454–63.
18. Beck J, Procopio G, Bajetta E, Keilholz U, Negrier S, Szczylik C, Bokemeyer C, Bracarda S, Richel DJ, Staehler M, Strauss UP, Mersmann S, Burock K, Escudier B. Final results of the European Advanced Renal Cell Carcinoma Sorafenib (EU-ARCCS) expanded-access study: a large open-label study in diverse community settings. Ann Oncol. 2011;22(8):1812–23.

19. Stadler WM, Figlin RA, McDermott DF, Dutcher JP, Knox JJ, Miller Jr WH, Hainsworth JD, Henderson CA, George JR, Hajdenberg J, Kindwall-Keller TL, Ernstoff MS, Drabkin HA, Curti BD, Chu L, Ryan CW, Hotte SJ, Xia C, Cupit L, Bukowski RM, ARCCS Study Investigators. Safety and efficacy results of the advanced renal cell carcinoma sorafenib expanded access program in North America. Cancer. 2010;116(5):1272–80.

20. Bukowski RM, Stadler WM, McDermott DF, Dutcher JP, Knox JJ, Miller Jr WH, Hainsworth JD, Henderson CA, Hajdenberg J, Kindwall-Keller TL, Ernstoff MS, Drabkin HA, Curti BD, Chu L, Ryan CW, Hotte SJ, Xia C, Cupit L, Figlin RA. Safety and efficacy of sorafenib in elderly patients treated in the North American advanced renal cell carcinoma sorafenib expanded access program. Oncology. 2010;78(5–6):340–7.

21. Escudier B, Pluzanska A, Koralewski P, Ravaud A, Bracarda S, Szczylik C, Chevreau C, Filipek M, Melichar B, Bajetta E, Gorbunova V, Bay JO, Bodrogi I, Jagiello-Gruszfeld A, Moore N, AVOREN Trial Investigators. Bevacizumab plus interferon alfa-2a for treatment of metastatic renal cell carcinoma: a randomised, double-blind phase III trial. Lancet. 2007;370(9605):2103–11.

22. Escudier B, Bellmunt J, Négrier S, Bajetta E, Melichar B, Bracarda S, Ravaud A, Golding S, Jethwa S, Sneller V. Phase III trial of bevacizumab plus interferon alfa-2a in patients with metastatic renal cell carcinoma (AVOREN): final analysis of overall survival. J Clin Oncol. 2010;28(13):2144–50.

23. Rini BI, Halabi S, Rosenberg JE, Stadler WM, Vaena DA, Ou SS, Archer L, Atkins JN, Picus J, Czaykowski P, Dutcher J, Small EJ. Bevacizumab plus interferon alfa compared with interferon alfa monotherapy in patients with metastatic renal cell carcinoma: CALGB 90206. J Clin Oncol. 2008;26(33):5422–8.

24. Rini BI, Halabi S, Rosenberg JE, Stadler WM, Vaena DA, Archer L, Atkins JN, Picus J, Czaykowski P, Dutcher J, Small EJ. Phase III trial of bevacizumab plus interferon alfa versus interferon alfa monotherapy in patients with metastatic renal cell carcinoma: final results of CALGB 90206. J Clin Oncol. 2010;28(13):2137–43.

25. Hudes G, Carducci M, Tomczak P, Dutcher J, Figlin R, Kapoor A, Staroslawska E, Sosman J, McDermott D, Bodrogi I, Kovacevic Z, Lesovoy V, Schmidt-Wolf IG, Barbarash O, Gokmen E, O'Toole T, Lustgarten S, Moore L, Motzer RJ, Global ARCC Trial. Temsirolimus, interferon alfa, or both for advanced renal-cell carcinoma. N Engl J Med. 2007;356(22):2271–81.

26. Bellmunt J, Szczylik C, Feingold J, Strahs A, Berkenblit A. Temsirolimus safety profile and management of toxic effects in patients with advanced renal cell carcinoma and poor prognostic features. Ann Oncol. 2008;19(8):1387–92.

27. Motzer RJ, Escudier B, Oudard S, Hutson TE, Porta C, Bracarda S, RECORD-1 Study Group, et al. Efficacy of everolimus in advanced renal cell carcinoma: a double-blind, randomised, placebo-controlled phase III trial. Lancet. 2008;372(9637):449–56.

28. Lane BR, Abouassaly R, Gao T, Weight CJ, Hernandez AV, Larson BT, Kaouk JH, Gill IS, Campbell SC. Active treatment of localized renal tumors may not impact overall survival in patients aged 75 years or older. Cancer. 2010;116(13):3119–26.

29. Rothwell PM, Coull AJ, Silver LE, Fairhead JF, Giles MF, Lovelock CE, Redgrave JN, Bull LM, Welch SJ, Cuthbertson FC, Binney LE, Gutnikov SA, Anslow P, Banning AP, Mant D, Mehta Z, Oxford Vascular Study. Population-based study of event-rate, incidence, case fatality, and mortality for all acute vascular events in all arterial territories (Oxford Vascular Study). Lancet. 2005;366(9499):1773–83.

30. Denys K, Cankurtaran M, Janssens W, Petrovic M. Metabolic syndrome in the elderly: an overview of the evidence. Acta Clin Belg. 2009;64(1):23–34. Review.

31. Petersson I. Occurrence of osteoarthritis of the peripheral joints in European populations. Ann Rheum Dis. 1996;55:659–64.

32. http://www.afssaps.fr/Dossiers-thematiques/Interactions-medicamenteuses/Interactions-medicamenteuses-et-cytochromes/. Accessed on 15 Dec 2011.

Part VII
Rare Cancers

Chapter 22
Carcinoma of the Penis in the Elderly

Jérôme Rigaud and Olivier Bouchot

Abstract Squamous cell carcinoma of the penis is a rare tumor. There are no specific references in the literature concerning the management of carcinoma of the penis in the elderly, but the incidence is situated between 60 and 70 years. The most common histological type (95 % of cases) is squamous cell carcinoma. Physical examination of the penis is usually sufficient for the diagnosis. In case of doubt, a biopsy must be done. Treatment of the penis must be as conservative as possible with surgery with negative surgical margins or brachytherapy in selective cases. Preservation of voiding and sexual function and the psychological aspect must be taken into account in the treatment decision. Lymph node invasion is an independent prognostic factor for survival of this cancer. The first draining lymph nodes are superficial and deep inguinal lymph nodes, followed by pelvic lymph nodes. Indication for a therapeutic procedure on inguinal lymph nodes is based on clinical examination (presence or absence of palpable nodes) and the risk of lymph node involvement, which depends on the stage and grade of the penile lesion ($\geq$pT1bG2). Lymph node management must be systematic and bilateral, and must be performed at the time of diagnosis of penile cancer. Inguinal lymphadenectomy has a curative role in patients with lymph node metastasis (stage N1). Multimodal management combining chemotherapy, surgery, and possibly radiotherapy should be considered in patients with more extensive lymph node involvement (stage N2–N3).

Keywords Penile cancer • Elderly • Lymph node • Prognosis • Treatment • Surgery Chemotherapy • Brachytherapy

J. Rigaud, M.D. (✉) • O. Bouchot, M.D.
Department of Urology, Nantes University Hospital,
Nantes, France
e-mail: jrigaud@chu-nantes.fr; obouchot@chu-nantes.fr

J.-P. Droz, R.A. Audisio (eds.), *Management of Urological Cancers in Older People*,
Management of Cancer in Older People,
DOI 10.1007/978-0-85729-999-4_22, © Springer-Verlag London 2013

Introduction

Squamous cell carcinoma of the penis is a rare tumor in Europe, whose prognosis and survival are influenced by metastatic lymph node invasion.

Few large-scale series, mostly retrospective, have been reported in the literature, and no randomized prospective study or Cochrane Database review has been performed.

There are no specific references in the literature concerning the management of carcinoma of the penis in the elderly. However, carcinoma of the penis is classically a disease of the elderly with an incidence that increases with age. The peak incidence is situated between 60 and 70 years. Consequently, all of our knowledge concerning carcinoma of the penis is applicable to the elderly, although comorbidities must obviously be taken into account.

Epidemiology

The incidence of carcinoma of the penis varies from one country to another. In Europe and the USA, the incidence is estimated to be 1 per 100,000 men [1]. Variations of incidence are observed between the various countries of Europe and the rest of the world with higher rates in Hispanic populations, Brazil, and Uganda [2].

The diagnosis is often delayed by about 12 months and, in some cases, the cancer is only diagnosed at a locally invasive stage and/or at the stage of regional or systemic metastatic disease.

Risk Factors

Circumcision exerts a preventive role when it is performed during the neonatal period or before puberty, but not when it is performed in adults. Early circumcision is associated with a 3- to 5-fold decreased risk of carcinoma of the penis [3].

Risk factors (odds ratio > 10) are mainly related to maceration and poor local hygiene secondary to phimosis. Other risk factors include:

- Chronic inflammation (balanoposthitis, lichen sclerosus et atrophicus)
- Photodynamic therapy using psoralen and ultraviolet A radiation

Sexual practices (multiple partners, early age at first sexual intercourse) and history of condylomata are associated with a 3- to 5-fold increased risk of carcinoma of the penis [4].

Human papillomavirus (HPV) DNA has been identified in 70–100 % of cases of penile intraepithelial neoplasia and in 40–50 % of invasive tumors. HPV-16 and HPV-18 subtypes are involved in 50 % of cases of carcinoma of the penis. No guidelines are currently available concerning HPV-16 and HPV-18 vaccination in men, while awaiting the results of HPV vaccination in women [5].

Despite the strong correlation between HPV and carcinoma of the penis, no correlation is observed between HPV infection and tumor grade.

The main risk factor in elderly men therefore appears to be maceration due to phimosis that is more frequent and more often neglected than in younger patients. However, phimosis per se does not constitute a precursor lesion, but a precursor condition that predisposes to development of a cancer due to maceration and poor hygiene. Elderly men with acquired phimosis associated with discharge or bleeding must therefore be carefully evaluated. Carcinoma of the penis is also a relatively common incidental finding during circumcision for phimosis. In this setting, treatment of the cancer is performed during a second operation, after taking a biopsy and after informing the patient.

Histology

Precursor Lesions

Precursor lesions progress to carcinoma of the penis in the absence of treatment in about 30 % of cases [6]. These lesions must be identified and treated before the appearance of carcinoma.

HPV-Related Precursor Lesions

Some forms of carcinoma of the penis have been associated with HPV (human papillomavirus) infection. They are correlated with early age at first sexual intercourse and a large number of partners. HPV serotypes 8, 16, and 18 are particularly involved in carcinogenesis via transformation of HPV-related skin lesions. When HPV-related lesions are identified, the patient's partner must also be assessed (presence of other STDs, cervical assessment). The HPV-related oncogenic profile increases the risk of relapse, including long-term relapse. In Europe, one-half of all carcinomas of the penis are related to HPV infection. This proportion varies from one country to another, with a peak of 2/3 of cases in South America.

- *Bowen disease and erythroplasia of Queyrat.* These lesions are essentially observed in men over the age of 50. Clinically, the lesion is solitary and well demarcated with centrifugal extension. Bowen disease consists of leukoplakia lesions, while erythroplasia of Queyrat involves the mucosa.
- *Bowenoid papulosis.* Clinically, Bowenoid papulosis consists of multiple white, pink, or brown maculopapular lesions with possible perineal extension. Bowenoid papulosis is more common in young men and immunodepressed (HIV) subjects. Histological examination demonstrates keratinocytic atypias (irregular size of

nuclei and cells, hyperchromatic nuclei, and mitotic figures), irregular architecture, dyskeratosis (disorder of maturation), and parakeratotic hyperkeratosis.

Precursor Lesions Not Related to HPV

Other precursor lesions include penile intraepithelial neoplasia secondary to neglected lichen sclerosus et atrophicus caused by irritation. Physical examination reveals leukoplakia and erythroplakia associated with verrucous epithelial hyperplasia.

Balanitis xerotica obliterans is a form of lichen sclerosus involving the glans, extending to the meatus, and then to the navicular fossa causing stricture.

Histological examination demonstrates cytonuclear atypias limited to the basal cell layer of the epithelium with acanthosis but no signs of HPV lesions.

Cancers

Several histological types of carcinoma are observed: the most common histological type (95 % of cases) is squamous cell carcinoma (superficial, or ulcerative and invasive), but we also observed basaloid carcinoma, verrucous carcinoma (warty or condylomatous), sarcomatoid carcinoma, melanoma, sarcoma, adenosquamous carcinoma, and mixed carcinomas, etc.

The two most frequent sites are the glans (48 % of cases) and the prepuce (25 % of cases).

Two main forms of squamous cell carcinoma are observed with a different clinical course and prognosis:

- Exophytic papillary lesion with rare and late lymph node invasion
- Invasive ulcerative lesion, which is rapidly associated with lymph node invasion and which has a poorer prognosis

The prognosis of squamous cell carcinoma depends on the depth of infiltration, histoprognostic grade, and the presence of lymphovascular emboli or perineural invasion (TNM classification) [7].

TNM Classification

The TNM classification was revised in 2009 (Table 22.1) with division of stage T1 into substages T1a and T1b according to the presence or absence of lymphovascular invasion. Clinical and pathological lymph node staging has also been revised. It was also proposed to modify stage T2 by distinguishing invasion of the corpus spongiosum (T2a) which has a better prognosis from invasion of the corpora cavernosa (T2b) [8], but this proposal was not adopted in the final version.

Table 22.1 2009 TNM classification

T primary tumor	
pTx	Primary tumor cannot be assessed
T0	No evidence of primary tumor
Tis	Carcinoma in situ
Ta	Noninvasive verrucous carcinoma
T1	Tumor invades subepithelial connective tissue
T1a	Tumor invades subepithelial connective tissue without lymphovascular invasion and is not poorly differentiated or undifferentiated (T1 G1–2)
T1b	Tumor invades subepithelial connective tissue with lymphovascular invasion, or is poorly differentiated or undifferentiated (T1 G3–4)
T2	Tumor invades corpus spongiosum or cavernosum
T3	Tumor invades urethra
T4	Tumor invades other adjacent structures
cN regional lymph nodes (clinical: palpation or imaging)	
Nx	Regional (inguinal) lymph nodes cannot be assessed
N0	No palpable or visibly enlarged inguinal lymph nodes
N1	Palpable mobile unilateral inguinal lymph node
N2	Palpable mobile multiple or bilateral inguinal lymph nodes
N3	Fixed inguinal nodal mass or pelvic lymphadenopathy unilateral or bilateral
pN regional lymph nodes (pathological: biopsy or resection)	
pNx	Regional (inguinal) lymph nodes cannot be assessed
pN0	No regional lymph node metastasis
pN1	Intranodal metastasis in a single inguinal lymph node
pN2	Metastasis in multiple or bilateral inguinal lymph nodes
pN3	Metastasis in pelvic lymph node(s), unilateral or bilateral, or extranodal extension of regional lymph node metastasis
M distant metastases	
Mx	Distant metastasis cannot be assessed
M0	No distant metastasis
M1	Distant metastasis
Histopathological grading	
Gx	Grade of differentiation cannot be assessed
G1	Well differentiated
G2	Moderately differentiated
G3–4	Poorly differentiated/undifferentiated

Management of Carcinoma of the Penis

Diagnostic Assessment

Physical Examination

Physical examination of the penis is usually sufficient and must comprise assessment of tumor topography, the number and size of tumors, presence or absence of corpus spongiosum and corpus cavernosum invasion, the ulcerated or invasive appearance, the length of healthy penile tissue proximal to the tumor, and invasion of the urethra or adjacent structures.

Radiological Assessment

Complementary investigations can be performed in doubtful cases or to ensure more accurate staging:

- *Ultrasound.* Ultrasound can demonstrate invasion of the corpus cavernosum or tunica albuginea when the tumor arises in the glans. It can facilitate assessment of very large lesions.
- *Penile MRI.* MRI is the most sensitive examination to identify cavernous or urethral extension, but does not provide any additional information to physical examination in stage T1 lesions. Carcinoma of the penis has a low-intensity signal on T1- and T2-weighted sequences, with moderate gadolinium enhancement. When performed during a pharmacological erection test, MRI allows more accurate staging of corpora cavernosa invasion and can help to determine whether or not conservative surgery is possible.

Biopsy

Biopsy of the lesion is unnecessary when there is no doubt about the diagnosis, but should always be proposed in the presence of a suspicious precursor lesion or a doubt concerning a possible cancer.

Wide local excision should be preferred for limited lesions, ensuring healthy surgical margins and precise labeling of the operative specimen.

Treatment Options

Treatment of carcinoma of the penis has two essential aspects in addition to cancer eradication: preservation of voiding and sexual function is essential, and the psychological aspect related to damage to the body image and self-esteem. These two aspects must be taken into account in the treatment decision, even in elderly patients, and must be discussed with the patient.

Local Conservative Management

Stage pTis or pTa tumors can be treated locally by cytotoxic creams (5-fluorouracil or imiquimod 5 %) or photodynamic therapy.

YAG or CO_2 laser excision can also be performed with good functional results: no urinary impact and cosmetic preservation. Quality of life is excellent (better than after partial amputation) with very rapid return of sexual activity. Complications are early postoperative pain and minor bleeding. Local recurrence is observed in 18.3 % of cases following this technique.

Surgery

- *General principles.* The principles of surgical resection of carcinoma of the penis are determined by the size and site of the tumor, preoperative staging, and the surgical margins. Surgery must be as conservative as possible. Negative surgical margins are mandatory, as the risk of recurrence is multiplied by three in the case of positive margins [9]. Resection must be extended if frozen section or definitive histological examination demonstrates positive surgical margins, regardless of the type of procedure performed, in order to ensure negative surgical margins.
- *Surgical techniques.* Various procedures can be performed, adapted to the size and extension of the tumor:

  - *Wide local excision*: No standardized surgical technique has been defined, as it depends on technical possibilities, according to the size and site of the tumor.
  - *Circumcision*: It is reserved to tumors confined to the prepuce and not involving the corona of the glans.
  - *Glans resurfacing*: It is performed for lesions situated on the glans; specific procedures can be proposed, such as total or partial glansectomy with skin graft.
  - *Partial amputation*: The remaining length of the penis must be at least 4 cm so that the patient can urinate easily or can ensure penetration. The main complication is meatal stricture (7–10 %). Glans or penis reconstruction can be performed. Quality of life scores indicate a satisfactory postoperative quality of life.
  - *Total amputation*: It is indicated in the case of tumor of the shaft of the penis or a very advanced lesion of the glans, and requires perineal urethrostomy. Reconstruction by phalloplasty techniques provides good psychological and cosmetic results, but urethroplasties can cause major morbidity. Emasculation or complete resection of the corpora cavernosa is not performed routinely, but only when absolutely necessary.

Radiotherapy

- *External radiotherapy.* External radiotherapy is rarely used due to the difficulties of positioning of the penis during treatment. It can be indicated as palliative treatment for locally advanced or metastatic tumor at a dose of 50–60 Grays.
- *Brachytherapy.* Brachytherapy can be proposed for tumors of the glans or balanopreputial sulcus situated away from the urethra and the urethral meatus, without invasion of the tunica albuginea of the corpora cavernosa, and not exceeding

40 mm. Penile MRI is performed for local staging before this type of treatment. Prior to brachytherapy, patients must undergo biopsy to obtain histological evidence of carcinoma and circumcision to avoid radiation-induced edema, but the tumor is left in situ.

Brachytherapy consists of temporary implantation of radioactive material (Iridium-192 wires) in the tumor using an implantation cage, delivering a total dose of 60–65 Gy. Brachytherapy ensures good local control with a local recurrence rate of 20 % and a regional lymph node recurrence rate of 10 %. Long-term surveillance is essential, as late recurrences may be observed. About 90 % of patients are satisfied with the functional results.

The most common complications are meatal stricture (17 %), necrosis (18 %), and pain [10]. Brachytherapy-induced necrosis requires local dressings, and biopsy must not be performed to avoid interfering with healing. The risk of complications is correlated with the volume treated and the isodose on dosimetry.

Therapeutic Indications

Therapeutic indications are summarized in Table 22.2 [11, 12].

Local Recurrence

Treatment of the primary tumor must be as conservative as possible, but conservative management is associated with a risk of local recurrence estimated to be between 15 and 30 % regardless of the type of treatment (brachytherapy, laser, or local resection). Recurrence occurs during the first 2 years. Glansectomy is associated with the lowest local recurrence rate (2 %) [13].

Recurrence after initial conservative management should preferably be treated by conservative salvage surgery whenever possible. Total or partial amputation may be indicated for deep invasion.

Predictive factors for local recurrence after surgery are: the site of the tumor on the glans and positive margins [14]. However, tumor size is not a predictive factor of positive margins. It should be stressed that local recurrence has no significant impact on specific survival when it is managed correctly.

Management of Lymph Nodes

Lymph node invasion is an independent prognostic factor for survival of this cancer. Lymph node invasion is a nonrandom, sequential process, depending on the anatomy of the penile lymphatic drainage and always precedes hematogenous metastatic

Table 22.2 Treatment strategies for penile cancer

Type of lesion	Treatment options	Level of evidence	Grade of recommendation
Tis, Ta, T1a	CO$_2$ or YAG laser	2b	C
	Wide local excision	2b	C
	Glansectomy	2b	C
T1b or T2 of the glans	Wide local excision	2b	B
	Glansectomy	2b	B
	Partial amputation	2b	B
	External radiotherapy/ brachytherapy	2b	B
T2 of the body of the penis	Partial amputation	2b	B
T3	Total amputation	2b	B
T4	Neoadjuvant chemotherapy and amputation in responders	3	C
Local recurrence	Conservative surgery	2b	B
	Partial or total amputation	2b	B

spread. The first draining lymph nodes are superficial and deep inguinal lymph nodes, followed by pelvic lymph nodes. No skip lesions are observed with this cancer.

Inguinal lymph node management is therefore the cornerstone of treatment of penile cancer. About 60 % of patients, regardless of stage, have palpable lymph nodes, and about one-half (45 %) of these palpable nodes correspond to lymph node metastases, while the remaining nodes are simply inflammatory. About 20 % of patients without palpable nodes have micrometastases [15]. The prognosis of penile cancer essentially depends on the presence or absence of inguinal lymph node involvement. Inguinal lymphadenectomy plays an important role in the treatment strategy for penile cancer with clinical lymph node invasion and for tumors without palpable lymph nodes but at high risk of subclinical metastases.

Predictive Factors of the Risk of Lymph Node Involvement

The risk of lymph node metastases depends on the stage of the primary tumor, its histological grade, the presence of venous and lymphatic emboli, and the presence of palpable lymph nodes. Two classifications were previously used in the literature to classify tumors as a function of the risk of lymph node involvement. However, according to the most recent guidelines, the indication for a therapeutic procedure on inguinal lymph nodes is based on clinical examination (presence or absence of palpable nodes) and the risk of lymph node involvement, which depends on the stage and grade of the penile lesion ($\geq$pT1bG2) [11, 12].

Nomograms have been proposed to determine the risk of lymph node involvement and to adapt treatment, but with a predictive value of 80 %. They are rarely used, as they have never been validated.

Diagnostic Assessment

Clinical Examination

About 60 % of patients have palpable lymph nodes, regardless of stage. Clinical examination defines the size and number of lymph nodes, the presence of unilateral or bilateral involvement, and adherence to underlying tissues or skin.

About 45 % of palpable lymph nodes correspond to lymph node metastases, while the remainder corresponds to inflammatory lymph nodes. The false-negative rate of clinical examination is 18–23 % and is higher in the presence of abdominal obesity.

After treatment of the primary tumor, palpable inguinal lymph nodes can be treated by antibiotics for 4 weeks followed by another clinical assessment of lymph node status in order to define the final cN stage for each patient.

Aspiration Cytology

Ultrasound-guided (10 MHz transducer) fine-needle aspiration cytology of palpable lymph nodes now appears to be the preferred technique, as it is simple, associated with a low risk and can be performed as an outpatient procedure. The aspirated product is smeared in thin layers on a slide, dried, and then sent in the histology department. When this examination is positive, lymphadenectomy should be performed immediately without waiting for reassessment after a course of antibiotics.

Aspiration cytology only has a predictive value when it is positive, but can be used to guide lymph node management. Aspiration cytology has a sensitivity of 93 % and a specificity of 91 % for palpable lymph nodes. This technique has a sensitivity of 39 % and a specificity of 100 % for the detection of impalpable lymph nodes visualized by ultrasound [16, 17]. It also increases the micrometastasis detection rate in the sentinel node technique [18].

Ultrasound

Ultrasound with a high-resolution transducer can detect architectural changes of lymph nodes that appear before any increase in size. These changes may consist of asymmetrical thickness or focal lobulation of the lymph node cortex, and loss of the hilum. The diagnostic performance is improved by a combination of ultrasound and fine-needle aspiration cytology for suspicious lymph nodes.

Computed Tomography

No imaging examination has yet been shown to be superior to clinical examination for the detection of lymph nodes. Abdomen and pelvis computed tomography is recommended when clinical examination is difficult (obese patients) or in the presence of clinical inguinal lymph node involvement (for evaluation of pelvic lymph nodes). Imaging is not essential in patients with no palpable inguinal lymph nodes. Imaging may fail to diagnose micrometastases in cN0 patients.

Computed tomography is nevertheless able to detect iliac node involvement in patients with more than two persistent inguinal lymph nodes after antibiotic therapy [19]. Similarly, no pelvic lymph node involvement is demonstrated in the absence of palpable inguinal lymph nodes.

Magnetic Resonance Imaging (MRI)

MRI has not been shown to be superior to computed tomography for the detection of inguinal lymphadenopathy. However, this examination has the advantage of being nonirradiating and, like CT, is indicated in the case of difficult palpation and suspicious inguinal lymph nodes in order to detect iliac node involvement.

Positron Emission Tomography (PET)

^{18}F-FDG PET ([18]fluorine-labeled fluorodeoxyglucose) is a promising examination for lymph node and metastatic staging of penile cancer. The value of ^{18}F-FDG PET is currently limited by its inability to detect micrometastases.

A first study based on 20 patients demonstrated a sensitivity of 75 % for lymph node detection [20]. Subsequently, several studies have confirmed these results with a sensitivity of 40–91 %, a specificity of 97–100 %, a positive predictive value of 67–100 %, a negative predictive value of 91–96 %, and an accuracy of 89 % [21, 22].

^{18}F-FDG PET provides more precise distant staging in the presence of palpable inguinal lymph nodes. It is therefore optional, but recommended in patients with palpable lymph nodes (cN+), but is not recommended in the absence of palpable inguinal lymph nodes (cN0).

Sentinel Node Technique

The principle of the sentinel node technique is to identify and specifically resect the first draining inguinal lymph nodes. Dynamic lymphoscintigraphy is performed on the day before the operation with injection of a radioactive tracer into the tumor and detection of the first draining lymph node(s) by a gamma camera. During the operation, double detection of the sentinel lymph node is performed by detection of the radioactive tracer using a gamma probe then, after incision, by visualization of patent blue dye injected around the tumor at the beginning of the operation.

The technique was standardized by Horenblas and coworkers with a false-negative rate of 4.8 % and a complication rate of 6 % [18]. The sentinel node technique is more effective in cN0 patients than in cN+patients. It is therefore not recommended in patients with palpable lymph nodes [23]. This technique has been shown to be reproducible in two expert centers with a short specific learning curve [24], but few centers use this technique in routine practice in France.

Treatment Options

Surgery (Lymphadenectomy)

Inguinal lymph node surgery is the only reliable way to diagnose lymph node involvement, but it especially has a curative and prognostic role in patients with penile cancer at high risk of lymph node involvement.

- *Total inguinal lymphadenectomy.* This procedure consists of resection of all superficial and deep inguinal lymph nodes. The limits of total inguinal lymph- adenectomy are the superficial fascia anteriorly, the inguinal ligament superiorly, the anteromedial border of the sartorius muscle laterally, the anterolateral border of the adductor longus muscle medially, the apex of the femoral triangle inferi- orly, and the anterior plane of the femoral pedicle posteriorly (Fig. 22.1). Inguinal lymphadenectomy is performed via a transverse skin incision (Gibson incision), parallel to and 3 cm below the groin.
- *Modified inguinal lymphadenectomy.* The technique was described by Catalona in 1988. It consists of resection of the superomedial group of superficial inguinal lymph nodes situated superiorly and medially to the arch of the great saphenous vein over the femoral vein (Fig. 22.1) [25]. This technique, indicated for cN0 patients (no palpable nodes), has significantly decreased the short-term and medium-term complications related to lymphadenectomy. However, the decreased extent of lymphadenectomy increases the false-negative rate.
- *Morbidity of inguinal lymphadenectomy.* The morbidity of inguinal lymphadenec- tomy remains a major problem of this surgery because it is considerable, but varies as a function of the type of lymphadenectomy. In a series comparing the complica- tions of 118 modified lymphadenectomies and 58 superficial and deep (total) lymphadenectomies, the authors reported 6.8 and 41.4 % of early complications, and 3.4 and 43.1 % of late complications, respectively [26]. The most frequent early complications of modified lymphadenectomy were skin necrosis and lymphocele, and the most frequent late complication was lymphoedema of the lower limbs.
- *Iliac lymphadenectomy.* Iliac lymphadenectomy must remove all internal iliac, external iliac, and common iliac lymph nodes. It is indicated in the case of:

  - Iliac nodes visualized by staging imaging
  - ≥2 metastatic inguinal lymph nodes
  - Capsular effraction of a lymph node

In these situations, the probability of pelvic lymph node involvement is 23 % when 2 or 3 inguinal lymph nodes are involved and 56 % when more than 3 nodes are involved [27].

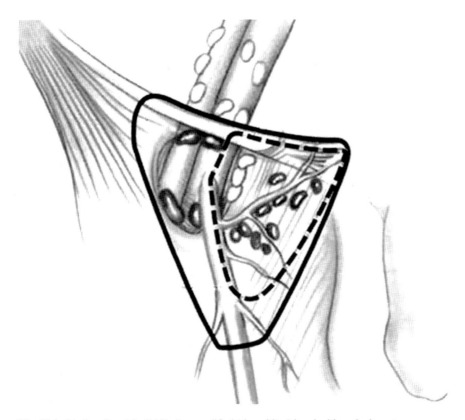

Fig. 22.1 Limits of total (*solid line*) or modified (*dotted line*) inguinal lymphadenectomy

Chemotherapy

No chemotherapeutic agent is currently approved (marketing authorization) for use in penile cancer. However, chemotherapy may be useful as adjuvant therapy for stages pN2 and pN3. In contrast, there are no solid arguments in favor of chemotherapy before lymphadenectomy (neoadjuvant) or after lymphadenectomy (adjuvant).

- *Neoadjuvant chemotherapy.* The only indications for neoadjuvant chemotherapy at the present time are locally advanced (cN3) and metastatic (M+) penile cancer. In the presence of fixed lymph node involvement, the objective of treatment is to reduce the tumor bulk before possibly proposing inguinal lymphadenectomy [28]. In 1996, Pizzocaro et al. reported their experience of the use of bleomycin, vincristine, and methotrexate in five patients with fixed inguinal lymph node metastases. Three patients obtained a partial response sufficient to allow secondary inguinal lymphadenectomy. These 3 patients were alive and recurrence-free 20, 27, and 72 months after surgery.

Leijte published a retrospective analysis of 20 patients who received preoperative chemotherapy to reduce the size of unresectable masses [29]. Twelve patients

(60 %) obtained an objective response, and nine of them were able to be operated. Eight patients obtained long-term recurrence-free survival (mean, 20.4 months). As this series was based on a period of 34 years, several different protocols were used. The protocol most frequently used was the BMP combination (bleomycin, methotrexate, cisplatin). It was associated with severe toxicity, with three treatment-related deaths.

Bermejo performed a retrospective analysis of ten patients who received neoadjuvant chemotherapy prior to surgery, over a period of 15 years [30]. Three patients received a BMP protocol, two received paclitaxel and carboplatin, and five received the TIP protocol (paclitaxel, ifosfamide, cisplatin). Among the five patients who received the TIP protocol, three obtained a pN0 complete response with a 5-year survival of 40 % and a median survival of 26 months.

More recently, Pizzocaro treated six patients by TPF (paclitaxel, cisplatin, and 5-fluorouracil) neoadjuvant chemotherapy for unresectable tumor (two cases) or lymph node recurrence (four cases) [31]. Three patients died from their disease within 1 year, and the other 3 patients were alive without recurrence at 25, 27, and 46 months.

Finally, Pagliaro, in a phase II study, evaluated neoadjuvant chemotherapy comprising four cycles of TIP for patients with penile cancer and stage N2 or N3 lymph node involvement, and M0 [32]. Overall, 30 patients were included in the study: an objective response was observed in 50 % of cases and a complete response was observed in 10 % of cases. With a median follow-up of 34 months, 30 % of patients were live without recurrence.

These various results of neoadjuvant chemotherapy suggest that a combination of neoadjuvant chemotherapy and inguinal lymphadenectomy would allow an improvement of the overall survival and recurrence-free survival of penile cancer patients with lymph node involvement. Even a partial response to chemotherapy may allow surgery, although it is often associated with severe morbidity [29, 30, 33]. A possible disadvantage of this approach would be to delay surgical treatment in patients who fail to respond to chemotherapy

- *Adjuvant chemotherapy.* Many candidate molecules were evaluated in the first studies evaluating the efficacy of chemotherapy in penile cancer. These studies were based on the results obtained in the treatment of head and neck, vulva, and anal canal squamous cell carcinoma. Responses to bleomycin and methotrexate were reported.

The largest published series by Haas was a phase II clinical trial conducted in 40 patients using the BMP combination (bleomycin, methotrexate, and cisplatin) [34]. These patients had either unresectable inguinal lymphadenopathy or visceral metastases. Thirteen (33 %) responses were observed, including 5 (13 %) complete responses. However, the toxicity of the BMP protocol was considerable, with 5 treatment-related deaths and 9 patients in whom treatment had to be discontinued because of adverse effects.

In another pilot study reported by Pizzocaro, based on 12 patients treated by bilateral total inguinal lymphadenectomy followed by chemotherapy comprising bleomycin, vincristine, and methotrexate, 11 patients remained recurrence-free throughout follow-up (mean follow-up, 42 months) [33]. Although this study was based on a small sample size, it demonstrated the probable survival gain related to adjuvant chemotherapy in locally advanced cancers. Concordant results were also reported by Hakenberg with a BMP protocol [35]. Of the 8 patients treated by lymphadenectomy followed by adjuvant chemotherapy, 3 remained recurrence-free throughout follow-up (mean follow-up, 54 months). One death related to the toxicity of treatment was observed.

Radiotherapy

Adjuvant radiotherapy to inguinal lymph nodes appears to have a probable role in local control of nodal disease: neoadjuvant radiotherapy for unresectable lymph nodes or adjuvant radiotherapy following surgery. Chemotherapy can be coprescribed in these two settings to provide multimodal chemoradiotherapy, which can consolidate local control and treat disease in the process of dissemination. However, these multimodal strategies have not been evaluated in penile cancer.

One of the problems raised by radiotherapy is the poor tolerance of the inguinal region to radiation, particularly a high risk of skin necrosis. These complications are exacerbated in the setting of adjuvant radiotherapy after lymphadenectomy.

Few studies have evaluated the efficacy of neoadjuvant radiotherapy on micrometastases and clinical lymphadenopathy. Ravi studied the effect of inguinal radiotherapy delivered before lymphadenectomy in patients with one or more clinical inguinal lymph nodes larger than 4 cm. Capsular effraction of the lymph node was detected on histological examination in 33 % (14/43) of nonirradiated patients and 9 % (3/34) of irradiated patients. Series evaluating the impact of prophylactic irradiation of inguinal lymph nodes in cN0 patients have reported identical progression rates (about 20 %) to those observed after modified inguinal lymphadenectomy, illustrating the limited efficacy of radiotherapy on micrometastases.

Therapeutic Indications

Timing of Management

Lymph node management must be systematic and bilateral, and must be performed at the time of diagnosis of penile cancer, as appropriate initial management achieves better survival results than treatment at the time of local progression [36].

Immediate lymph node management is unequivocally indicated in patients with palpable nodes. However, treatment is more controversial in patients without palpable inguinal lymph nodes (cN0), as 82 % of these cN0 patients do not have lymph node metastasis, even subclinical metastasis. In contrast, in a series of 40 high-risk cN0

Table 22.3 Treatment strategies for lymph node metastases

Lymph nodes		Treatment options	Level of evidence	Grade of recommendation
No palpable lymph nodes	*Type of penile lesion*			
	pTis, pTaG1, pT1aG1	Surveillance	2a	B
	≥pT1b G2	Sentinel node	2a	B
		Bilateral modified lymphadenectomy	2a	B
Palpable lymph nodes	*Fine-needle aspiration cytology*			
	Negative	Surveillance and to remake aspiration cytology	2a	B
		Bilateral modified lymphadenectomy	2a	B
	Positive	Total inguinal lymphadenectomy on cN+side	2a	B
		Modified inguinal lymphadenectomy on cN0 side		
Fixed lymph nodes		Neoadjuvant chemotherapy	2a	B
		Total lymphadenectomy in good responders		
		Radiotherapy or palliative management in nonresponders		
Pelvic lymph nodes		Pelvic lymphadenectomy if:	2a	B
		2 or more inguinal lymph node metastases		
		Capsular effraction		
		Pelvic lymph node metastases detected on CT		
		Neoadjuvant or adjuvant chemotherapy		

patients, Kroon reported a 3-year survival of 84 % following early lymphadenectomy versus 35 % in the case of watchful waiting and deferred lymphadenectomy [36].

Type of Lymph Node Management

The standard treatment for lymph nodes in penile cancer is surgical lymphadenectomy. Inguinal lymphadenectomy provides a survival gain in cN1–cN2 patients and in cN0 patients. However, within the group of cN0 patients, it is important to define the subgroup at high risk of subclinical metastases which, according to the latest guidelines, are those patients with stage ≥pT1bG2 penile cancer.

Inguinal lymphadenectomy has a curative role in patients with lymph node metastasis (stage N1). Multimodal management combining chemotherapy, surgery, and possibly radiotherapy should be considered in patients with more extensive lymph node involvement (N2–N3) (Table 22.3) [11, 12, 37, 38].

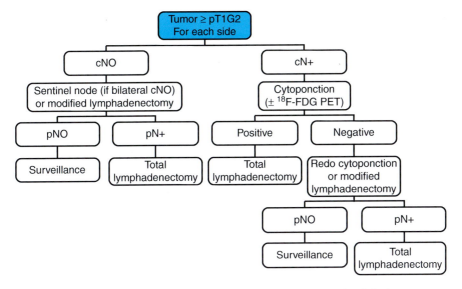

Fig. 22.2 Type of inguinal lymphadenectomy for each side according to the clinical status

Indication for the Type of Inguinal Lymphadenectomy

The therapeutic indication is primarily based on clinical examination: the presence or absence of palpable nodes, and the risk of lymph node involvement, which depends on the stage and grade of penile cancer (≥pT1bG2).

When modified inguinal lymphadenectomy confirms lymph node involvement (frozen section or definitive examination), it must be systematically completed by total or radical lymphadenectomy on the side of lymph node invasion.

In the elderly, the management of lymph node must be equivalent, but comorbidities must obviously be taken into account. In fact, chemotherapy is not always possible, and the morbidity of inguinal lymphadenectomy could alter the quality of life and the return at the initial stage.

Lymphadenectomy must always be bilateral, and the type of lymphadenectomy depends on the clinical findings on each side. Therapeutic indications of lymph node are summarized in Fig. 22.2.

Local Recurrence

In case of secondary apparition of inguinal lymph node without any first treatment, a total bilateral inguinal lymphadenectomy is indicated.

In case of recurrence of inguinal lymph node with adapted first treatment, a total inguinal lymphadenectomy is indicated on the side of recurrence, and chemotherapy (adjuvant or neoadjuvant) must be discussed.

Prognosis

The prognosis of penile cancer essentially depends on the presence or absence of inguinal lymph node involvement.

Treatment of the primary penile tumor must be as conservative as possible, but conservative management is associated with a risk of local recurrence estimated to be between 15 and 30 %. However, local recurrence has no significant impact on specific survival when it is managed correctly.

Inguinal lymphadenectomy plays an essential role in the treatment of documented inguinal lymph node metastases and is curative in about 80 % of patients with 1 or even 2 inguinal lymph node metastases. The mean 5-year overall survival was 85 % for pN0 patients and 40 % for pN + patients (Table 22.1). For pN + patients, the 5-year overall survival was 70–80 % for pN1 (only 1 lymph node invaded), 30–40 % for pN2, and 0–10 % for pN3 (Table 22.2).

The local recurrence rate was 5–10 % for pN0 and 20–30 % for pN + after local therapy with lymphadenectomy alone without chemotherapy. The mean time to recurrence was 10 months and the 5-year recurrence-free survival was 75–85 % for pN0 and 30–45 % for pN + [39].

References

1. Barnholtz-Sloan JS, Maldonado JL, Pow-sang J, Giuliano AR. Incidence trends in primary malignant penile cancer. Urol Oncol. 2007;25(5):361–7.
2. Bray F, Sankila R, Ferlay J, Parkin DM. Estimates of cancer incidence and mortality in Europe in 1995. Eur J Cancer. 2002;38(1):99–166.
3. Misra S, Chaturvedi A, Misra NC. Penile carcinoma: a challenge for the developing world. Lancet Oncol. 2004;5(4):240–7.
4. Nordenvall C, Chang ET, Adami HO, Ye W. Cancer risk among patients with condylomata acuminata. Int J Cancer. 2006;119(4):888–93.
5. Gerend MA, Barley J. Human papillomavirus vaccine acceptability among young adult men. Sex Transm Dis. 2009;36(1):58–62.
6. Renaud-Vilmer C, Cavelier-Balloy B, Verola O, Morel P, Servant JM, Desgrandchamps F, et al. Analysis of alterations adjacent to invasive squamous cell carcinoma of the penis and their relationship with associated carcinoma. J Am Acad Dermatol. 2010;62(2):284–90.
7. Cubilla AL. The role of pathologic prognostic factors in squamous cell carcinoma of the penis. World J Urol. 2009;27(2):169–77.
8. Leijte JA, Gallee M, Antonini N, Horenblas S. Evaluation of current TNM classification of penile carcinoma. J Urol. 2008;180(3):933–8. discussion 8.
9. Lont AP, Gallee MP, Meinhardt W, van Tinteren H, Horenblas S. Penis conserving treatment for T1 and T2 penile carcinoma: clinical implications of a local recurrence. J Urol. 2006;176(2):575–80. discussion 80.
10. de Crevoisier R, Slimane K, Sanfilippo N, Bossi A, Albano M, Dumas I, et al. Long-term results of brachytherapy for carcinoma of the penis confined to the glans (N- or NX). Int J Radiat Oncol Biol Phys. 2009;74(4):1150–6.
11. Pizzocaro G, Algaba F, Horenblas S, Solsona E, Tana S, Van Der Poel H, et al. EAU penile cancer guidelines 2009. Eur Urol. 2010;57(6):1002–12.

12. Rigaud J, Avances C, Camparo P, Culine S, Durand X, Iborra F, et al. Recommandations en Onco-Urologie 2010: tumeurs malignes du pénis. Prog Urol. 2010;20 Suppl 4:S280–9.
13. Smith Y, Hadway P, Biedrzycki O, Perry MJ, Corbishley C, Watkin NA. Reconstructive surgery for invasive squamous carcinoma of the glans penis. Eur Urol. 2007;52(4):1179–85.
14. Meijer RP, Boon TA, van Venrooij GE, Wijburg CJ. Long-term follow-up after laser therapy for penile carcinoma. Urology. 2007;69(4):759–62.
15. Solsona E, Iborra I, Ricos JV, Monros JL, Dumont R, Casanova J, et al. Corpus cavernosum invasion and tumor grade in the prediction of lymph node condition in penile carcinoma. Eur Urol. 1992;22(2):115–8.
16. Saisorn I, Lawrentschuk N, Leewansangtong S, Bolton DM. Fine-needle aspiration cytology predicts inguinal lymph node metastasis without antibiotic pretreatment in penile carcinoma. BJU Int. 2006;97(6):1225–8.
17. Kroon BK, Horenblas S, Deurloo EE, Nieweg OE, Teertstra HJ. Ultrasonography-guided fine-needle aspiration cytology before sentinel node biopsy in patients with penile carcinoma. BJU Int. 2005;95(4):517–21.
18. Leijte JA, Kroon BK, Valdes Olmos RA, Nieweg OE, Horenblas S. Reliability and safety of current dynamic sentinel node biopsy for penile carcinoma. Eur Urol. 2007;52(1):170–7.
19. Lont AP, Kroon BK, Gallee MP, van Tinteren H, Moonen LM, Horenblas S. Pelvic lymph node dissection for penile carcinoma: extent of inguinal lymph node involvement as an indicator for pelvic lymph node involvement and survival. J Urol. 2007;177(3):947–52. discussion 52.
20. Scher B, Seitz M, Reiser M, Hungerhuber E, Hahn K, Tiling R, et al. 18 F-FDG PET/CT for staging of penile cancer. J Nucl Med. 2005;46(9):1460–5.
21. Graafland NM, Leijte JA, Valdes Olmos RA, Hoefnagel CA, Teertstra HJ, Horenblas S. Scanning with 18 F-FDG-PET/CT for detection of pelvic nodal involvement in inguinal node-positive penile carcinoma. Eur Urol. 2009;56(2):339–45.
22. Souillac I, Rigaud J, Ansquer C, Marconnet L, Bouchot O. Prospective evaluation of (18) F-fluorodeoxyglucose positron emission tomography-computerized tomography to assess inguinal lymph node status in invasive squamous cell carcinoma of the penis. J Urol. 2012;187(2):493–7.
23. Hungerhuber E, Schlenker B, Frimberger D, Linke R, Karl A, Stief CG, et al. Lymphoscintigraphy in penile cancer: limited value of sentinel node biopsy in patients with clinically suspicious lymph nodes. World J Urol. 2006;24(3):319–24.
24. Leijte JA, Hughes B, Graafland NM, Kroon BK, Olmos RA, Nieweg OE, et al. Two-center evaluation of dynamic sentinel node biopsy for squamous cell carcinoma of the penis. J Clin Oncol. 2009;27(20):3325–9.
25. Catalona WJ. Modified inguinal lymphadenectomy for carcinoma of the penis with preservation of saphenous veins: technique and preliminary results. J Urol. 1988;140(2):306–10.
26. Bouchot O, Rigaud J, Maillet F, Hetet JF, Karam G. Morbidity of inguinal lymphadenectomy for invasive penile carcinoma. Eur Urol. 2004;45(6):761–5 discussion 5–6.
27. Culkin DJ, Beer TM. Advanced penile carcinoma. J Urol. 2003;170(2 Pt 1):359–65.
28. Protzel C, Hakenberg OW. Chemotherapy in patients with penile carcinoma. Urol Int. 2009;82(1):1–7.
29. Leijte JA, Kerst JM, Bais E, Antonini N, Horenblas S. Neoadjuvant chemotherapy in advanced penile carcinoma. Eur Urol. 2007;52(2):488–94.
30. Bermejo C, Busby JE, Spiess PE, Heller L, Pagliaro LC, Pettaway CA. Neoadjuvant chemotherapy followed by aggressive surgical consolidation for metastatic penile squamous cell carcinoma. J Urol. 2007;177(4):1335–8.
31. Pizzocaro G, Nicolai N, Milani A. Taxanes in combination with cisplatin and fluorouracil for advanced penile cancer: preliminary results. Eur Urol. 2009;55(3):546–51.
32. Pagliaro LC, Williams DL, Daliani D, Williams MB, Osai W, Kincaid M, et al. Neoadjuvant paclitaxel, ifosfamide, and cisplatin chemotherapy for metastatic penile cancer: a phase II study. J Clin Oncol. 2010;28(24):3851–7.

33. Pizzocaro G, Piva L. Adjuvant and neoadjuvant vincristine, bleomycin, and methotrexate for inguinal metastases from squamous cell carcinoma of the penis. Acta Oncol. 1988;27(6b):823–4.

34. Haas GP, Blumenstein BA, Gagliano RG, Russell CA, Rivkin SE, Culkin DJ, et al. Cisplatin, methotrexate and bleomycin for the treatment of carcinoma of the penis: a Southwest Oncology Group study. J Urol. 1999;161(6):1823–5.

35. Hakenberg OW, Nippgen JB, Froehner M, Zastrow S, Wirth MP. Cisplatin, methotrexate and bleomycin for treating advanced penile carcinoma. BJU Int. 2006;98(6):1225–7.

36. Kroon BK, Horenblas S, Lont AP, Tanis PJ, Gallee MP, Nieweg OE. Patients with penile carcinoma benefit from immediate resection of clinically occult lymph node metastases. J Urol. 2005;173(3):816–9.

37. Protzel C, Alcaraz A, Horenblas S, Pizzocaro G, Zlotta A, Hakenberg OW. Lymphadenectomy in the surgical management of penile cancer. Eur Urol. 2009;55(5):1075–88.

38. Heyns CF, Fleshner N, Sangar V, Schlenker B, Yuvaraja TB, van Poppel H. Management of the lymph nodes in penile cancer. Urology. 2010;76(2 Suppl 1):S43–57.

39. Marconnet L, Rigaud J, Bouchot O. Long-term followup of penile carcinoma with high risk for lymph node invasion treated with inguinal lymphadenectomy. J Urol. 2010;183(6):2227–32.

Chapter 23
Lymphomas of the Testis in Elderly Patients

Catherine Thieblemont, Claire Benet, and Josette Briere

Abstract Primary testicular lymphoma (PTL) is the most common malignant testicular tumor in men older than 50 years. Among them, diffuse large B-cell subtype is the most frequent. Other lymphoma subtypes are very rare. Typical clinical presentation is a painless unilateral testicular mass. Constitutional symptoms such as fever, weight loss, anorexia, and night sweats are rare at diagnosis. Treatment is complex and requires a multidisciplinary approach. The therapeutic strategy will be dependent on the initial characteristics of the patient, particularly the International Prognostic Index (IPI) including characteristics of the tumor (stage, histology) and characteristics of the patients (performance status, age, and comorbidity). The orchidectomy will provide the diagnosis and is part of the treatment. The specificity of the outcome of PTL-DLBCL is a high risk of extranodal relapse, particularly CNS relapse and contralateral testis, even in cases with localized disease at diagnosis. These particular features remain the most therapeutic challenges in the treatment of PTL. Therefore, management of the patients should be carefully discussed in terms of adjuvant therapy after orchidectomy, including immunotherapy with R-CHOP or R-CHOP-like regimen, CNS prophylaxis, and radiotherapy for the opposite testis.

Keywords Lymphoma • Testis • Elderly • Diffuse large-B cell lymphoma

C. Thieblemont, M.D., Ph.D. (✉)
Department of Hemato-Oncology, Hôpital Saint-Louis,
Paris, France
e-mail: catherine.thieblemont@sls.aphp.fr

C. Benet, M.D. • J. Briere, M.D., Ph.D.
Department of Pathology, Hôpital Saint-Louis,
Paris, France
e-mail: claire.benet@sls.aphp.fr; josette.briere@sls.aphp.fr

J.-P. Droz, R.A. Audisio (eds.), *Management of Urological Cancers in Older People*,
Management of Cancer in Older People,
DOI 10.1007/978-0-85729-999-4_23, © Springer-Verlag London 2013

Introduction

Lymphoma is a cancer with an increased incidence in the Western world. Among them, the primary testicular non-Hodgkin's lymphoma (PTL) is a very rare disease, accounting for 1–2 % of non-Hodgkin's lymphomas and less than 5 % of testicular malignancies [1–5]. However, a very important clinical sign to underline is that PTL is the most common malignant testicular tumor in men older than 50 years [4, 6]. This is important for the clinician as a diagnostic warning in front of testicular mass in elderly patients and also regarding the treatment. In terms of therapeutic management, therapeutic cutoff between young and elderly patients with lymphoma is usually set at 60 years because this breakpoint is globally relevant for therapeutic strategies and particularly intensive treatments such as high-dose chemotherapy plus autologous stem cell transplantation (HDT/ASCT). This procedure is preferentially proposed to patients less than 60 years old with an aggressive presentation of the disease. In this chapter, we described the presentation of PTL, the diagnostic and staging procedures, and the therapeutic strategies in elderly patients.

Epidemiology

PTL is a rare disease. The median age of PTL occurrence is described at 65 years old [5, 7, 8]. No epidemiologic factor has been related to the incidence of testicular lymphoma. In patients with immunodeficiency virus infection, PTL occurs at an early age (median, 37 years) and is associated with a worse prognosis [4].

Histology

PTL arises in the testis. Involvement of the testis by systemic lymphoma defines secondary testicular lymphoma. PTL represents a heterogeneous disease, and various histologic subtypes may occur including diffuse large B-cell lymphoma (DLBCL), Burkitt lymphoma, and follicular lymphoma, lymphoblastic lymphoma, and T-cell lymphoma [9–11]. Very rare entities such as Hodgkin's lymphoma and plasmocytoma have been mentioned in this site [9–11]. Recently, it has been described a new subtype of B-cell lymphoma named unclassifiable with features intermediate between DLBCL and Burkitt lymphoma [12] that may occur in the testis. In adult, PTL of DLBCL subtype (PTL-DLBCL) is the most frequent histological subtype of PTL representing 80–90 % of the PTL [6]. The other subtypes are unfrequent and are excluded from our purpose.

Gross Features

Tumors vary in size but are frequently quite large. The median diameter is approximately 6 cm. The majority of the tumors have a homogenous texture and diffusely replace the testis, although multinodular growth has been noted. Foci of hemorrhage and necrosis may be seen. The tumor may extend into the epididymis, spermatic cord, or adjacent soft tissues [13, 14].

Microscopic Features

The typical aspect of PTL-DLBCL consists of a diffuse infiltration with large lymphoid cells with oval to round, vesicular nuclei with fine chromatin into tissue spaces producing wide separation of the normal structures. However, the seminiferous tubules may be preserved, atrophic, or completely obliterated. Spermatogenic arrest, interstitial fibrosis, and tubular hyalinization are commonly seen. The tubules may be surrounded by the reticulin fibers producing a loose, open network of peritubular fibers [14, 15].

Immunohistochemistry (IHC)

PTL-DLBCL expresses B-cell markers such as CD19, CD20, CD22, and CD79a [12] (Fig. 23.1). Using gene expression profiling, DLBCL has been further subclassified into germinal-center B-cell-like DLBCL (GCB-like DLBCL) and activated B-cell-like DLBCL (ABC-like DLBCL) [16]. Based on three markers, CD10, BCL6, and MUM1-IRF4, it is possible to make these distinctions between GCB versus non-GCB DLBCL by IHC. PTL-DLBCL subtype is more likely to be non-GCB subtype as reported in two series [7, 17]. Al-Abbadi et al. found that 89 % (16/18 cases) of PTL belong to the non-GCB DLBCL subgroup and all exhibited high-proliferative activity [17]. In the series reported by Hasselblom, 24 cases out of 35 (69 %) exhibit a non-GCB profile.

Molecular Features

The use of cytogenetics, fluorescence in situ hybridization, and array comparative genomic hybridization has shown that genetic alterations in PTL-DLBCL often comprise complex abnormalities, including translocations, trisomies, amplifications, and deletions. The more commonly observed abnormalities include 3q27

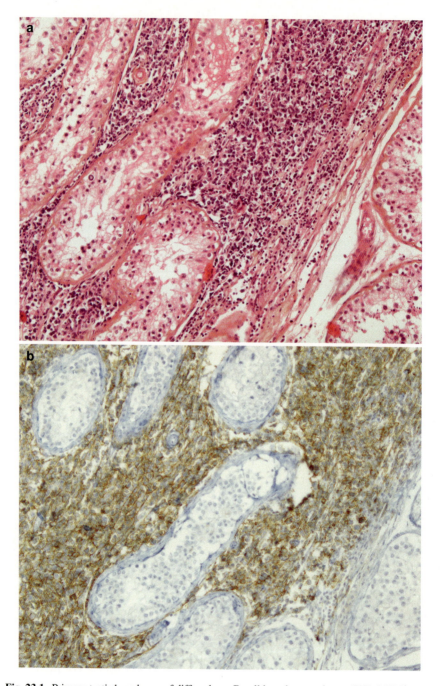

Fig. 23.1 Primary testis lymphoma of diffuse large B-cell lymphoma subtype (PTL-DLBCL). (**a**) H&E staining of PTL-DLBCL. (**b**) Strong CD20 expression in PTL-DLBCL. (**c**) Proliferative index of PTL-DLBCL is usually important as illustrated here by the Ki67 expression (>80 % in this case)

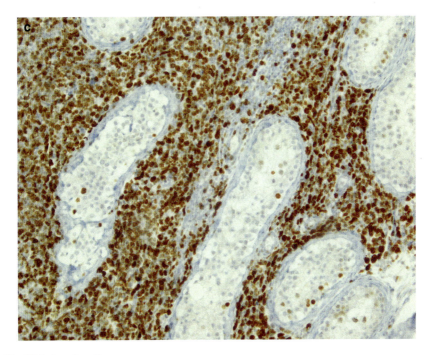

Fig. 23.1 (continued)

abnormalities and 6q deletions [18]. Although deletion of 6q is considered a second-ary chromosomal abnormality, in some cases, a primary pathologic role is suggested by the observation that it occurs as the sole cytogenetic abnormality [18]. Several studies have shown that 6q deletions are more frequent in tumors with an activated B-cell type gene expression profile than in those with a GC profile [19, 20].

Clinical Presentation

PTL-DLBCL arises in the testis and presents in adult patients with a median age in the sixth decade. The most common presentation is a unilateral painless enlarge-ment of the testis, with a rapid progression. The history of testicular swelling is generally several weeks. Patients present usually with a good performance status, without B symptoms [6–8, 21].

The disease is localized, but bilateral involvement has been described in 8 % of the patients [13, 21]. Involvement of the scrotum and regional retroperitoneal lymph nodes may develop in the course of the disease. Full staging at this time is based on the Ann Arbor staging system describing I through IV stages [22]. A specific attention should be paid to particular predilection areas for dissemina-tion. PTL-DLBCL is associated with a high risk of extranodal dissemination, which includes the bone marrow, the Waldeyer ring, the skin, the lung, and the central nervous system [3, 5, 21, 23].

Serum lactate dehydrogenase (LDH) or β2-microglobulin (β2MG) levels above normal values are observed in less than 10–20 % of the patients. Serum β-human-chorionic gonadotropin and serum α-fetoprotein are rarely elevated [3].

Diagnostic and Initial Staging Procedures

Orchidectomy is the first procedure that not only provides histological tissue for diagnosis but also removes a potential sanctuary site as the blood-testis barrier makes testicular tumors more difficult to access for the chemotherapeutic agents [21].

For initial staging procedures, the following exams are mandatory: history and physical exam (including lymph node regions, eye, and ENT areas); liver and spleen evaluation; complete blood counts; and basic biochemical studies, including evaluation of renal and liver function, seric levels of lacticodeshydrogenase and β-2 microglobulin, serum protein immunofixation, HIV, HCV, and HBV serology. CT of the chest, abdomen, and pelvis is mandatory, as well as the ultrasonography of the opposite testis. The value of positron emission tomography (PET) scan is recommended as any other DLBCL for the evaluation of extension and assessment of therapeutic response. Bone marrow aspirate and biopsy are highly recommended. Cerebrospinal fluid analysis including standard cytology and flow cytometry is highly recommended because of the high risk of meningeal dissemination.

Treatment

Treatment for PTL-DLBCL should not be distinguished from other DLBCL, except that the risk of relapse in the opposite testis and in CNS site should be specifically taken into account. To define the best treatment for patients with DLBCL, whatever the location, clinical risk groups have been identified to classify patients and to predict response to treatment and survival. The International Prognostic Index (IPI) including five parameters (age, performance status, stage, LDH level, and involvement of extranodal site) was the first established and the most commonly used, stratifying patients into four groups (low, low-intermediate, high-intermediate, and high) [24], and further validated in the rituximab era [25].

Systemic Therapy: R-CHOP and R-CHOP-Like

For nearly three decades, the standard of care for patients with DLBCL was the association cyclophosphamide, vincristine, doxorubicin, and prednisone (CHOP), established in 1976 as a regimen that induces the highest rate of overall response, the best overall survival with the less toxicity in patients with advanced NHL, compared to the so-called second and third generation regimens [26, 27]. Still, the cure rate with CHOP was suboptimal, with 3-year progression-free survival (PFS) and overall survival (OS) rates of about 40 and 50 %, respectively [26].

The addition of rituximab to CHOP (R-CHOP) has been a major improvement in terms of response rate as well as in survivals, with 5- and 10-year PFS and OS, respectively, at 54 and 36.5 % and at 58 and 43.5 %, without increasing the toxicity [28]. More intensive regimens (R-EPOCH, R-ACVBP) have been proposed for young patients less than 60 years old [29, 30]. These regimens are based on nearly the same drugs but with higher dosages and/or shorter recycling. R-EPOCH combined infused agents including etoposide 50 mg/m^2/day, D1–D4 (96 h); doxorubicin 10/m^2/day, D1–D4 (96 h); and vincristine 0.4/m^2/day, D1–D4 (96 h), associated with bolus agents including cyclophosphamide 750 mg/m^2/day day 5 and prednisone 60 mg/m^2/bid D1–D5. R-ACVBP is given every 14 days. It combines doxorubicin 75 mg/m^2 D1, cyclophosphamide 1,200 mg/m^2 intravenously on D1, vindesine 2 mg/m^2 on D1 and D5, bleomycin 10 mg on D1 and D5, and prednisone 60 mg/m^2 orally from D1 to D5. ACVBP has demonstrated superiority to CHOP in two randomized studies in young patients with DLBCL [29, 31].

Treatment Adapted to IPI Risk Factors

The age-adjusted IPI (aaIPI) risk score will determine the intensity of the treatment for each given patient with PTL-DLBCL. This score is based on three parameters: serum LDH level, stage, and performance status.

Using six cycles of R-CHOP, subgroup of patients with very favorable prognosis (IPIaa=0 and no bulky disease) will achieve 3-year event-free survival rates of >90 % and overall survival of 97 % [32]. The use of PET/CT scan may help in the future to decrease doses even more in patients with chemosensitive disease. It is very important to underline that even for the patients that have been treated by orchidectomy and that have no more macroscopic disease after the surgery, treatment must be completed by immunochemotherapy such as R-CHOP and specific treatment related to the testicular location (see below prophylaxis).

In the subgroup of patients with poor prognosis (IPIaa≥1), more intense regimens have been carefully evaluated in elderly patients by different groups. The German DSHNHL group has demonstrated in the pre-rituximab era that interval reduction from 3 (CHOP-21) to 2 weeks (CHOP-14) improves the complete remission rate (77 % vs. 63 %, $p=0.03$) and the outcome with 3-year PFS and OS, respectively, at 53.4 % versus 42.5 %, $p=0.03$ and 64.3 % versus 49 %, $p=0.04$ (median follow-up of 40 months) in patients less than 75 without increasing the toxicity [33]. Their subsequent protocol, the RICOVER-60 trial, assessed whether combining CHOP-14 with rituximab could further improve outcomes of elderly patients (61–80 years, stage I–IV) [34]. These patients were randomized to receive six or eight cycles of CHOP-14 with or without eight applications of rituximab. Of 1,222 patients, six cycles of CHOP-14 plus eight injections of rituximab yielded the best results in terms of response rates and survivals (EFS, PFS, and OS). If R-CHOP-14 is superior to CHOP-14, the question of whether or not it should replace the standard R-CHOP-21 is not solved. The GELA randomized study comparing dose-dense R-CHOP-14 versus R-CHOP-21 was recently reported for the first interim analysis with comparable results between the two arms [35].

Prophylactic Scrotal Radiotherapy for the Opposite Testis

Evidence from retrospective reports [2, 5, 13] suggests that radiotherapy to the contralateral testis could reduce the risk of treatment failure at this site. Prophylactic irradiation to the contralateral testis should be proposed at the end of chemoimmunotherapy, at the dose of 25–30 Gy [21].

Prophylactic Procedures for Central Nervous System (CNS)

CNS relapses, in both brain parenchyma and meninges, remain a major problem in PTL-DLBCL, since they are definitively more frequent than in other aggressive lymphomas. Five- and ten-year risks are evaluated at 20 and 35 % [5]. Therefore, routine central nervous system prophylaxis is recommended. However, the best way to achieve this is still a matter of debate, as central nervous system relapses occur even in patients who had received standard CNS prophylaxis with intrathecal methotrexate, 12 mg total dose, weekly [36, 37]. Moreover, CNS relapses in PTL-DLBCL occur more frequently in brain parenchyma than in meninges making this intrathecal chemotherapy inefficient [9, 36]. On the other hand, PTL occurs usually in elderly patients, and many of them may not tolerate aggressive CNS prophylaxis such as systemic high-dose methotrexate or cytarabine chemotherapy regimens.

Evolution and Prognostic Factors

PTL-DLBCL is an aggressive disease. Before rituximab era, 5- and 10-year PFS were described as a declined survival from 48 to 33 %, respectively [5]. Even in the subset of patients with stage I disease, the PFS was similar with rates at 5 and 10 years of 54–36 % in the subset of stage I patients [5].

The addition of rituximab to CHOP chemotherapy may have improved outcome by preventing relapses with better control of microscopic systemic disease that might have been present since the onset of the disease. The benefit of the addition of rituximab in the treatment of PTL was recently questioned by the

Table 23.1 Relapse features in PTL-DLBCL

	Hasselblom et al. [7]	Lagrange et al. [8]	Zucca et al. [5]	Fonseca et al. [23]	Vittolo et al. [21]
n	23	61	373	51	53
Study type	Retrospective	Retrospective	Retrospective	Retrospective	Prospective
Median follow-up, months (range)	45 (34–88)	38 (1–147)	91.2	32.4	65
Failing patients	8	32	195	41	9
CNS relapse	6	9	56	13	3
Contralateral testis (with or without nodal site)	1	4	43	6	0
Extranodal sites other than testis or CNS	1	2	83	6	4

PTL-DLBCL primary testicular lymphoma of diffuse large B-cell lymphoma subtypes

population-based retrospective study, which showed no difference in the outcome of patients with PTL treated before and after the rituximab era, using the year 2000 as the cut point [2]. However, this retrospective study was limited by the lack of information regarding treatment delivered and what proportion of patients actually received rituximab-containing chemotherapy regimens.

In the most recent prospective trial [21], Vitolo et al. reported a series of 53 patients with PTL at stage I or II. The patients were treated with 6–8 courses of rituximab added to cyclophosphamide, doxorubicin, vincristine, and prednisone (R-CHOP) every 21 days (R-CHOP21); four doses of intrathecal methotrexate (IT-MTX); and radiotherapy (RT) to the contralateral testis (30 Gy) for all patients and to regional lymph nodes (30–36 Gy) for stage II disease. With a median follow-up of 65 months, the 5-year PFS rate was 74 % (95 % CI, 59–84 %). The 5-year OS rate was 85 % (95 % CI, 71–92 %), with a 5-year cumulative incidence of lymphoma progression or death as a result of lymphoma (TTP) of 8 % (95 % CI, 7–29 %). These results showed an excellent local and systemic control of the disease, and radiotherapy avoided contralateral testis relapse. However, CNS relapses occurred in three (4 %) patients, with an isolated CNS relapses in two patients and a concurrent meningeal and lymph nodal relapses in one patient.

The incidence of CNS relapses in both brain parenchyma and meninges is more common in PTL than in any other aggressive lymphomas (Table 23.1). This complication is usually observed during the first 2 years of follow-up in nodal DLBCL [36], whereas late CNS relapses have been reported in PTL [5, 9, 23, 37, 38]. In the results reported by Zucca et al. [5], 5- and 10-year risks of CNS relapse of 20 and 35 % were observed. In this study, the cumulative incidence of CNS relapse at 5 years was only 6 %.

Several variables have been reported as prognostic factors in PTL-DLBCL including age, performance status, systemic symptoms, tumor burden, 0.9 cm spermatic cord involvement, lactate dehydrogenase serum level, histologic grade, vascular invasion, degree of sclerosis, and stage of disease [39]. These prognostic factors are similar than nodal DLBCL and reflect the importance of tumor mass.

Conclusions

The most common histologic type of PTL is the diffuse large B-cell subtype. It usually presents as a painless unilateral testicular mass in men over 50 years old. Constitutional symptoms such as fever, weight loss, anorexia, and night sweats are rare at diagnosis. Treatment is complex and requires a multidisciplinary approach. The therapeutic strategy will be dependent on the initial characteristics of the patient. The orchidectomy, especially in early-stage disease, is advantageous because it provides tissue for pathologic evaluation and removes a sanctuary site, as the blood-testis barrier makes testicular tumors difficult to be accessible to systemic chemotherapy. The specificity of the outcome of PTL-DLBCL is a high risk of extranodal relapse, particularly CNS relapse and contralateral testis, even in cases with localized disease at diagnosis. These particular features remain the most therapeutic challenges in the treatment of PTL. Therefore, management of the patients should be carefully discussed in terms of chemotherapy associated or not with immunotherapy depending of histological subtype, CNS prophylaxis, and radiotherapy for the opposite testis.

References

1. Booman M, Douwes J, Glas AM, de Jong D, Schuuring E, Kluin PM. Primary testicular diffuse large B-cell lymphomas have activated B-cell-like subtype characteristics. J Pathol. 2006;210(2):163–71.
2. Gundrum JD, Mathiason MA, Moore DB, Go RS. Primary testicular diffuse large B-cell lymphoma: a population-based study on the incidence, natural history, and survival comparison with primary nodal counterpart before and after the introduction of rituximab. J Clin Oncol. 2009;27(31):5227–32.
3. Moller MB, d'Amore F, Christensen BE. Testicular lymphoma: a population-based study of incidence, clinicopathological correlations and prognosis. The Danish Lymphoma Study Group, LYFO. Eur J Cancer. 1994;30A(12):1760–4.
4. Shahab N, Doll DC. Testicular lymphoma. Semin Oncol. 1999;26(3):259–69.
5. Zucca E, Conconi A, Mughal TI, et al. Patterns of outcome and prognostic factors in primary large-cell lymphoma of the testis in a survey by the International Extranodal Lymphoma Study Group. J Clin Oncol. 2003;21(1):20–7.
6. Zucca E, Roggero E, Bertoni F, Cavalli F. Primary extranodal non-Hodgkin's lymphomas. Part 1: gastrointestinal, cutaneous and genitourinary lymphomas. Ann Oncol. 1997;8(8):727–37.
7. Hasselblom S, Ridell B, Wedel H, Norrby K, Sender Baum M, Ekman T. Testicular lymphoma – a retrospective, population-based, clinical and immunohistochemical study. Acta Oncol. 2004;43(8):758–65.
8. Lagrange JL, Ramaioli A, Theodore CH, et al. Non-Hodgkin's lymphoma of the testis: a retrospective study of 84 patients treated in the French anticancer centres. Ann Oncol. 2001;12(9):1313–9.

9. Ferry JA, Harris NL, Young RH, Coen J, Zietman A, Scully RE. Malignant lymphoma of the testis, epididymis, and spermatic cord. A clinicopathologic study of 69 cases with immunophenotypic analysis. Am J Surg Pathol. 1994;18(4):376–90.

10. Heller KN, Teruya-Feldstein J, La Quaglia MP, Wexler LH. Primary follicular lymphoma of the testis: excellent outcome following surgical resection without adjuvant chemotherapy. J Pediatr Hematol Oncol. 2004;26(2):104–7.

11. Kremer M, Ott G, Nathrath M, et al. Primary extramedullary plasmacytoma and multiple myeloma: phenotypic differences revealed by immunohistochemical analysis. J Pathol. 2005;205(1):92–101.

12. Swerdlow S, Campo E, Harris N, et al. WHO classification of tumors of haematopoietic and lymphoid tissues. Lyon: IARC Press; 2008.

13. Doll DC, Weiss RB. Malignant lymphoma of the testis. Am J Med. 1986;81(3):515–24.

14. Paladugu RR, Bearman RM, Rappaport H. Malignant lymphoma with primary manifestation in the gonad: a clinicopathologic study of 38 patients. Cancer. 1980;45(3):561–71.

15. Turner RR, Colby TV, MacKintosh FR. Testicular lymphomas: a clinicopathologic study of 35 cases. Cancer. 1981;48(9):2095–102.

16. Alizadeh AA. Distinct types of diffuse large B cell lymphoma identified by gene expression profiling. Nature. 2000;403:503–11.

17. Al-Abbadi MA, Hattab EM, Tarawneh MS, Amr SS, Orazi A, Ulbright TM. Primary testicular diffuse large B-cell lymphoma belongs to the nongerminal center B-cell-like subgroup: a study of 18 cases. Mod Pathol. 2006;19(12):1521–7.

18. Bosga-Bouwer AG, Kok K, Booman M, et al. Array comparative genomic hybridization reveals a very high frequency of deletions of the long arm of chromosome 6 in testicular lymphoma. Genes Chromosomes Cancer. 2006;45(10):976–81.

19. Bea S, Zettl A, Wright G, et al. Diffuse large B-cell lymphoma subgroups have distinct genetic profiles that influence tumor biology and improve gene-expression-based survival prediction. Blood. 2005;106(9):3183–90.

20. Rickert CH, Dockhorn-Dworniczak B, Simon R, Paulus W. Chromosomal imbalances in primary lymphomas of the central nervous system. Am J Pathol. 1999;155(5):1445–51.

21. Vitolo U, Ferreri AJ, Zucca E. Primary testicular lymphoma. Crit Rev Oncol Hematol. 2008;65(2):183–9.

22. Edge SB, Compton CC. The American Joint Committee on Cancer: the 7th edition of the AJCC cancer staging manual and the future of TNM. Ann Surg Oncol. 2010;17(6):1471–4.

23. Fonseca R, Habermann TM, Colgan JP, et al. Testicular lymphoma is associated with a high incidence of extranodal recurrence. Cancer. 2000;88(1):154–61.

24. The International Non-Hodkin's Lymphoma Prognostic Factors Project. A predictive model for aggressive non-Hodgkin's lymphoma. N Eng J Med. 1993;329:987–94.

25. Sehn LH, Berry B, Chhanabhai M, et al. The revised International Prognostic Index (R-IPI) is a better predictor of outcome than the standard IPI for patients with diffuse large B-cell lymphoma treated with R-CHOP. Blood. 2007;109(5):1857–61.

26. Fisher RI, Gaynor ER, Dahlberg S, et al. Comparison of a standard regimen (CHOP) with three intensive chemotherapy regimens for advanced non-Hodgkin's lymphoma. N Engl J Med. 1993;328(14):1002–6.

27. McKelvey E, Gottlieb J, Wilson II, et al. Hydroxyldaunomycin (adriamycin) combination chemotherapy in malignant lymphoma. Cancer. 1976;38:1484–93.

28. Coiffier B, Lepage E, Briere J, et al. CHOP chemotherapy plus rituximab compared with CHOP alone in elderly patients with diffuse large-B-cell lymphoma. N Engl J Med. 2002;346(4):235–42.

29. Tilly H, Lepage E, Coiffier B, et al. Intensive conventional chemotherapy (ACVBP regimen) compared with standard CHOP for poor-prognosis aggressive non-Hodgkin lymphoma. Blood. 2003;102(13):4284–9.

30. Wilson WH, Grossbard ML, Pittaluga S, et al. Dose-adjusted EPOCH chemotherapy for untreated large B-cell lymphomas: a pharmacodynamic approach with high efficacy. Blood. 2002;99(8):2685–93.

31. Reyes F, Lepage E, Ganem G, et al. ACVBP versus CHOP plus radiotherapy for localized aggressive lymphoma. N Engl J Med. 2005;352(12):1197–205.
32. Pfreundschuh M, Trumper L, Osterborg A, et al. CHOP-like chemotherapy plus rituximab versus CHOP-like chemotherapy alone in young patients with good-prognosis diffuse large-B-cell lymphoma: a randomised controlled trial by the MabThera International Trial (MInT) Group. Lancet Oncol. 2006;7(5):379–91.
33. Pfreundschuh M, Trumper L, Kloess M, et al. Two-weekly or 3-weekly CHOP chemotherapy with or without etoposide for the treatment of elderly patients with aggressive lymphomas: results of the NHL-B2 trial of the DSHNHL. Blood. 2004;104(3):634–41.
34. Pfreundschuh M, Schubert J, Ziepert M, et al. Six versus eight cycles of bi-weekly CHOP-14 with or without rituximab in elderly patients with aggressive CD20+ B-cell lymphomas: a randomised controlled trial (RICOVER-60). Lancet Oncol. 2008;9(2):105–16.
35. Delarue R, Haioun C, Broussais-Guillaumot F, et al. Efficacy and safety of prophylactic use of darbepoetin alfa in patients with diffuse large B-cell lymphoma (DLBCL) treated with immunochemotherapy: results of the interim analysis of the LNH03-6B GELA study. Paper presented at the American Society of Hematology, New Orleans, 2009.
36. Boehme V, Schmitz N, Zeynalova S, Loeffler M, Pfreundschuh M. CNS events in elderly patients with aggressive lymphoma treated with modern chemotherapy (CHOP-14) with or without rituximab: an analysis of patients treated in the RICOVER-60 trial of the German High-Grade Non-Hodgkin Lymphoma Study Group (DSHNHL). Blood. 2009;113:3896–902.
37. Crellin AM, Hudson BV, Bennett MH, Harland S, Hudson GV. Non-Hodgkin's lymphoma of the testis. Radiother Oncol. 1993;27(2):99–106.
38. Seymour JF, Solomon B, Wolf MM, Janusczewicz EH, Wirth A, Prince HM. Primary large-cell non-Hodgkin's lymphoma of the testis: a retrospective analysis of patterns of failure and prognostic factors. Clin Lymphoma. 2001;2(2):109–15.
39. Sussman EB, Hajdu SI, Lieberman PH, Whitmore WF. Malignant lymphoma of the testis: a clinicopathologic study of 37 cases. J Urol. 1977;118(6):1004–7.

Chapter 24
Upper Urinary Tract Tumors in Elderly Patients

Fabio Campodonico

Abstract Upper urinary tract tumor is a rare disease, accounting for 6–7 % of all primary malignant tumors of the kidney, and they occur in association with primary bladder cancer in only 2–4 % of patients. The most common symptoms at presentation are gross painless hematuria, occurring in 70–80 % of patients. In elderly patients, from 10 to 15 % of upper urinary tract tumors are diagnosed as an incidental disease after a computed tomography. The prognosis is well correlated to tumor stage. Compared with younger patients, a corresponding increase in stage and grade in the elderly was found at disease diagnosis. Recent studies report a worse disease-specific survival in older patients who have undergone nephroureterectomy. However, these outcomes reported in advanced age may be linked to a selection bias since patients have significant comorbidities and lower performance status leading to a suboptimal treatment, either surgical or chemotherapic when indicated. Specifically, for elderly patients, treatment should be planned on the basis of an accurate preoperative assessment.

Keywords Upper urinary tract • Transitional cell cancer • Renal pelvis • Ureter • Nephroureterectomy • Ureterectomy • Ureteroscopy • Elderly • Urologic oncology Ureteral cancer • Kidney cancer • Urinary cytology

Epidemiology and Etiology

Although bladder and upper urinary tract tumors share the common histology of transitional cells and are part of the same anatomic system, their incidence is very unequal. Upper urinary tract tumor is a rare disease, accounting for 6–7 % of all

F. Campodonico, M.D.
Department of Urology, Galliera Hospital,
Genova, Italy
e-mail: fabio.campodonico@galliera.it

J.-P. Droz, R.A. Audisio (eds.), *Management of Urological Cancers in Older People*,
Management of Cancer in Older People,
DOI 10.1007/978-0-85729-999-4_24, © Springer-Verlag London 2013

primary malignant tumors of the kidney, and they occur in association with primary bladder cancer in only 2–4 % of patients [1]. The most involved part of the ureter is the lower third, in 60–74 % of cases. Ureteral tumors are twice as common in men as in women with the peak incidence occurring in the fifth decade.

The tumor biology shows evidence of the different occurrence rates in the urinary tract. The bladder is the most common site of transitional cell tumors. The prolonged contact between urine that stores carcinogens and the urinary mucosa is the hypothesized mechanism of carcinogenesis. Following this paradigm, the ureter is the most unusual site for the onset of tumor occurrence because of rapid urine passage, whereas the renal pelvis is four times more involved in tumor occurrence because urine contact time is longer. According to this observation, it is accepted that the risk factors for bladder cancer, excluding bladder schistosomiasis, are the same as for upper tract carcinoma. In elderly patients, the contact time between urine carcinogens and mucosa is by far the longest. Mostly in elderly patients, another mechanism of urothelial carcinogenesis peculiar to the upper tract is implicated. The inflammation of the collecting tubules consequent to the exposure of nephrotoxins and tubulointerstitial nephritis is reported to be associated with end-stage renal disease or nonfunctional kidneys. These pathologic conditions allow the development of urothelial cancer of the renal pelvis after an extended period of time [2].

Cigarette smoking is by far the most relevant risk factor for urothelial cancer of the upper urinary tract. Smokers have an overall 3.1-fold increase in risk that increases to 7.2 times risk for those with a long-term smoking habit (>45 year). In general, smoking is associated with seven of ten upper urinary tract cancers in men and four of ten cancers in women. The cancer risk is highest in the ureter followed by the renal pelvis and then the bladder [3].

The well-known risk association between analgesic consumption and urothelial cancer of the renal pelvis is related to the evidence that phenacetin yields carcinogenic metabolic relatives. A latency period of up to 25 year of exposure has been suggested, thus indicating a somewhat higher risk in the elderly. The removal of phenacetin from the analgetic market in Scandinavia, Australia, and New Zealand has dramatically decreased the incidence of analgetic-related nephropathy that is considered the pathologic substrate of urothelial carcinogenesis. However, the metabolic derivatives of phenacetin, acetaminophen, and paracetamol are the current drugs of choice in the Western world, thus requiring uninterrupted epidemiologic monitoring.

Occupational exposure to chemical substances is also involved in urothelial carcinogenesis because of the direct contact between these products or their metabolites excreted through the urinary system. The most risk-linked occupations include working with dyestuff products, rubber, plastics, textiles and leather, hair dressing chemicals, and pesticides [4].

Patients previously treated with chemotherapeutic schedules containing cyclophosphamide or under treatment with this drug for autoimmune diseases also have a significant risk of developing an upper urinary tract urothelial cancer after several years.

Presentation, Diagnosis, and Staging

Symptoms

The most common symptom at presentation is gross painless hematuria, occurring in 70–80 % of patients. In general, a total hematuria that does not decrease with bladder washing suggests onset of bleeding from the upper urinary tract. Flank pain is reported by only a third of patients and usually depends on the development of hydronephrosis due to obstruction of the ureter by the ureteral tumor or blood clots. The passage of vermiform clots in the urine, although not common, is a typical clinical sign that suggests an upper urinary tract transitional cell tumor. Occasionally, a urothelial tumor of the kidney may present as a large renal mass similar to renal cell cancer associated with hematuria; in this case, urine cytology can be useful if samples are collected when hematuria disappears.

In elderly patients, from 10 to 15 % of upper urinary tract tumors are diagnosed as an incidental disease after a computed tomography (CT) scan is performed for other reasons, usually gastroenterologic or vascular studies.

Sometimes older patients present hematuria after a fall because the trauma is associated with a preexisting tumor of the upper urinary tract.

A palpable flank mass may be occasionally detected in advanced, often metastatic disease in minority of patients. Conversely, a persistent microscopic hematuria not related to an infective, phlogistic, or prostatic cause requires a staged investigation with cytology, cystoscopy, or radiologic imaging.

Diagnosis

As recently recommended by the European Association of Urology, CT urography is used as an alternative to conventional intravenous urography (IVU) [5]. A CT scan offers more information than IVU, especially in an invasive tumor of the upper urinary tract, and it can differentiate tumor from blood clots, ureteritis cystica, air bubbles, vascular impressions, overlying bowel gas, radiolucent calculi and artifacts, and filling defects especially in the renal calyces. It is important to perform thin CT slices (3–5 mm) before and after intravenous contrast administration because urothelial tumors are usually hypovascular, compared with renal carcinomas (Fig. 24.1).

Flexible cystoscopy is useful to exclude the bladder onset and show the bleeding ureteral orifice in order to plan the subsequent ureteroscopy. Ureteroscopy is generally performed to see and biopsy the endophytic lesion directly or to take multiple biopsies and collect selective urine for cytology in case of non-evident tumor (carcinoma in situ [Cis] or non-tumoral lesion). Ureteroscopy and magnetic resonance imaging are useful diagnostic tools in patients with an allergy to the contrast medium or in patients with poor renal function.

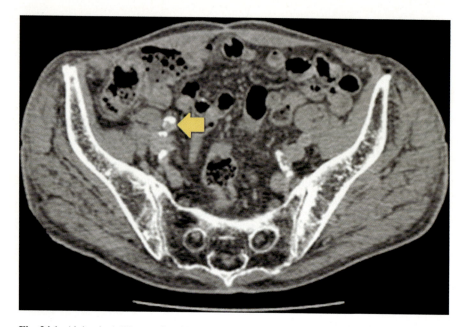

Fig. 24.1 Abdominal CT scan showing a ureteral tumor (*arrow*)

In elderly patients not suitable for surgery due to severe comorbidities or refusal of surgery, cytology and urinary fluorescence in situ hybridization (FISH) can predict the prognosis of the disease. A negative cytology and FISH test more likely indicate a low-stage/low-grade disease (Ta-G1) or Ta-G2, whereas a positive cytology and a high-risk pattern urinary FISH are likely associated with a more invasive disease (Cis, T1, or high-grade disease) [6].

Staging

Staging for upper urinary tract is similar to that used for bladder cancer. The most relevant exception is that superficial and muscular layer invasion in the renal pelvis are not distinguished.

The most widely accepted staging classification is the TNM system (1997) [7].
Primary Tumor (T)

- Tx tumor not assessed
- T0 no evidence of primary
- Ta tumor limited to the mucosa
- Tis, also *Cis*, flat tumor, high grade, limited to the mucosa
- T1 involvement of the subepithelial connective tissue
- T2 invasion of the muscularis

- T3 (for renal pelvis only) invasion beyond the muscularis into peripelvic fat or renal parenchyma
- T3 (for the ureter) invasion beyond the muscularis into periureteral fat
- T4 invasion of the neighboring organs or through the kidney into the perinephric fat

Regional Lymph nodes (N)

- Nx no information on nodal status
- N0 no evidence of tumor within the examined nodes
- N1 tumor present in one node, ≤2 cm diameter
- N2 tumor present in one node, >2 cm to <5 cm diameter, or multiples nodes <5 cm
- N3 metastasis in a lymph node >5 cm

Distant Metastases (M)

- Mx no information on M
- M0 absence of metastases
- M1 metastasis present

Histopathologic Grade (G)

- GX grade not assessed
- G1 well differentiated
- G2 moderately differentiated
- G3 poorly differentiated

The prognosis is well correlated to tumor stage. Patients with tumors confined to the mucosa have a 5-year survival rate of 100 %; with the involvement of the lamina propria (T1), rates range from 80 to 95 %. Survival rates with the invasion of the muscle wall range from 40 to 80 %; with spread to periureteral fat, rates are 15–33 % [8]. However, there is somewhat of a difference between survival for T3 of the ureter and T3 of the renal pelvis; the ureteral T3 tumors have a worse survival rate (24 %) compared with the renal pelvis (54 %) [9]. In a recent study, Stanley et al. investigated the effect of advancing age on disease extent and survival in a cohort of 12,639 patients with upper urinary tract urothelial tumors. Compared with younger patients, a corresponding increase in stage and grade in the elderly was found at disease diagnosis. After analysis adjusted for stage, grade, and treatment type, older patients still showed a worse disease-specific survival, with a hazard ratio of 2.64 [10]. However, such large cohort studies based on the Surveillance, Epidemiology and Results database from the National Cancer Institute do not take into account important variables in elderly patients such as general comorbidities, performance status, and residual renal function after nephroureterectomy [11]. Specifically, for elderly patients, treatment should be planned on the basis of an accurate preoperative assessment, tailored to the individual American Society of Anesthesiologists (ASA) grade, tumor stage, and type of surgery [12].

Pathology

Most upper urinary tract tumors are transitional cell carcinomas. They can occur as solitary or multiple tumors at presentation, or they may appear before, after, or synchronous with a carcinoma of the bladder. The invasive cancers are often poorly differentiated urothelial tumors, especially in elderly patients. A small percentage of renal pelvic tumors are squamous cell carcinomas, sometimes associated with a calculus long after inducing squamous metaplasia, leukoplakia, and subsequent cancer, but it is never the sequence commonly observed in the bladder [13].

Treatment (Surgical and Conservative)

Nephroureterectomy

The traditional surgery for pelvic and ureteric carcinoma dates for decades has been nephroureterectomy. It is indicated for invasive disease, poorly differentiated non-muscle-invasive tumors, or in the case of multifocal disease as well as in case of a well-documented Cis of the ureter. The rationale for the operation is based on the high rate of stump recurrence after partial or subtotal ureterectomy. A historical series showed a recurrence rate of the ureter ranging from 2.5 to 8 % in low-grade tumors to 30 % in high-grade tumors [14, 15]. The recurrence at the ureter is likely to be advanced and can be fatal. Elderly patients were generally less likely to undergo lymphadenectomy to shorten time intervention and avoid surgical complications, taking into consideration the lower life expectancy [16]. The higher cancer-specific mortality of elderly patients reported in several studies may be secondary to suboptimal use of nephroureterectomy, patient selection, delay of intervention, and omitted chemotherapy. However, the worse outcomes reported in advanced age may be linked to a selection bias since elderly patients are treated with relatively more advanced disease [17].

The operative incision is influenced by personal choice. We prefer a double incision, the first step anteriorly, with an umbilical-pubic line to remove the ureter with the bladder cuff and perform pelvic lymphadenectomy. Then the patient is moved to the lateral lumbotomic position to perform a lumbotomy along the prolongation of the 11th rib, which is partially resected (Fig. 24.2). A regional retroperitoneal lymphadenectomy can be easily performed if needed. In patients with a tumor of the high ureter or renal pelvis, not requiring pelvic node dissection, we also do a single extended prolonged lumbotomic incision to shorten the operating time.

The radical nephroureterectomy is performed in the same way as radical nephrectomy except for the need to remove the entire ureter with the bladder cuff. Generally, the adrenal gland can be left if the tumor does not involve the renal parenchyma. The surgical specimen has to be removed "en bloc" without any urine spillage, which can be obtained from the bladder cuff opening by securing the cutting line with stay sutures.

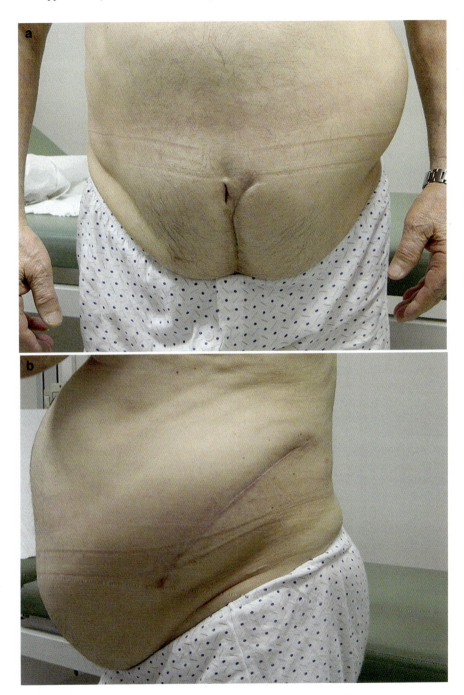

Fig. 24.2 Midline suprapubic incision (**a**) and lumbotomic incision (**b**) for left ureteral tumor nephroureterectomy

When a radical nephrectomy is performed for a presumed parenchymal renal tumor and histology shows a transitional cell carcinoma, a second operation is needed to remove the ureteric stump including the bladder cuff.

Ureterectomy (partial ureterectomy) can be performed in selected cases. Each individual case may be very different, requiring the surgeon to be familiar with the technical principles but also be able to improvise as needed. The indication for partial ureterectomy is a localized low-grade biopsy-proven single lesion. For tumors in the upper third, the resection can be simply performed by including a sufficient safety margin and by repairing the organ with a tension-free end-to-end anastomosis. To ensure the tension-free condition, it is sometimes necessary to mobilize the kidney from its upper pole attachments. For tumors of the middle third, an end-to-end anastomosis is suitable as well. However, if the resected portion of the ureter is too long, it is also possible to perform a transureteroureterostomy. For the lower third of the ureter, a direct bladder implant with or without a psoas hitch technique is the choice. Cancerous tumors in the lower ureter tend to be smaller and less invasive than in the renal pelvis.

Conservative Treatment

The rationale for endoscopic and percutaneous treatment is the renal-sparing approach. From the long-term follow-up of patients who have undergone nephrectomy (for renal cancer or organ donation), the risk of hypertension or renal failure is very low and generally mild in clinical relevance. Thus, renal-sparing therapy for upper tract urothelial cancer should be well justified. The most typical indication is the solitary kidney. An elderly patient treated with nephroureterectomy with subsequent hemodialysis has high risk of dying of renal failure or having a poor quality of life. The 5-year survival rate for patients >65 year of age on hemodialysis ranges from 10 to 20 % [18]. Thus, in a solitary kidney, even in the case of a high-grade tumor, if resectable, the treatment of choice should be organ conserving. For patients with comorbidities and an increasing ASA score, an endoscopic approach should also be considered. The endoscopic management of urothelial cancer is more feasible for tumors located in the ureter than tumors located in the renal pelvis. The risk of ureteral perforation during operative endoscopy can be minimized by the use of the neodymium: yttrium aluminum garnet laser at reduced power setting (25 W) and working with a tangential application of the energy [19]. However, patients should be made aware that a conservative approach is not the gold standard and the risk of failure of disease control is higher than surgery.

Chemotherapy and Immunotherapy

Upper tract Cis can be treated with a topical course of bacillus Calmette-Guérin (BCG) instillations. Studies reported short number series, but the recurrence rate was apparently reduced in >50 % of patients for 1–2 year [20]. The toxicity reported was similar as seen for bladder instillations. We use two modalities to perform ureteral and renal pelvis instillation: by stenting the patient and using bladder instillation for a ureteral reflux of BCG and by placing an indwelling catheter connected to the BCG solution that is administered during a 1-h interval. The literature reported a schedule of six instillations (as the inductive course for bladder Cis) if any significant toxicity occurs.

Systemic Chemotherapy

Metastatic urothelial cancer is sensitive to chemotherapy. Response rates of 70 % are reported, and in a neoadjuvant setting (for bladder cancer), the complete response rates are >30 %. The standard drug combination is cisplatin plus gemcitabine. This schedule has some limitations especially in elderly patients. The main dose-limiting toxicity of cisplatin is nephrotoxicity that peaks 2 week after starting the schedule and is generally reversible. The dose-limiting toxicity for gemcitabine is myelosuppression. Thus, in some elderly patients with poor renal function, it is at least possible to offer a single-agent treatment with gemcitabine (palliative chemotherapy).

Adjuvant Radiotherapy

Radiotherapy of upper urinary tract tumors can reduce the risk of local relapse but does not influence the development of metastasis [21].

Surveillance

Most recurrences occur in the first 3 year following the initial diagnosis. The follow-up should be tailored according to the patient's condition and the stage and grade of the primary disease. Cystoscopy and cytology can be performed at intervals according to the risk group. Up to 40 % of patients who have an upper tract primary tumor later develop a urothelial cancer in the bladder [22]. The upper urinary tract can be monitored with regular cytology and ureteroscopy. Because retrograde pyelography is less sensitive, ureteroscopy is the best tool to survey the upper tract at 6-month intervals. An abdominal CT scan can also be done yearly to monitor the contralateral urinary unit.

References

1. Jemal A, Siegel R, Xu J, et al. Cancer statistics 2010. CA Cancer J Clin. 2010;60:277–300.
2. Fleshner N. Demographics and epidemiology of urothelial cancer of the renal pelvis and ureter. In: Droller MJ, editor. American Cancer Society atlas of clinical oncology urothelial tumors. Hamilton, London: BC Decker Inc; 2004. p. 318–23.

3. Zincke H, Aguilo JJ, Farrow GM, et al. Significance of urinary cytology in the early detection of transitional cell cancer of the upper tract. J Urol. 1976;116:781.

4. Robbins SE, Droller M. Transitional cell carcinoma of the upper urinary tract: incidence, etiology, epidemiology and genetics. In: Hamdy FC, Basler JW, Neal DE, Catalona WJ, editors. Management of urologic malignancies. London: Churchill Livingstone; 2002. p. 349–53.

5. Babjuk M, Oosterlinck W, Sylvester R, et al. EAU guidelines on non-muscle-invasive urothelial carcinoma of the bladder, the 2011 update.Eur Urol. 2011;59:997–1008.

6. Maffezzini M, Campodonico F, Capponi G, et al. Prognostic significance of fluorescence in situ hybridization in the follow-up of non-muscle-invasive bladder cancer. Anticancer Res. 2010;30:4761–5.

7. American Joint Committee on Cancer. Renal pelvis and ureter. In: Manual for staging of cancer. 5th ed. Philadelphia: Lippincott-Raven; 1997. p. 235–7.

8. Huben RP, Mounzer AM, Murphy G. Tumor grade and stage as prognostic variables in upper tract urothelial tumors. Cancer. 1988;62:2016–20.

9. Guinan P, Volgelzang NJ, Randazzo R, et al. Renal pelvic transitional cell carcinoma: the role of the kidney in tumor-node-metastasis staging. Cancer. 1992;69:1773–5.

10. Stanley AY, Clayton WS, Chamie K, et al. Effect of age on transitional cell carcinoma of the upper urinary tract: presentation, treatment, and outcomes. Urology. 2011;78:87–92.

11. Cloutier V, Capitanio U, Zini L, et al. Thirty-day mortality after nephrectomy: clinical implications for informed consent. Eur Urol. 2009;56:998–1005. (Comment on Eur Urol 2009; 56: 998–1003).

12. Pope D, Ramesh H, Gennari R, et al. Pre-operative assessment of cancer in the elderly (PACE): a comprehensive assessment of underlying characteristics of elderly cancer patients prior to elective surgery. Surg Oncol. 2007;15:189–97.

13. Melamed MR, Reuter VE. Pathology and staging of urothelial tumors of the kidney and ureter. Urol Clin North Am. 1993;20:333–47.

14. Zincke H, Neves RJ. Feasibility of conservative surgery for transitional cell carcinoma of the upper urinary tract. Urol Clin North Am. 1984;11:717–24.

15. Steffens J, Nagel R. Tumors of the renal pelvis and the ureter. Br J Urol. 1988;61:277–83.

16. Shariat SF, Godoy G, Lotan Y, et al. Advanced patient age is associated with inferior cancer-specific survival after radical nephroureterectomy. BJU Int. 2009;105:1672–7.

17. Chromecki TF, Ehdaie B, Novara G, et al. Chronological age is not an independent predictor of clinical outcomes after radical nephroureterectomy. World J Urol. 2011;29(4):473–80.

18. Fenton S, Desmeules M, Copleston P, et al. Renal replacement therapy in Canada: a report from the Canadian Organ Replacement Register. Am J Kidney Dis. 1995;25:134–50.

19. Carson C. Endoscopic treatment of upper and lower urinary tract lesions using lasers. Semin Urol. 1991;9:185–91.

20. Oldbring J, Glifberg I, MIkulowski P, et al. Carcinoma of the renal pelvis and ureter following bladder carcinoma: frequency, risk factors and clinicopathological findings. J Urol. 1989;141: 1311–3.

21. Schoenberg MP, van Arsdalen KN, Wein AJ. The management of transitional cell carcinoma in solitary renal units. J Urol. 1991;146:700–3.

22. Cozad SC, Smalley SR, Austenfeld M, et al. Adjuvant radiotherapy in high stage transitional cell carcinoma of the renal pelvis and ureter. Int J Radiat Oncol Biol Phys. 1992;24:743–5.

Chapter 25
Adrenal Tumors in the Elderly

Jean-Louis Peix and Jean-Christophe Lifante

Abstract The frequency and the types of adrenal tumors in the general population are well described, but it is difficult to define the frequency and types of adrenal diseases in the elderly. We performed a multicenter retrospective study between 2005 and 2010 in collaboration with the French Association of Endocrine Surgery (AFCE) and the French Association of Surgery (AFC) for describing adrenal tumors in patients over 70 years of age. Pheochromocytomas are the most frequent tumors in these patients. The distribution of adrenal diseases in cases of incidentaloma in elderly patients does not differ from that reported for younger patients. The most frequent diagnoses are nonfunctioning adenomas followed by pheochromocytomas and cortisol-secreting adenomas. Malignant tumors are rare. The diagnosis of metastases is the most probable if the patient has had a past history of cancer, especially in cases of lung carcinoma, breast carcinoma, melanoma, or lymphoma. Adrenal disease in the elderly seems to be similar to that observed in younger patients. In both populations, the same problems are present concerning the determination of the nature of indeterminate adrenal masses. Surgery should be reserved for patients with secreting masses or very suspicious adrenal tumors after meticulous screening.

Keywords Adrenal • Elderly • Surgery • Pheochromocytoma • Incidentaloma • Adrenal cortical carcinoma

J.-L. Peix, M.D. • J.-C. Lifante, M.D., Ph.D. (✉)
Department of General and Endocrine Surgery, Centre Hospitalier Lyon Sud,
Pierre Bénite, France
e-mail: jean-louis.peix@chu-lyon.fr; jean-christophe.lifante@chu-lyon.fr

J.-P. Droz, R.A. Audisio (eds.), *Management of Urological Cancers in Older People*,
Management of Cancer in Older People,
DOI 10.1007/978-0-85729-999-4_25, © Springer-Verlag London 2013

Introduction

Adrenal tumors are rare and are typically revealed in two ways: abnormal hormone secretion, such as Cushing's syndrome, or by coincidental discovery known as an incidentaloma. The frequency and the types of adrenal tumors in the general population are well described, but it is difficult to define the frequency and types of adrenal diseases in the elderly. Furthermore, the literature is limited in this field. In this chapter, we reported the recent study performed by the French Association of Surgery and the Francophone Association of Endocrine Surgery in an attempt to describe adrenal disease in the elderly.

The AFCE Study [1]

We performed a multicenter retrospective study between 2005 and 2010 in collaboration with the French Association of Endocrine Surgery (AFCE) and the French Association of Surgery (AFC). Patients were enrolled from 15 centers that were performing adrenal surgery. During the study period, 153 patients underwent adrenalectomies for adrenal tumors. We excluded Cushing's syndrome patients who underwent bilateral adrenalectomies because this disease involves the hypophysis and not the adrenal glands.

Among these 153 patients, 41 (27 %) presented with pheochromocytomas, 36 (23 %) with nonsecreting adenomas, 21 (14 %) with adenomas with hypercorticism, and 19 (12 %) with adrenal metastases. Eleven (7 %) patients had malignant adrenal carcinomas, and 9 (6 %) patients had aldosteronomas. Sixteen patients had a separate type of rare tumor (4 myelolipomas, 4 hematomas, 1 lymphoma, 2 angiomas, 1 echinococcus infection, 3 nonsecreting hyperplasias, and 1 adrenal cyst) (Fig. 25.1). Among these 153 patients, 54 presented incidentalomas without symptoms. Of these 54 incidentalomas, hormone assays and pathology examinations revealed 36

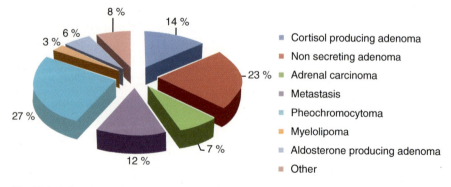

Fig. 25.1 Adrenal tumors in the elderly

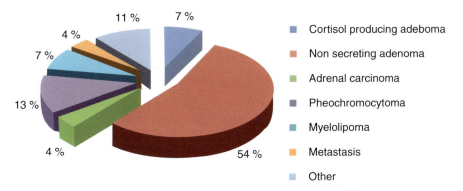

Fig. 25.2 Adrenal incidentaloma in the elderly

nonsecreting adenomas (54 %), 7 (13 %) pheochromocytomas, 4 (11 %) cortisol-secreting adenomas, 4 (11 %) myelolipomas, 2 (4 %) metastases, 2 (4 %) malignant adrenal carcinomas, and 6 other rare tumors (2 hematomas, 2 angiomas, 1 adrenal hyperplasia, and 1 echinococcus infection) (Fig. 25.2).

Comments

Adrenal tumors are rare in the general population, and we have found that the distribution of adrenal tumors in the elderly does not differ from that of the general population. Pheochromocytomas are the most frequent tumors in patients over 70 years of age. Nevertheless, in the literature, pheochromocytomas were reported to be less frequent in the elderly than in patients under the age of 60 [2]. Pheochromocytomas are most likely more difficult to diagnose in patients older than 60 because the condition is often masked by arteriosclerosis and is frequently fatal before a correct diagnosis can be made. Furthermore, in a study by Sutton et al., older patients with pheochromocytomas had less florid symptomatology than did younger patients. Cardiomegaly and left ventricular hypertrophy are characteristic of pheochromocytomas in elderly patients [3, 4]. The diagnosis is all the more difficult to make because there could be decreased cardiovascular responsiveness to catecholamines with age, and thus, classical symptoms are less evident in the elderly [5].

The second type of adrenal tumor found in the elderly is a benign adenoma. Most of these tumors are nonsecreting adenomas (23 %) followed by cortisol-secreting adenomas (14 %) and Conn's adenomas (6 %). The second subset of benign adenomas found in our study contained cortisol-secreting adenomas. Few reports have described Cushing's syndrome in the elderly. However, dementia and depression can lead to hypercortisolism during old age [6]. Therefore, classical signs of Cushing's syndrome, such as HTA, diabetes, and depression or dementia but also important loss of weight when they appear brutally, should make think to Cushing's syndrome. Aldosterone adenomas account for 6 % of adrenal diseases described in

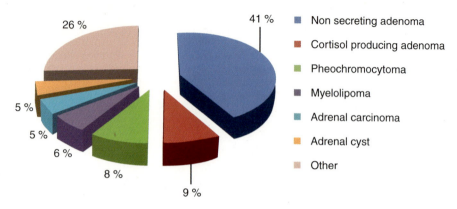

Fig. 25.3 Diagnosis of adrenal incidentalomas in the general population

our study. The age of onset of primary hyperaldosteronism is usually between 20 and 60 years. Aldosterone-producing adenomas are the most common cause of primary hyperaldosteronism and accounts for more than 90 % of all cases. Additionally, primary hyperaldosteronism constitutes the most frequent cause of arterial hypertension. Despite the occurrence of primary hyperaldosteronism in young patients, many case reports of the disease in the elderly can be found in the literature. This diagnosis should be considered when aggravation of arterial hypertension or recent arterial hypertension occurs in an elderly patient [7].

Interestingly, some adrenal tumors are discovered via imaging when patients are asymptomatic; these tumors are known as incidentalomas in the literature. Incidentalomas are occurring with increased frequency due to the greater availability of CT scans. In recent studies, an adrenal incidentaloma was found in 4.5 % of CT scans [8]. In autopsies, adrenal incidentalomas are found in 8.7 % of cases, and the frequency of occurrence increases with age, obesity, diabetes, and arterial hypertension. Based on radiological series, incidentalomas are found in almost 5 % of patients who receive CT scans [9]. According to reports in the literature concerning all age groups, nonfunctioning adenomas account for 35–71 % of the incidentalomas, cortisol-producing adenomas for 13–7.9 %, pheochromocytomas for 11–5.6 %, and aldosterone-producing adenomas for 1.2–3 %. Concerning malignant tumors, incidentalomas represent adrenal carcinomas in 5 % (range, 4–11 %) of cases and metastasis in approximately 2 % [9, 10]. These results are similar to those reported for the general population in our study conducted by the AFCE and AFC [1] (Fig. 25.3). There are no reports in the literature concerning incidentalomas in the elderly. We report the results of a study conducted by the AFCE and AFC concerning the elderly population. We found that the distribution of adrenal diseases in cases of incidentaloma in elderly patients does not differ from that reported for younger patients. The most frequent diagnoses are nonfunctioning adenomas followed by pheochromocytomas and cortisol-secreting adenomas. Malignant tumors are rare. The diagnosis of metastases is the most probable if the patient has had a past history of cancer, especially in cases of lung carcinoma, breast carcinoma, melanoma, or lymphoma. In these patients, the frequency of adrenal metastases in incidentaloma cases varies from 45 to 73 %. Adrenal carcinomas are rare in the elderly and account for approximately 4 % of incidentaloma cases. In the study conducted with the AFCE, we found that adrenal carcinoma also accounted for approximately 4 % of incidentaloma cases in the general population. Our data are far from approaching the rate of 11 % reported by Mantero et al. [11]. In the recent prospective study from Sweden, no adrenal carcinomas were found among 226 incidentalomas that were followed for 2 years. If this diagnosis seems rare in young patients, it is even rarer in elderly patients. For these reasons, we propose that the management of adrenal incidentalomas in elderly patients should not differ from that employed in younger patients. Therefore, we suggest that physicians answer the following three questions when treating patients: Is the tumor secreting? Is the tumor malignant? Should the patient receive surgical intervention? [1, 9–11]

Is the Tumor Secreting?

Patients with incidentalomas should be screened for both catecholamine excess and hypercortisolism except in those patients for whom imaging data are typical of myelolipoma or adrenal cyst. Primary hyperaldosteronism should only be considered in cases of arterial hypertension or hypokalemia. For screening of pheochromocytoma, we suggest the measurement of metanephrine and normetanephrine in the plasma, which has a sensitivity of 99 %. An elevation of more than fourfold above the normal level confirms the pheochromocytoma diagnosis [9–11].

Screening for hypercortisolism requires the measurement of UFC, and we recommend the systematic 1-mg overnight dexamethasone suppression test for the diagnosis of mild hypercortisolism. Androgenic secretion should only be considered when the patient exhibits indicative clinical signs.

Is the Tumor Malignant?

Imaging is useful to characterize adrenal tumors. The size and appearance of an adrenal mass, as determined by CT scan, may help distinguish between benign and malignant lesions. For a mass with a spontaneous density of less than 10 UH, the diagnosis of a benign tumor can be confirmed with a sensitivity range from 66 to 100 %. When a spontaneous density ranges between 10 and 50 UH, the measurement of tumor washout using an enhanced CT scan is necessary. Lipid-poor adenomas represent 10–40 % of adenomas and typically demonstrate rapid washout with an absolute washout of more than 60 % (sensitivity of 86–100 %, specificity of 83–92 %) and a relative washout of more than 40 % (sensitivity of 82–97 %, specificity of 92–100 %) [9, 10]. Obviously, the presence of venous thrombosis, lymph node metastasis, or distant metastasis suggests a malignant tumor. Magnetic resonance imaging is as effective as CT scans in the diagnosis of benign adrenal tumors. However, this technique does not have any advantage when compared with CT scan. In current practice, magnetic resonance imaging is only used when the incidentaloma has been discovered initially on an MRI. The FDG PET scan is also being assessed, and as published recently, it will become a new tool for the future assessment of adrenal masses [9].

Should the Patient Receive Surgical Intervention?

All secreting and malignant tumors must be resected. The difficulty exists in determining the benign or malignant nature of the tumor in a suspicious adrenal mass. Therefore, we continue to operate on patients with indeterminate adrenal masses to diagnose tumors, particularly when they are larger than 4 cm. The surgical strategy remains the same than in younger patients [1, 9, 10].

Adrenal disease in the elderly seems to be similar to that observed in younger patients. In both populations, the same problems are present concerning the determination of the nature of indeterminate adrenal masses. Surgery should be reserved for patients with secreting masses or very suspicious adrenal tumors after meticulous screening.

References

1. Ochoa S, Lifante JC, et al. Enquête AFCE. In: Mathonnet M, Peix JL, Sebag F, editors. Chirurgie des glandes surrénales Rapport présenté au 113e congrès de chirurgie 2011. Paris: Arnette; 2011. p. 229–39.
2. Cooper ME, Goodman D, Frauman A, Jerums G, Louis WJ. Phaeochromocytoma in the elderly: a poorly recognised entity? Br Med J. 1986;293:1474–5.
3. Mizuta E, Hamada T, Taniguchi S, Shimoyama M, Nawada T, Miake J, Kaetsu Y, Peili L, Ishiguro K, Ishiguro S, Igawa O, Shigemasa C, Hisatome I. Small extra-adrenal pheochromocytoma causing severe hypertension in an elderly patient. Hypertens Res. 2006;29:635–8.
4. Sutton MG, Sheps SG, Lie JT. Prevalence of clinically unsuspected pheochromocytoma. Review of a 50-year autopsy series. Mayo Clin Proc. 1981;56:354–60.
5. Somana S, Marilier S, Mazen E, de la Vega MF, Camus A, Popitean L, Pfitzenmeyer P, Manckoundia P. Psychobehavioral disorders, orthostatic hypotension, and falls related to a pheochromocytoma in a very elderly subject: a case report. J Am Geriatr Soc. 2010;58:1611–2.
6. Guldiken S, Guldiken B. Subclinical Cushing's syndrome is a potential cause of metabolic dementia and rapidly progressive Alzheimer-type dementia. Med Hypotheses. 2008;71:703–5.
7. Tamura Y, Adachi J, Chiba Y, Mori S, Takeda K, Kasuya Y, Murayama T, Sawabe M, Sasano H, Araki A, Ito H, Horiuchi T. Primary aldosteronism due to unilateral adrenal microadenoma in an elderly patient: efficacy of selective adrenal venous sampling. Intern Med. 2008;47:37–42.
8. Muth A, Hammarstedt L, Hellström M, Sigurjónsdóttir HÁ, Almqvist E, Wängberg B, Adrenal Study Group of Western Sweden. Cohort study of patients with adrenal lesions discovered incidentally. Br J Surg. 2011;98:1383–91.

9. Tabarin A, Bardet S, Bertherat J, Dupas B, Chabre O, Hamoir E, Laurent F, Tenenbaum F, Cazalda M, Lefebvre H, Valli N, Rohmer V, French Society of Endocrinology Consensus. Exploration and management of adrenal incidentalomas. French Society of Endocrinology Consensus. Ann Endocrinol (Paris). 2008;69:487–500.

10. Terzolo M, Stigliano A, Chiodini I, Loli P, Furlani L, Arnaldi G, Reimondo G, Pia A, Toscano V, Zini M, Borretta G, Papini E, Garofalo P, Allolio B, Dupas B, Mantero F, Tabarin A, Italian Association of Clinical Endocrinologists. AME position statement on adrenal incidentaloma. Eur J Endocrinol. 2011;164:851–70.

11. Arnaldi G, Masini AM, Giacchetti G, Taccaliti A, Faloia E, Mantero F. Adrenal incidentaloma. Braz J Med Biol Res. 2000;33:1177–89.

Chapter 26
Retroperitoneal Tumors in the Elderly

Pierre Meeus and Helen Boyle

Abstract Retroperitoneal tumors are rare tumors. Most of them are malignant. They are often diagnosed at an advanced stage because symptoms appear when the lesions are quite big. Obtaining good cross-sectional imaging and a preoperative biopsy is important to make an accurate diagnosis and to decide on the treatment. Sarcomas are the most frequent malignant tumors and require aggressive surgery. Careful assessment of the patient's general condition is necessary to decide on the best treatment options. There are no specific guidelines for their management in elderly patients.

Keywords Retroperitoneal • Sarcoma • Lymphoma • Elderly • Surgery

Introduction

Retroperitoneal tumors are rare tumors. They are often diagnosed at an advanced stage because symptoms are nonspecific and usually only appear when the lesions are quite big. They can also be an incidental finding on a scan performed for another reason.

Retroperitoneal tumors usually originate outside the retroperitoneal organs. More than 70 % of these tumors are malignant. A third of them are sarcomas. The other frequent tumors are lymphomas and metastases [1].

P. Meeus, M.D. (✉)
Department of Surgery, Center Léon-Bérard,
Lyon, France
e-mail: pierre.meeus@lyon.unicancer.fr

H. Boyle, M.D.
Department of Medicine, Center Léon-Bérard,
Lyon, France
e-mail: helen.boyle@lyon.unicancer.fr

J.-P. Droz, R.A. Audisio (eds.), *Management of Urological Cancers in Older People*,
Management of Cancer in Older People,
DOI 10.1007/978-0-85729-999-4_26, © Springer-Verlag London 2013

The most frequent benign tumors are schwannomas, neurofibromas, paragangliomas, angiomyolipomas, and lipomas. They are usually diagnosed incidentally.

This chapter will review the most frequent retroperitoneal tumors in elderly patients. The issue of primary kidney tumors will not be addressed here as there is a specific chapter on them in this book.

Anatomy of the Retroperitoneum

The retroperitoneum is the anatomical space that extends from the diaphragm to the pelvis [2]. It is bounded anteriorly by the posterior layer of peritoneum and posteriorly by the fascia transversalis. It can be further divided into several spaces as the anterior pararenal space, between the peritoneum and the Gerota's fascia and the posterior pararenal space between the Zuckerkandl fascia and the transversalis fascia.

The great vessels (aorta and vena cava) are situated in the median axes and are bordered by the psoas muscles.

The retroperitoneum communicates inferiorly with the pelvis and the paravesical space.

These anatomical considerations are important as they are the basis for the surgical management of retroperitoneal tumors.

Symptoms

Symptoms usually occur when the tumor is quite large, and they are usually nonspecific: abdominal swelling, abdominal discomfort, early satiety, etc. Most patients have a palpable mass. Some patients are asymptomatic, and the tumor is discovered incidentally on a radiological exam performed for another reason.

Retroperitoneal Sarcomas

They represent a third of all retroperitoneal tumors [3]. Mean age at diagnosis is 55–60 years. The sex ratio is one. Most frequent symptoms are back or abdominal pain.

It is important to perform a CT scan with intravenous contrast to distinguish a retroperitoneal mass from an intraperitoneal lesion.

Histological proof is mandatory to make the diagnosis. It can be obtained by a preoperative needle biopsy that should be performed by a posterior approach to avoid peritoneal seeding [4, 5].

The need for a biopsy and the technique should be discussed at a multidisciplinary meeting with a surgeon and a radiologist. A biopsy must be performed if a neoadjuvant treatment is to be administered (chemotherapy or conformational radiotherapy).

The main treatment of retroperitoneal sarcomas is surgery. French cancer centers have published their recommendations on the management of retroperitoneal sarcomas. A CT scan should be performed to define the localization of the tumor and its relationship with adjacent structures. Density of the mass should be reported. A needle biopsy should be obtained.

An MRI should be performed when the lesion is close to the spine, when a neurological tumor is suspected, or when there are neurological symptoms suggesting nerve/cord compression or involvement [6].

The biopsy should be directed to the most suspicious zone and be performed by a posterior, extraperitoneal approach. The biopsy route should be protected and tattooed.

Once the pathology is obtained, the case must be discussed at a multidisciplinary meeting to decide on the treatment strategy that might involve neoadjuvant chemotherapy.

Because of the size of the tumors and their localization, vascular reconstruction, bone resection, etc., may be needed to ensure complete en bloc resection, and this must be planned carefully before hand [7]. The organs that are more often removed during surgery are the kidney, the colon, the spleen, and the pancreas [8–11].

Complete resection is one of the most important prognostic factors for overall survival [12]. Histological subtype is also an independent prognostic factor [13].

Despite complete en bloc resections, 5-year local relapse rates reach 50 %. The two main prognostic factors for local relapse are positive margins and histological subtype.

Neoadjuvant chemotherapy can be used in patients with intermediate or poorly differentiated sarcomas. Some authors favor this strategy because renal function is better before nephrectomy and preoperative chemotherapy makes surgery easier by decreasing the tumor volume. However, there is no prospective data to support this, and decision should be made in multidisciplinary meetings on a case to case basis.

When surgery is not possible (vascular mesenteric involvement, sarcomatosis), chemotherapy plays a major role.

There is no benefit on progression-free survival or on overall survival from adjuvant chemotherapy.

Radiotherapy is difficult to perform, especially after surgery, because of its toxicity when the dose to the small bowel reaches 45 Gy. In fact, the bowel is "trapped" in the resection zone and receives a high dose of radiation. However, several groups support the use of pre- or postoperative radiotherapy. Results from randomized trials would help better define its use. An EORTC trial (EORTC62092) testing the role of preoperative radiotherapy is currently ongoing [14].

Retroperitoneal Liposarcomas

They are the most common retroperitoneal sarcomas. There are four histological subgroups: well differentiated, dedifferentiated, myxoid, and round cell. The presence of a dedifferentiated component is associated with a poor prognosis. Dedifferentiated and well-differentiated components can coexist in large liposarcomas at initial presentation or at relapse. A biopsy may not be needed if the scans are reviewed in a specialized center and are suggestive of the diagnosis [15].

Surgery is the only curative treatment: en bloc resection often requires removal of the kidney and the homolateral colon. The mass should not be dissected because it leads to tumor seeding (R2 resection) and recurrence in 100 % of cases.

Some teams perform tumor enucleation in selected cases: elderly patients, patients with impaired renal function, and well-differentiated liposarcomas [16].

Despite optimal surgery, 5-year relapse rates approach 50 %. Margin positivity and histological subtype are major factors associated with relapse. There are no indications for adjuvant chemotherapy. Perioperative radiotherapy can be given. Preoperative radiotherapy using conformational techniques seems the most interesting and the less toxic option.

It is important to remember that surgery still plays a role in treating local recurrences and can also be performed in palliative situations (decompressive surgery for sarcomatosis).

Retroperitoneal Leiomyosarcomas

Leiomyosarcomas arise from smooth muscle of large vessels or embryonic remnants (Wolffian ducts). Retroperitoneal leiomyosarcomas are more frequent in women in the fifth and sixth decade. They can involve the inferior vena cava, the genital veins, and the renal veins.

Presence of necrosis and vascular involvement on the MRI are important factors for the diagnosis.

Surgery must be aggressive with resection of vascular structures and adjacent organs to obtain negative margins, even in the aorta. Vascular surgery is a main part of the procedure with resection and reconstruction [17, 18].

Neoadjuvant chemotherapy can reduce tumor size but does not change the type of surgery. Both local recurrences and metastases are frequent.

Sarcomas of the inferior vena cava are real challenges because of the type of resection and the type of replacement needed [18]. Multidisciplinary discussion is necessary to define the treatment strategy. If there is a complete thrombosis of the inferior vena cava, replacement is not necessary. Absence of replacement reduces the risk of thrombosis and pulmonary embolism. However, if the renal veins are involved, replacement is mandatory.

Other Sarcomas

The third most common type of retroperitoneal sarcoma is malignant peripheral nerve sheath tumors (MPNST). Other types of sarcomas are quite rare: rhabdomyosarcomas and angiosarcomas. Chondrosarcomas and synaviolosarcomas are even less frequent [1].

The diagnostic procedures are the same as for other sarcomas. Surgery is the main treatment; neoadjuvant chemotherapy can be given in some cases.

Other Retroperitoneal Tumors

Hematological Malignancies

Primary retroperitoneal lymphomas are quite rare. However, lymphomas are the most frequent retroperitoneal hematological malignancy. In elderly patients, non-Hodgkin's lymphomas are the most frequent [19].

CT-guided biopsy allows diagnosis in most cases. It is important to have sufficient material to perform microscopic examination, flow cytometry, immunophenotyping, and molecular studies.

Preoperative biopsy of all retroperitoneal masses avoids useless surgery. However, mini-invasive surgery may be needed in some cases, to obtain a correct diagnosis.

Treatment is based on chemotherapy. There are several retrospective studies on lymphomas suggesting that elderly patients tend to have aggressive lymphomas [20].

A specific phase II trial has shown that R-mini CHOP (rituximab, cyclophosphamide, doxorubicin, vincristine, and prednisone) in patients over 80 yields a 2-year overall survival rate of 59 % (49–67 %) [21]. Twelve patients out of the 149 died of treatment toxicity. In the univariate analysis, poor performance status, age-adjusted IPI score of 2–3, number of extra-nodal sites > 1, serum albumin ≤ 35 g/L, tumor mass > 10 cm, and IADL score < 4 were associated with worse survival. In the multivariate analysis, only serum albumin level ≤ 35 g/L was significant (hazard ratio 3.2, 95 % CI 1.4–7.1; $p=0.0053$).

A phase III trial compared CHOP to R-CHOP, administered every 3 weeks, in patients with large B cell diffuse lymphoma aged between 60 and 80. It showed a benefit in event-free survival, progression-free survival, disease-free survival, and overall survival for patients treated with rituximab [22]. Median overall survival (OS) was not reached for R-CHOP patients compared with 3.1 years (95 % CI, 2.2 to not reached) for CHOP patients ($p=0.0073$). The 5-year OS rate was 58 % (95 % CI, 50.8–64.5 %) in R-CHOP patients compared with 45 % (95 % CI, 39.1–53.3 %) in CHOP patients.

Another phase III trial in this population compared six to eight cycles of CHOP +/–rituximab [23]. Cycles were administered every 2 weeks. Maximum survival benefit was obtained with six cycles of R-CHOP compared to six cycles of CHOP. There was no extra benefit with the addition of two cycles of chemotherapy. The 3-year OS rate was 78.1 % (73.2–83.0) for six cycles of R-CHOP 14.

Interim results of a phase III trial R-CHOP 14 to R-CHOP 21 in that population have not shown a benefit with the 2-week administration. Long-term results are still pending [24].

Extramedullary plasmocytomas are characterized by a monoclonal proliferation of plasma cell. They are rare. The diagnosis is made only after excluding multiple myeloma. Peak incidence occurs in the sixth and seventh decade. They are more frequent in males. Retroperitoneal plasmocytomas are very rare; they usually arise in the perirenal region. Diagnosis is made on needle biopsy. Treatment is not well codified as these are exceptional [25].

Neurogenic Tumors

Neurogenic tumors represent around 10 % of primary retroperitoneal tumors. They are more frequent in younger patients. They can originate from the nerve sheath (schwannomas, neurofibromas, neurofibromatosis, and malignant peripheral nerve sheath tumors), ganglionic cells (ganglioneuromas, ganglioneuroblastomas, neuroblastomas), or paraganglionic cells (paragangliomas, pheochromocytomas) [2].

Needle biopsy guides the diagnosis. Surgery is performed depending on the symptoms.

Multidisciplinary discussions are mandatory before treatment: patients must be informed of potential sequela especially for schwannomas of the femoral nerve.

Germ Cell Tumors and Sex Cord Tumors

Germ cell tumors are rare in elderly patients [2]. The retroperitoneum can be involved either by a primary extragonadal retroperitoneal tumor or by metastases from a testicular primary. Seminomas can occur in older patients; nonseminomatous germ cell tumors are excessively rare over 60.

Sex cord tumors (granulosa tumor or less frequently Sertoli-Leydig tumors) occur mainly in women.

Metastases

Metastatic involvement of retroperitoneal lymph nodes can occur in the evolution of many malignancies, such as cervical carcinomas, bladder and prostate cancers [2]. Sometimes no primary is identified. Treatment is based on chemotherapy.

Benign Lesions

Lipomatosis consists of homogeneous, mature, adult white fat cells separated by fibrous septa. They occur mainly in the pelvis and along the perirectal spaces. They are less frequent in the abdominal retroperitoneum [2].

CT scan and MRI show excess fat in the pararenal spaces and in the mesos. There is no specific treatment, a part from symptom management.

Retroperitoneal fibrosis is a rare disease characterized by the presence of a retroperitoneal tissue consisting of chronic inflammation and marked fibrosis [26]. It is often idiopathic. Its pathogenesis is not completely elucidated and is probably multifactorial (genetic, immunological, and environmental). It is 2–3 times more frequent in men; mean age at diagnosis is 50–60 years. However, it can occur in older patients. It usually surrounds the infrarenal aorta and the origin of the iliac arteries.

There are some cases of secondary retroperitoneal fibrosis caused by drugs, malignancies, infections, radiotherapy, surgery, and so on.

Clinical symptoms are nonspecific: local symptoms include back or abdominal pain, lower limb edema, deep vein thrombosis, constipation, and so on. There can also be systemic manifestations such as fatigue, low-grade fever, nausea, anorexia, weight loss, and myalgias. Some patients also have manifestations of autoimmune disease.

C-reactive protein and erythrocyte sedimentation rate can be increased. Diagnosis is made on CT or MRI imaging. These studies can help distinguish between idiopathic and secondary fibrosis. A histological examination is needed if the localization is atypical or if there is a suspicion of malignancy or infection.

Treatment of idiopathic retroperitoneal fibrosis is based on steroids. Immunosuppressants or tamoxifen can be used in steroid refractory patients.

Ureteral stenting or surgery may be needed to relieve ureteral obstruction.

When the fibrosis develops around an aneurismal aorta, surgery is usually performed when the aortic diameter exceeds 50 mm. Endovascular techniques can be used.

Specific Problems in Elderly Patients

Diagnosis of retroperitoneal masses follows the same steps as in younger patients. It is mandatory to obtain good quality cross-sectional imaging and a preoperative biopsy.

If the diagnosis is sarcoma, multidisciplinary assessment is important. It should concern technical aspects such as surgical procedure, use of neoadjuvant chemotherapy, and also evaluation of patients' general condition. Surgery of retroperitoneal sarcomas is often quite challenging and can require vascular replacement, a nephrectomy, and so on. This can be a problem in elderly patients who have more frequent vascular problems and/or impaired renal function than younger patients. They also tend to be malnourished. It is important to make sure a patient can undergo such a surgery. There are no specific guidelines for the management of retroperitoneal sarcomas in the elderly as the disease is rare. However, if surgery is decided, it must be performed as a complete en bloc resection after careful assessment of patients' health. The preoperative assessment in elderly cancer patients (PACE) developed by the SIOG (International Society of Geriatric Oncology) is one of the tools that can help guide decision. Age alone should not preclude radical surgery [27].

Chemotherapy for advanced soft tissue sarcomas is single-agent doxorubicin [28]. It can be administered to elderly patients if cardiac function is adequate.

Chemotherapy for lymphomas has been specifically studied in elderly patients and these adapted protocols should be used.

Conclusions

Retroperitoneal tumors are rare tumors. Most of them are malignant. The important point is to make an accurate histological diagnosis before deciding on the treatment.

There are no specific guidelines for their management in elderly patients. Sarcomas are the most frequent malignant tumors and require aggressive surgery. Careful assessment of the patient's general condition is necessary to decide on the best treatment options.

References

1. Mullinax JE, Zager JS, Gonzalez RJ. Current diagnosis and management of retroperitoneal sarcoma. Cancer Control. 2011;18(3):177–87. Review.
2. Rajiah P, Sinha R, Cuevas C, Dubinsky TJ, Bush Jr WH, Kolokythas O. Imaging of uncommon retroperitoneal masses. Radiographics. 2011;31(4):949–76.
3. Strauss DC, Hayes AJ, Thomas JM. Retroperitoneal tumours: review of management. Ann R Coll Surg Engl. 2011;93(4):275–80.
4. Gangopadhyay M, Bhattacharyya NK, Ray S, Chakrabarty S, Pandit N. Guided fine needle aspiration cytology of retroperitoneal masses – our experience. J Cytol. 2011;28(1):20–4.
5. Stattaus J, Kalkmann J, Kuehl H, Metz KA, Nowrousian MR, Forsting M, Ladd SC. Diagnostic yield of computed tomography-guided coaxial core biopsy of undetermined masses in the free retroperitoneal space: single-center experience. Cardiovasc Intervent Radiol. 2008;31(5):919–25.
6. Elsayes KM, Staveteig PT, Narra VR, Chen ZM, Moustafa YL, Brown J. Retroperitoneal masses: magnetic resonance imaging findings with pathologic correlation. Curr Probl Diagn Radiol. 2007;36(3):97–106.
7. Tseng WW, Wang SC, Eichler CM, Warren RS, Nakakura EK. Complete and safe resection of challenging retroperitoneal tumors: anticipation of multi-organ and major vascular resection and use of adjunct procedures. World J Surg Oncol. 2011;9:143.
8. Bonvalot S, Miceli R, Berselli M, Causeret S, Colombo C, Mariani L, Bouzaiene H, Le Péchoux C, Casali PG, Le Cesne A, Fiore M, Gronchi A. Aggressive surgery in retroperitoneal soft tissue sarcoma carried out at high-volume centers is safe and is associated with improved local control. Ann Surg Oncol. 2010;17(6):1507–14.

9. Tseng WH, Martinez SR, Tamurian RM, Chen SL, Bold RJ, Canter RJ. Contiguous organ resection is safe in patients with retroperitoneal sarcoma: an ACS-NSQIP analysis. J Surg Oncol. 2011;103(5):390–4. doi:10.1002/jso.21849. Epub 2010 Dec 28.
10. Hassan I, Park SZ, Donohue JH, Nagorney DM, Kay PA, Nasciemento AG, Schleck CD, Ilstrup DM. Operative management of primary retroperitoneal sarcomas: a reappraisal of an institutional experience. Ann Surg. 2004;239(2):244–50.
11. Pisters PW. Resection of some – but not all – clinically uninvolved adjacent viscera as part of surgery for retroperitoneal soft tissue sarcomas. J Clin Oncol. 2009;27(1):6–8.
12. Anaya DA, Lev DC, Pollock RE. The role of surgical margin status in retroperitoneal sarcoma. J Surg Oncol. 2008;98(8):607–10.
13. Bonvalot S, Rivoire M, Castaing M, Stoeckle E, Le Cesne A, Blay JY, Laplanche A. Primary retroperitoneal sarcomas: a multivariate analysis of surgical factors associated with local control. J Clin Oncol. 2009;27(1):31–7.
14. Van De Voorde L, Delrue L, van Eijkeren M, De Meerleer G. Radiotherapy and surgery – an indispensable duo in the treatment of retroperitoneal sarcoma. Cancer. 2011;117(19):4355–64.
15. Lahat G, Madewell JE, Anaya DA, Qiao W, Tuvin D, Benjamin RS, Lev DC, Pollock RE. Computed tomography scan-driven selection of treatment for retroperitoneal liposarcoma histologic subtypes. Cancer. 2009;115(5):1081–90.
16. Smith CA, Martinez SR, Tseng WH, Tamurian RM, Bold RJ, Borys D, Canter RJ. Predicting survival for well-differentiated liposarcoma: the importance of tumor location. J Surg Res. 2012;175(1):12–7.
17. O'Sullivan PJ, Harris AC, Munk PL. Radiological imaging features of non-uterine leiomyosarcoma. Br J Radiol. 2008;81(961):73–81.
18. Cho SW, Marsh JW, Geller DA, Holtzman M, Zeh 3rd H, Bartlett DL, Gamblin TC. Surgical management of leiomyosarcoma of the inferior vena cava. J Gastrointest Surg. 2008;12(12):2141–8.
19. Chen L, Kuriakose P, Hawley RC, Janakiraman N, Maeda K. Hematologic malignancies with primary retroperitoneal presentation: clinicopathologic study of 32 cases. Arch Pathol Lab Med. 2005;129(5):655–60.
20. Thieblemont C, Grossoeuvre A, Houot R, Broussais-Guillaumont F, Salles G, Traullé C, Espinouse D, Coiffier B. Non-Hodgkin's lymphoma in very elderly patients over 80 years. A descriptive analysis of clinical presentation and outcome. Ann Oncol. 2008;19(4):774–9.
21. Peyrade F, Jardin F, Thieblemont C, Thyss A, Emile JF, Castaigne S, Coiffier B, Haioun C, Bologna S, Fitoussi O, Lepeu G, Fruchart C, Bordessoule D, Blanc M, Delarue R, Janvier M, Salles B, André M, Fournier M, Gaulard P, Tilly H, Groupe d'Etude des Lymphomes de l'Adulte (GELA) investigators. Attenuated immunochemotherapy regimen (R-miniCHOP) in elderly patients older than 80 years with diffuse large B-cell lymphoma: a multicentre, single-arm, phase 2 trial. Lancet Oncol. 2011;12(5):460–8.
22. Mounier N, Heutte N, Thieblemont C, Briere J, Gaulard P, Feugier P, Ghesquieres H, Van Den Neste E, Robu D, Tilly H, Bouabdallah R, Safar V, Coiffier B, Groupe d'Etude des Lymphomes de l'Adulte (GELA). Ten-year relative survival and causes of death in elderly patients treated with R-CHOP or CHOP in the GELA LNH-985 trial. Clin Lymphoma Myeloma Leuk. 2012;12(3):151–4.
23. Pfreundschuh M, Schubert J, Ziepert M, Schmits R, Mohren M, Lengfelder E, Reiser M, Nickenig C, Clemens M, Peter N, Bokemeyer C, Eimermacher H, Ho A, Hoffmann M, Mertelsmann R, Trümper L, Balleisen L, Liersch R, Metzner B, Hartmann F, Glass B, Poeschel V, Schmitz N, Ruebe C, Feller AC, Loeffler M, German High-Grade Non-Hodgkin Lymphoma Study Group (DSHNHL). Six versus eight cycles of bi-weekly CHOP-14 with or without rituximab in elderly patients with aggressive CD20+ B-cell lymphomas: a randomised controlled trial (RICOVER-60). Lancet Oncol. 2008;9(2):105–16.
24. Delarue R, Tilly H, Salles G, Gisselbrecht C, Mounier N, Fournier M, Molina TJ, Caroline Bonmati C, Ghesquieres H, Blanc M, Germain D, Girard L, Haioun C, Bosly A. R-CHOP14 compared to R-CHOP21 in elderly patients with diffuse large B-Cell lymphoma: results of the interim analysis of the LNH03-6B GELA study. ASH Annual Meeting Abstracts, J Clin Oncol. 2009;27(114):406.

25. Hong W, Yu XM, Jiang MQ, Chen B, Wang XB, Yang LT, Zhang YP. Solitary extramedullary plasmacytoma in retroperitoneum: a case report and review of the literature. World J Gastroenterol. 2009;15(19):2425–7.
26. Vaglio A, Salvarani C, Buzio C. Retroperitoneal fibrosis. Lancet. 2006;367(9506):241–51.
27. PACE participants, Audisio RA, Pope D, Ramesh HS, Gennari R, van Leeuwen BL, West C, Corsini G, Maffezzini M, Hoekstra HJ, Mobarak D, Bozzetti F, Colledan M, Wildiers H, Stotter A, Capewell A, Marshall E. Shall we operate? Preoperative assessment in elderly cancer patients (PACE) can help. A SIOG surgical task force prospective study. Crit Rev Oncol Hematol. 2008;65(2):156–63.
28. Lorigan P, Verweij J, Papai Z, Rodenhuis S, Le Cesne A, Leahy MG, Radford JA, Van Glabbeke MM, Kirkpatrick A, Hogendoorn PC, Blay JY, European Organisation for Research and Treatment of Cancer Soft Tissue and Bone Sarcoma Group Study. Phase III trial of two investigational schedules of ifosfamide compared with standard-dose doxorubicin in advanced or metastatic soft tissue sarcoma: a European organisation for research and treatment of cancer soft tissue and bone sarcoma group study. J Clin Oncol. 2007;25(21):3144–50.

Index

Printed by Printforce, the Netherlands